Patients as Policy Actors

Critical Issues in Health and Medicine

Edited by Rima D. Apple, University of Wisconsin–Madison,
and Janet Golden, Rutgers University, Camden

Growing criticism of the U.S. health care system is coming from consumers, politicians, the media, activists, and healthcare professionals. Critical Issues in Health and Medicine is a collection of books that explores these contemporary dilemmas from a variety of perspectives, among them political, legal, historical, sociological, and comparative, and with attention to crucial dimensions such as race, gender, ethnicity, sexuality, and culture.

For a list of titles in the series, see the last page of the book.

Patients as Policy Actors

Edited by
Beatrix Hoffman, Nancy Tomes,
Rachel Grob, and Mark Schlesinger

Rutgers University Press

New Brunswick, New Jersey, and London

Library of Congress Cataloging-in-Publication Data

Patients as policy actors / edited by Beatrix Hoffman . . . [et al.].
    p. ; cm. — (Critical issues in health and medicine)
    Includes bibliographical references and index.
    ISBN 978–0–8135–5050–3 (hardcover : alk. paper) — ISBN 978–0–8135–5051–0
(pbk. : alk. paper)
    1. Patient advocacy—United States.   2. Medical policy—United States.   I. Hoffman,
Beatrix Rebecca.   II. Series: Critical issues in health and medicine.
    [DNLM: 1. Patient-Centered Care—trends—United States.   2. Health Care Reform—
trends—United States.   3. Health Policy—United States.   4. Patient Advocacy—United
States. W 84.7]
    R727.45.P455   2011
    362.1068—dc22

                                                                              2010041970

A British Cataloging-in-Publication record for this book is available from the British Library.

This collection copyright © 2011 by Rutgers, The State University of New Jersey

Individual chapters copyright © 2011 in the names of their authors

Visit our Web site: http://rutgerspress.rutgers.edu

Manufactured in the United States of America

In appreciation of the generous spirit of collaboration and mutual support fostered by the Robert Wood Johnson Investigator Awards in Health Policy Program, the authors dedicate this book to David Mechanic, Lynn Rogut, and Cynthia Church.

Contents

Part III   How Patients Matter   193

Patients as Policy Actors

Introduction

Patients as Policy Actors

As health care once again returns to the forefront of national attention, this book comes bearing an urgent message: any and all new measures adopted to reform the U.S. health care system must serve patients' interests. That point might seem so obvious that it hardly needs a volume to elaborate on it. But the harsh reality is that for all the talk of patient rights and consumer choices, Americans' health care needs have not been well served by the policy-making process in the United States. One of the most puzzling aspects of contemporary U.S. health politics is the patient conundrum: patients seem everywhere visible yet wield little independent or effective power. This book not only helps explain why that conundrum exists, but also suggests ways to escape it.

In the United States, too much emphasis is placed on treating patients as isolated, individual consumers. This market-based view of the health system assumes that medical care is a product like any other, and that individual consumers can and should make choices about health coverage and care based on economic self-interest. The contributors to *Patients as Policy Actors* challenge this definition of patient/consumer empowerment and seek to define, explore, and promote more democratic models of patient participation. Participatory models of patient action that were such a vibrant element of policy discourse during the 1960s and 1970s have largely disappeared in recent years. In this volume, we revisit and revitalize this tradition of inclusivity at a time when new national leadership in the United States shows a greater receptivity toward citizen participation in policy making.

Since the 1970s, patients, both as individuals and in groups, have become far more vocal in expressing their needs and preferences. What the physician-ethicist Jay Katz described in 1984 as the "silent world of doctor and patient," characterized by the latter's "surrender to silent and blind trust" in the former, seems far distant from today's reality. Inspired by civil rights, feminist, and consumer activism, a variety of patient empowerment movements have fomented a noisy revolt against medical authority.[1] Declaring themselves patient no more, they have invented new terms for themselves—consumers, clients, citizens, and survivors—in their search to be heard in the health care system.

Yet while grassroots activism has brought about important changes, patient advocates have found it difficult to present a strong, united front in national policy deliberations. Other groups, among them the medical profession, hospital administrators, insurance companies, and pharmaceutical firms, have been far better organized and influential in determining broad policy directions. These powerful stakeholders, who sometimes call themselves patient advocates, primarily promote measures that advance their own economic and professional interests. Meanwhile, the collective voice of patients, whether expressed through lobbying, town meetings, academic research, or opinion polling, remains muted and fragmented.

Even so, health care professionals and policy makers increasingly consider patient voices important, in large part because the health care system serves people so poorly. Neither direct government regulation nor market-based managed competition has succeeded in improving quality and access while holding down costs. As these strategies have faltered, policy makers have looked to harnessing the power of patient choice to discipline and improve a dysfunctional, disorganized health care system.

The idea that the patient should be "the source of control," as the Institute of Medicine asserted in 2001, is now widely espoused as a guiding policy principle. Two paradigms—patient-centered medicine and consumer-driven health care—have emerged as roadmaps for how patients should exercise greater control over their care. Patient-centered medicine attempts to enhance patients' involvement in clinical decision making, while consumer-driven health care focuses on economic choice. In different ways, both paradigms assume that consumers empowered to act on their needs and preferences will change the health care system for the better.[2]

Of the two paradigms, patient-centered medicine is the more broadly (although not completely) accepted, because it builds on established traditions of informed consent and collaborative healing.[3] Consumer-driven health care, heavily promoted during the second George W. Bush administration, remains more controversial and has yet to be widely adopted.[4] Although both approaches have drawn new attention to the role that empowered patients can play in restructuring a dysfunctional health care system, they tend to put the cart before the horse: they assume that patients can have a corrective influence on health care trends in the absence of concrete evidence that such a capacity exists. That is, for all the lip service that has been paid to the importance of patients and consumers, the role they have actually had or could have in transforming the doctor-patient relationship, medical institutions, or health care policy remains little investigated and little understood.

The desire to understand the role that patients do, can, and should have in health care policy making is the driving force behind this book. We wrestle here with fundamental questions. To what extent has U.S. health policy—defined as decisions made by government or health care institutions that affect the delivery of medical care—been shaped from below as well as from above? To what extent should and can patient voices and actions directly influence health care policy?

We begin with the recognition that when policy discussions have acknowledged the importance of patient actors, it has largely been in a negative context. Ironically, given the nation's commitment to democratic politics, consumer choice, and privatized medicine, there is a long tradition in the U.S. health care system of describing patients/consumers as stumbling blocks to health care efficiency. Over the past century, public demand and desire have taken the blame for the rising cost of medical care, in particular the proliferation of expensive technologies. Contemporary discussions echo the complaint made by one hospital leader in 1962: "Although the American public complains about the amount spent for hospital care, it shows no willingness to forgo such care."[5] Similarly, the great expense of emergency care, as well as emergency room overcrowding, have been explained as problems created by patients who refused to distinguish between urgent and nonurgent conditions. Giving the U.S. public what it wants, then, seems to carry a very high cost.

The empowered patient/consumer has been portrayed as a problem rather than an asset in health policy discussions in other ways. Patients who "know too much" are precisely the ones thought to demand too many services. When members of the public "hear of new advances," they "demand them right away," asserted a hospital official in 1960.[6] Today, physicians trade horror stories about patients who imagine symptoms they have read about on the Internet, or who demand particular medications they have seen in drug advertisements.[7]

One example of patient agency that has received special scrutiny as a force in high health care costs is the malpractice suit. Although more often blamed on greedy trial lawyers than on injured patients themselves, high malpractice costs are still portrayed as the product of an overly litigious public that expects too much from medicine. Conservative health policy analysts continue to insist that malpractice suits are to blame for the high cost of health care in the United States.[8]

The allegedly irrational consumer also wants full health care coverage and free choice of doctor but doesn't want to pay high insurance premiums—two desires that inevitably conflict in the U.S. health system as it is currently configured. Managed care was initially intended to be a less expensive form of health coverage, but patients resisted the new restrictions it placed on their access to doctors and hospitals. The resulting "backlash against managed care" led to some reforms, such as laws against "drive-by deliveries," but also, according to health policy analysts, cancelled out the cost savings promised by HMOs and drove insurance premiums even higher.[9]

Similarly, patient activism, such as the movements of breast cancer and AIDS patients/survivors, is often associated with irrationality in health policy circles. Critics complain that the public emotions raised by pink ribbons for breast cancer or Michael J. Fox's advocacy for Parkinson's disease sufferers are an unscientific or irrational basis for allocating research dollars.[10]

As patients have moved from the periphery to the center of policy attention, it is perhaps inevitable that they attract negative scrutiny. But although patient initiatives have secured the expansion of some kinds of choices and safeguards, especially for the educated and affluent, they have been offset by growing demands for cost containment and market discipline that have limited both physicians' and patients' autonomy. Hence, as one of us has written elsewhere, "to replace the doctor blaming of the 1970s with patient blaming" seems wrongheaded.[11]

As the contentious debate surrounding the passage of the 2010 Patient Protection and Affordable Care Act made evident, there is a deep sense of concern about the nation's health care future. Thus it seems all the more important to understand why the health care crisis has not only persisted but deepened over the same decades that the consumer/patient empowerment movement has profoundly reshaped the practice of U.S. medicine. We need an explicit and wide-ranging conversation about how patients have figured as policy actors, both in the recent past and in the present. This book, by bringing together many threads of ideas about patients in U.S. health policy, begins such a conversation.

In exploring the varied roles of the patient as policy actor, we build on many previous studies of patient empowerment movements. Since the 1970s, social scientists, historians, and health care professionals sympathetic to their aims have scrutinized these movements—one might even argue co-created them.[12] But like the fable of the blind men describing an elephant, these studies have yet to add up to a coherent picture of how patient empowerment has transformed institutions and policy. As occurs in the health care system they study, scholars tend to specialize in their focus: bioethicists on clinical decision making, psychologists on communication skills, political scientists on interest groups, sociologists on activist movements, economists on funding mechanisms, and historians on long-term changes in all of these. Working away in their own silos, scholars know that these different spheres of individual decision making and collective action interact and possibly even cancel each other out yet have little idea how this process happens. Some parts of the elephant have become clearer, but the beast itself remains a mystery.

This book represents an effort to see the elephant a little more clearly. The contributors have a longstanding interest in patients' role in the health care system. They come from a broad range of policy-relevant disciplines: psychology, political science, law, sociology, history, journalism, public health, and economics. With the support of the Robert Wood Johnson Foundation Investigator Awards in Health Policy Program, they have had the luxury of escaping their silos and pooling their insights into the complex ways that patients interact with health care institutions and influence policy outcomes.

To address these complexities, our volume includes a wide variety of patient actions and policy arenas. We deliberately define "action" in a broader and more nuanced fashion than have previous analyses, believing that this expansive conception more accurately represents the impact and potential of the patient-consumer voice in the health care system. Where most of the literature has focused on single-issue advocacy groups, we examine a continuum that includes not only self-consciously activist patients but also the unorganized, the unaware, and the unexpected. We conceive of influential patient actions not only as organizing and lobbying, but also as choosing practitioners, bringing lawsuits, and lodging complaints. Our actors also include those who act as proxies—interested parties other than patients who position themselves as channels for patient interests, including family members and professional groups.

The policy arenas considered here are similarly expansive. We define "policy" not simply as the decisions of elected officials and government agencies, but also as the choices made within the private sector by hospitals, insurance companies, and employers. Just as we look at a continuum of patient activation, ranging from unaware or unwilling actors to organized activists, we also examine a wide spectrum of policy venues, from public to private, from top down to bottom up, from research foundations to doctors' offices.

The diversity of perspectives is evident in the variety of terms that the contributors to this book choose to designate the users of health care. In some settings, people interacting with the health care system refer to themselves as "patients"; in others, they use more politically charged terms such as "consumer" or "survivor." These choices reflect the ongoing struggle to give sick people a greater sense of agency and dignity when dealing with health care institutions.

The structure of *Patients as Policy Actors* reflects our determination to broaden conceptions of patient action and to appreciate the complexity of its influence. Each section focuses on a different type of patient action and voice in the health care system.

Part 1, "Voices of the Silent," examines patients who have been silent or silenced and reflects on the implications of their silence, including the efforts of others to speak for them. Clinician and bioethicist Joseph Fins and his colleague Jennifer Hersh focus on how family members become surrogate advocates for patients who are completely silenced due to severe brain injury. Psychologist M. Robin DiMatteo and her coauthors discuss how communication barriers between patient and physician compromise the health care of low-income and minority individuals. Sociologists Elizabeth Mitchell Armstrong and Eugene Declercq examine childbirth advocacy, asking why women's voices are ignored in shaping childbirth policies and practices. Finally, legal scholars Lori Andrews and Julie Burger call attention to patients who unknowingly become research subjects when their body tissues are taken and sold without their knowledge or consent.

Part 2, "From Individual to Collective," looks at patients who speak more directly on their own behalf, both as individuals and in groups. These chapters raise important questions about how individual and collective identities can shape patients' roles as policy actors and suggest that patient voices can constitute a collective action in ways other than group self-mobilization.

The section begins with two historical case studies of patient and consumer activism. Nancy Tomes charts the transformative impact of psychiatric patient/survivor activism, and Beatrix Hoffman tells the story of poor women's attempts to change the health system via the National Welfare Rights Organization in the 1970s. Compared to the ex-mental patients that Tomes describes, welfare activists had very limited success, an observation that underlines the immense difficulties faced by low-income Americans seeking services and justice in a market-oriented health care system. Political economist Mark Schlesinger explores how to more effectively use mechanisms for collecting the complaints and grievances of individual patients to create a collective voice on their behalf. Conversely, legal scholar Marc A. Rodwin examines the drawbacks of a fragmented grievance system, showing how collective discontent with HMOs' denial of services was channeled into an individualized and isolated appeal process.

Part 3, "How Patients Matter," explores situations in which patient influence, both intended and unexpected, succeeded in changing policy. Journalist Amy Dockser Marcus writes of how individuals thrust into activism following a diagnosis of a rare cancer developed innovative methods of raising funds, launching educational campaigns, and persuading researchers to devote attention to rare cancers. Historian Julie Fairman describes how nurse practitioners were able to bring legitimacy to their new profession by emphasizing patient needs and preferences. Sociologist Rachel Grob discusses the role of parents' advocacy in the adoption of state genetic-screening laws for newborn babies and the unintended negative consequences they precipitated. Sociologist Steven Epstein closes this section with a wide-ranging examination of what it means to say that a social movement has achieved "success."

Finally, in the epilogue, the authors join to distill shared perspectives on how best to amplify the policy presence of patient actors and advocates. Our ultimate purpose in analyzing how patients become policy actors is to imagine what a more truly patient-centered health policy process might look like. To that end, we sought consensus on some principles that could be implemented using existing initiatives from the United States and abroad. We also drew upon our chapters to identify key challenges to patients' participation in policy deliberation. The epilogue ends with a discussion of how best to revitalize policy making so that the health care system better serves those who must use it, whether we call them patients, consumers, survivors, or citizens.

Patients' Power: A Historical Overview

Too often health care policy debates depend upon and reinforce overly simplified views of patients' experiences in the past. As the foundation for more informed discussion, we offer here a brief overview of the patient's role in medical care and patient empowerment movements in the United States, which also provides essential background for the chapters that follow.

Implied in the term "patient" is the idea that the sick do not act but are acted upon. The word has its root in the Latin for "hearing or enduring without complaint."[13] Although the ancients used different terms for the subjects of a physician's care, they agreed that the sufferer must be, above all, cooperative. The Greek physician Galen argued that complete patient obedience was a prerequisite for healing. In the Middle Ages, renowned physician Rhazes of Persia declared: "With a learned physician and an obedient patient, sickness soon disappears." Such expectations of patient compliance persisted for centuries, shaping the first Code of Ethics adopted in 1847 by the newly formed American Medical Association, whose section "Obligations of Patients to Their Physicians" called for full obedience by the patient.[14]

Yet patients always played a role in medical care, most significantly by reporting symptoms. Before tests and technology took physicians inside the body, the patient's description of his or her symptoms was their most reliable guide, and doctors tailored treatments to each individual. In the eighteenth century, for example, U.S. physicians put such faith in the patient's self-report that some diagnosed and treated people through the mail. Well into the late nineteenth century, good medicine depended upon the practitioners' ability to listen closely to the patient and to analyze the clues they had to the body's inner workings (pulse, excretions, skin tone, and the like). As a consequence, the sick expected their doctors to listen to them.[15]

Like the "expert patients" of today, middle-class Americans with chronic illnesses often became very knowledgeable about their conditions and cultivated communities of fellow sufferers with whom to share advice and support. Historian Sheila Rothman has described this pattern among people suffering from pulmonary tuberculosis in the first half of the nineteenth century. The letters of Deborah Fiske of Massachusetts, who died of that disease in 1844, reflect a woman who was "a wary and sophisticated consumer of medicine, questioning her doctors, changing them when she was dissatisfied with her own progress or their answers, and adapting their recommendations to her own circumstances." Fiske wrote to a friend in 1841: "We are indeed a complicated piece of mechanism, and I sometimes think physicians might as well prescribe for watches that are out of order by looking at them, feeling of them, and harking to their ticking, as to prescribe for us without *seeing* the parts that are diseased."[16]

Starting in the late 1800s, medical science's ability to do just that—to see into the body of the living person—began to diminish the importance accorded the patient's self-reported symptoms. Twentieth-century patients began to be measured and probed by new medical technologies that provided independent, seemingly more objective information about their bodies. An expanding array of laboratory tests allowed doctors to assay the components of blood, to test sputum for the tubercle bacillus, and to detect proteins indicative of kidney failure in urine. X-ray technology introduced a revolutionary method for seeing "the parts that are diseased."[17]

As doctors gained more scientific certainty, they expected more patient deference and compliance. Those expectations were particularly reflected in the restructuring of hospital care. The old-style hospital, in which patients had freely spit, entertained their friends, and smuggled in their own tobacco and liquor (as so vividly described by historian Charles Rosenberg) gave way to the well-ordered "doctor's workshop" designed with the physician's convenience in mind.[18]

Despite the growing gap between physicians' and patients' technical knowledge, patients did not take easily to a more passive role. Laypeople continued to believe that they had an unrivaled source of insight into their bodies by virtue simply of inhabiting them. Deeply ingrained American habits of questioning authority and valuing personal freedom did not collapse in the face of the germ theory or the X-ray. As scientific medicine gained enormous institutional power, countless Americans continued to patronize alternative healers, including midwives, homeopaths, herbalists, chiropractors, osteopaths, and mind healers.[19] Even patients who accepted the scientific authority of the mainstream medical profession still felt entitled to ask questions and to complain.

Long before the appearance of formal patients' bills of rights, laypeople often framed health care decisions in the language of citizenship. As one patient wrote about her choice of a surgeon in 1900, "I am an American and a Free American," which she felt entitled her to express her opinions. (She was threatening a malpractice suit.)[20]

But as physicians and hospitals offered more and better services, patient passivity became a necessary cost of getting well. A case in point is the medicalization of childbirth, so well chronicled by Judith Walzer Leavitt. In the face of the dangers of childbirth, women gradually traded off autonomy for the cold sterility of hospital birthing practices, a greater chance of survival, and pain control.[21] But even what would appear to be the ultimate form of surrender—the twilight-sleep regimen that rendered birthing women helpless and unconscious—came at least in part as a response to patient demands; as Leavitt shows, feminist activists in the 1910s formed a national organization in support of the anesthesia, arguing that women should have the power to choose pain relief.[22]

Still, as the hospital more fully replaced the home as the locus of U.S. medical care by the mid-twentieth century, its rules and routines increasingly encouraged patient passivity. The excruciating rituals of hospital life became immortalized in popular culture, as well as in the memories of the people who experienced them: the brief appearance of imperious physicians, humiliating patient observation by medical students, the degrading backless gown, the nurses' patronizing "How are we feeling today?" Visiting hours were extremely limited; parents, for example, could see their hospitalized children only during one or two official visiting hours each week.[23] In perhaps the most indicative example of enforced powerlessness, throughout the mid-twentieth century doctors frequently did not tell patients with terminal illnesses, especially cancer, of their diagnosis.[24]

As hospitals became more aware of patients' discontent, and at the same time sought to increase revenues, some began to approach the patient as a customer. In the competition for paying patients, post–World War II hospitals increasingly used questionnaires and surveys to gauge patient satisfaction. These efforts likely had less to do with improving quality than with quelling patient complaints. As one hospital journal put it in 1946, sharing opinions allowed the hospital customer to "get it off his chest": "The moments spent in reflection as he fills out his questionnaire have a tendency to free the patient of complaints which otherwise may be carried with him and broadcast to the profit of no one."[25] Although initially introduced to keep the customer quiet, patient questionnaires would evolve into more elaborate systems of opinion surveying that would become a means to improve the patient experience.[26]

Although the hospital's image took a drubbing in postwar popular culture, the opposite was true of the medical profession. Magazines and newspapers featured medical miracles and triumphs, while film and television created the popular character of the heroic physician.[27] All these media sent the same messages to patients: ask your doctor, listen to your doctor, see your doctor. Organizations such as the American Cancer Society sought to conquer disease with the weapon of an informed public able to recognize dangerous symptoms. But although individual Americans were increasingly expected to be educated about the seven warning signs of cancer, for example, their primary duty upon spotting one was immediately to see their doctor. [28] Once patients arrived at the doctor's office, they seemingly turned responsibility over to the physician.

Yet even at the height of medicine's so-called golden age, some patients resisted the model of unquestioning compliance. Although many people trusted their personal physician, they harbored deep suspicions of the medical profession in general, in particular the American Medical Association. Even at the height of cold-war enthusiasm for medical progress, a robust critique of the doctor business flourished in the 1950s and early 1960s, drawing on the long tradition of portraying as undemocratic the special legal and institutional powers granted the medical profession. As medicine became a more lucrative occupation, the contradictions between the values of the businessperson and the professional became increasingly clear.[29]

In addition, the United States had a long tradition of alternative forms of health care delivery and finance, including prepaid group practices, consumer cooperatives, and worker-owned hospitals and clinics, some dating back to the nineteenth century. Initiated by unions, consumers, or progressive physicians, their very existence challenged both the AMA's insistence on fee-for-service medical care and the development of for-profit health insurance coverage. Many of these programs were early examples of consumer/patient empowerment, requiring that the organization's governing structure include representatives of workers and consumers. In 1941 longtime health reform advocate Michael M. Davis praised consumer representation in medical plans, arguing that "those who pay the bills should have a share in the say," an argument that would reemerge in the consumer movement of the 1970s.[30]

After World War II, a transformed understanding of rights added a new dimension to patient/consumer critiques of U.S. medicine. Franklin D. Roosevelt's "Four Freedoms" speech and his proposal for a new economic bill of rights shortly before his death introduced notions of social and economic rights into the individualistic U.S. rights tradition.[31] The 1947 Nuremberg Code, a response to Nazi medical experimentation, promulgated the doctrines of patient consent and other ethical guidelines for medical research on human subjects, although its principles were not widely discussed or accepted in the United States until the 1960s and 1970s.[32] Civil rights activists in the 1940s and 1950s increasingly criticized segregation in U.S. health care, including separate hospitals for blacks and whites in the South and the AMA's exclusion of black physicians. While physicians led efforts against health care discrimination, the 1963 Supreme Court decision that desegregated hospitals, *Simkins v. Cone*, included two African American patients as plaintiffs.[33]

As the civil rights movement and other movements for self-determination broadened in the 1960s, the assault on medical paternalism gained momentum. Psychiatric patients were among the first to revolt against traditional concepts of patienthood. Emulating the techniques used by civil rights and antiwar protesters, ex-mental patients began to organize to change the health care system. They advanced the argument, then quite radical, that people who suffered from a disease had a unique expertise about its nature that had to be accorded equal status with the judgment of medical science.[34]

Using a similar critique of medical absolutism and insisting on the patient's special knowledge of her body, feminists in the 1970s addressed a wide range of women's health issues, including contraception and abortion, childbirth, and sexually transmitted diseases. Feminist health clinics and the blockbuster bestseller *Our Bodies, Ourselves* embodied the principles of lay expertise, self-help, and demedicalization. Perhaps more than any other health care social movement, feminist health activism transformed the relationship between patients and the medical system. "In 1969, a woman who placed herself under a doctor's care had the duty to do what she was told," notes movement historian Sandra Morgen. "Now she has the right to gather information and resources to make her own decisions about her sexuality, her reproductive life and health, even her treatment for breast cancer."[35]

Antipoverty groups argued that poor people and people of color should have a voice in their own health care; welfare activists pushed the American Hospital Association and its members to adopt a patients' bill of rights in the early 1970s (see Beatrix Hoffman's essay, this volume). In response to growing concerns about the misuse of medical authority, most notably in the infamous Tuskegee case, in which information and treatment were withheld from poor black men enrolled in a U.S. Public Health Service study of syphilis, the American Medical Association in 1980 changed its Code of Ethics to include language about patients rights ("A physician shall respect the rights of patients").[36]

A reinvigorated and newly confrontational consumer movement played a key role in legitimating the new patient groups of the 1970s. Drawing on youthful discontent within the medical profession as well as on the new legal activism of the era, the consumer movement associated with Ralph Nader developed a broad-ranging critique of the health care system. The consumer backlash against medical authority reached into popular culture, as books telling readers how to "manage" or "talk back to your doctor" flooded the market.[37]

In the 1970s and 1980s, activists created a new, powerful type of patient advocacy: movements organized around a single disease, populated by sufferers and survivors whose voices carried unique authority and persuasiveness. The breast cancer and AIDS movements are the best-known examples. Both mobilized millions of people, transformed cultural understanding of the diseases, and got concrete results in the form of quicker drug approval and more research funding.[38] A disability rights movement arose to challenge discrimination and demand the participation of disabled people in policy making, encapsulated by the activist slogan "Nothing about us without us."[39]

In the 1980s, this ferment of activism collided with the revolt against high taxes and big government that brought Ronald Reagan to the presidency. Efforts to contain costs through managed care brought about a shift in emphasis from patient rights to consumer discipline. Many of the chapters in this volume explore the sometimes contradictory trends toward patient empowerment and fiscal constraint that still shape the landscape of policy debate today.

Decades of patient activism have resulted in some types of patient/consumer voices becoming institutionalized in the health care system and in U.S. culture. The races and bike rides for the cure created by breast cancer and AIDS groups have become hugely popular (and some would argue unquestioned) mainstream events.[40] Hospitals, health-planning boards, and policy task forces acknowledge consumer perspectives by appointing representatives from the community.[41] Patient activism has had a major impact on federal health agencies, particularly in the areas of research and drug trials.[42]

Official attempts to incorporate consumer voices may represent examples of the success of patient movements (see Steven Epstein's chapter for a more detailed discussion of movement success), but they are a far cry from the direct consumer participation and even control of health care institutions envisioned by activists in the 1960s and 1970s. Similarly, the Obama administration's health care reform campaign sought the voices of consumers and patients through novel forms of communication, including televised town meetings and social networking sites like Facebook, but more to amass support (and, it turned out, opposition) than to involve patients and consumers in the shaping of the legislation.[43]

The 2009–2010 health reform debate, in which it seemed that citizen participation was defined by those who could win media attention by screaming the loudest, points to a central problem with patients as policy actors: some voices drown out others, and the interests of some patient/consumer groups may be different from or even inimical to others'. The empowerment of some individuals and groups takes place in the context of pervasive social and economic inequality. Differentials of power, income, resources, and access to media shape the ability of patient groups to affect policy. As a result, no movement or group has been able to define patient-consumer interests broadly or speak on behalf of all seekers of health care. It may be that there is no such thing as a unified patient voice, but in seeking to define and understand the multiplicity of patient/consumer voices in the United States, we believe this book goes some way toward illuminating the connections and convergences among them, and their potential power to improve health care for all.

Notes

1. Jay Katz, *The Silent World of Doctor and Patient* (New York: Free Press, 1984), xvi. For overviews of the patient rights movement, see Nancy Tomes, "Patients or Health-Care Consumers? Why the History of Contested Terms Matters," in *History and Health Policy*, ed. Rosemary Stevens, Charles Rosenberg, and L. R. Burns (New Brunswick, N.J.: Rutgers University Press, 2006), 83–110; and Nancy Tomes, "Patient Empowerment and the Dilemmas of Late-Modern Medicalisation," *Lancet* 369, 9562 (February 24, 2007): 698–700.

2. Institute of Medicine, Committee on Quality of Health Care in America, *Crossing the Quality Chasm: A New Health System for the 21st Century* (Washington, D.C.: National Academy Press, 2001), 8; Regina Herzlinger, *Market Driven Health Care* (Cambridge, Mass.: Perseus Books, 1997), 245.

3. See, e.g., Susan B Frampton and Patrick A. Charme, , eds., *Putting Patients First: Best Practices in Patient-Centered Care* (Hoboken, N.J.: Jossey-Bass, 2008).

4. Julie Kosterlitz, "Bush's Health Savings Accounts," *National Journal* 36, 4 (January 24, 2004): 248–249; M. Gregg Bloche, "Consumer-Directed Health Care," *New England Journal of Medicine* 355, 17 (2006): 1756–1759.

5. George Bugbee, "Interpreting Hospital Costs to the Public," 1962, Papers of George Bugbee, Box 16, American Hospital Association Resource Center.

6. J. Milo Anderson, *Proceedings: National Congress on Prepaid Health Insurance* (sponsored by the American Medical Association Council on Medical Service, May 13–14, 1960, Chicago), American Hospital Association Resource Center. Typescript.

7. E.g., Russell Shaw, "Web Fertile Ground for Hypochondriacs," *USA Today*, June 25, 2002, http://www.usatoday.com/tech/2002/06/24/cyberchondria.htm; Kurt C. Stange, "Time to Ban Direct-to-Consumer Prescription Drug Marketing," *Annals of Family Medicine* 5 (2007): 101–104, http://www.annfammed.org/cgi/content/full/5/2/101.

8. E.g., John Cornyn and Edwin Meese III, "Health Care and Medical Malpractice Reform: The Necessity of Reform in the Current Debate," January 28, 2010, www.heritage.org, accessed April 20, 2010; Tom Baker, *The Medical Malpractice Myth* (Chicago: University of Chicago Press, 2007).

9. Uwe E. Reinhardt, "The Predictable Managed Care Kvetch on the Rocky Road from Adolescence to Adulthood," *Journal of Health Politics, Policy, and Law* 24, 5 (October 1999): 897–910; David Mechanic, "The Managed Care Backlash: Perceptions and Rhetoric in Health Care Policy and the Potential for Health Care Reform," *Milbank Quarterly* 79, 1 (2001): 35–54.

10. Daniel Greenberg, "NIH Resists Research Funding Linked to Patient Load," *Lancet* 349, 9060 (April 26, 1997): 1229; Alexandra Matisoff, "National Institutes of Health: Who Decides How Much Goes Where?" *Nurse Week*, September 24, 1998, http://www.nurseweek.com/features/98–9/fund.html; Institute of Medicine, *Scientific Opportunities and Public Needs: Improving Priority Setting and Public Input at the National Institutes of Health* (Washington, D.C.: National Academy Press, 1998).

11. Tomes, "Patient Empowerment," 698.

12. A sample of representative works from the past three decades of scholarship includes Rudolf Klein and Janet Lewis, *The Politics of Consumer Representation: A Study of Community Health Councils* (London: Centre for Studies in Social Policy, 1976); Marie Haug and Bebe Lavin, *Consumerism in Medicine: Challenging Physician Authority* (Beverly Hills, Calif.: Sage Publications, 1983); James M. Hoefler, with Brian E. Kamoie, *Deathright: Culture, Medicine, Politics, and the Right to Die* (Boulder, Colo.: Westview Press, 1994); Susan L. Smith, *Sick and Tired of Being Sick and Tired: Black Women's Health Activism in America, 1890–1950* (Philadelphia: University of Pennsylvania Press, 1995); Steven Epstein, *Impure Science: AIDS, Activism, and the Politics of Knowledge* (Berkeley: University of California Press, 1996); Carol S. Weisman, *Women's Health Care: Activist Traditions and Institutional Change* (Baltimore: Johns Hopkins University Press, 1998); Barron Lerner, *The Breast Cancer Wars: Hope, Fear, and the Pursuit of a Cure in Twentieth-Century America* (New York: Oxford University Press, 2003).

13. Online Etymology Dictionary, http://www.etymonline.com/index.php?term=patient.

14. Susan P. Mattern, *Galen and the Rhetoric of Healing* (Baltimore: Johns Hopkins University Press, 2008), 146; David A. Axelrod and Susan Dorr Goold, "Maintaining

Trust in the Surgeon-Patient Relationship: Challenges for the New Millennium," *Archives of Surgery* 135 (2000): 55–61.

15. Charles E. Rosenberg, "The Therapeutic Revolution," in *The Therapeutic Revolution*, ed. Morris Vogel and Charles E. Rosenberg (Philadelphia: University of Pennsylvania Press, 1979), 3–25.

16. Sheila M. Rothman, *Living in the Shadow of Death: Tuberculosis and the Social Experience of Illness in American History* (New York: Basic Books, 1994), 105, 111.

17. Joel Howell, *Technology in the Hospital: Transforming Patient Care in the Early Twentieth Century* (Baltimore: Johns Hopkins University Press, 1996); Bettyann H. Kevles, *Naked to the Bone: Medical Imaging in the Twentieth Century* (New York: Basic Books, 1998).

18. Charles Rosenberg, *The Care of Strangers: The Rise of America's Hospital System* (New York: Basic Books, 1992).

19. Norman Gevitz, ed., *Other Healers: Unorthodox Medicine in America* (Baltimore: Johns Hopkins University Press, 1988); James C. Whorton, *Nature Cures: The History of Alternative Medicine in America* (New York: Oxford University Press, 2004); Robert D. Johnston, ed., *The Politics of Healing: Histories of Alternative Medicine in Twentieth-Century North America* (New York: Routledge, 2003).

20. Agnes McCabe to J. B. Kennedy, August 10, 1900, and Agnes McCabe to the Hon. James McMillan, December 9, 1900, Miscellaneous Correspondence, Johnstone Burnside Kennedy Papers, Manuscript Collection No. 851597 Aa 2, Bentley Historical Library, University of Michigan, Ann Arbor.

21. Judith Walzer Leavitt, *Brought to Bed: Childbearing in America, 1750–1950* (New York: Oxford University Press, 1988); 22. Judith Walzer Leavitt, "Birthing and Anesthesia: The Debate over Twilight Sleep," *Signs* 6 (1980): 147–164.

23. Howard A. Markel, "When Hospitals Kept Children from Parents," *New York Times*, January 1, 2008, http://www.nytimes.com/2008/01/01/health/01visi.html.

24. Alexander Morgan Capron, "The Once and Future Silent World," foreword to Katz, *The Silent World*, x–xi.

25. "The Patient's Voice," *Modern Hospital* 67 (July 1946): 64–65.

26. See Mark Schlesinger's essay in this volume.

27. Joseph Turow, *Playing Doctor: Television, Storytelling, and Medical Power* (New York: Oxford University Press, 1989).

28. Leslie Reagan, "Engendering the Dread Disease: Women, Men, and Cancer," *American Journal of Public Health* 87, 11 (November 1997): 1779–1787; Kristen Gardner, *Early Detection: Men, Women, and Awareness Campaigns in the Twentieth-Century United States* (Chapel Hill: University of North Carolina Press, 2006).

29. Paul Starr, *The Social Transformation of American Medicine* (New York: Basic Books, 1984); Deborah Stone, "The Doctor as Businessman: The Changing Politics of a Cultural Icon," *Journal of Health Politics, Policy, and Law* 22, 2 (1997): 533–556; Nancy Tomes, *The Medicine Shop*, forthcoming.

30. Klein, *For All These Rights*, 160. See also Alan Derickson, *Workers' Health, Workers' Democracy: The Western Miners' Struggle* (Ithaca, N.Y.: Cornell University Press, 1989); Jennifer Klein, *For All These Rights: Business, Labor, and the Shaping of America's Public-Private Welfare State* (Princeton, N.J.: Princeton University Press, 2003).

31. Cass R. Sunstein, *The Second Bill of Rights: FDR's Unfinished Revolution—and Why We Need It More Than Ever* (New York: Basic Books, 2006).

32. Ruth R. Faden, Tom L. Beauchamp, and Nancy M. P. King, *A History and Theory of Informed Consent* (New York: Oxford University Press, 1986).

33. David Barton Smith, *Health Care Divided: Race and Healing a Nation* (Ann Arbor: University of Michigan Press, 1999); P. Preston Reynolds, "Hospitals and Civil Rights, 1945–1963: The Case of *Simkins v. Moses H. Cone Memorial Hospital*," *Annals of Internal Medicine* 126, 11 (June 1997): 898–906.

34. Tomes, "Patients or Health Care Consumers?"; Carol T. Mowbray and Mark C. Holter, "Mental Health and Mental Illness: Out of the Closet?" *Social Service Review* 76, 1 (March 2002): 135–179.

35. Sandra Morgen, *Into Our Own Hands: The Women's Health Movement in the United States, 1969–1990* (New Brunswick, N.J.: Rutgers University Press, 2002), 11.

36. AMA Code of Ethics, http://www.amaassn.org/ama/pub/category/2512.html.

37. Naomi Rogers, "Caution: The AMA May Be Dangerous to Your Health: The Student Health Organizations (SHO) and American Medicine, 1965–1970," *Radical History Review* 80 (2001): 5–34; Sidney M. Wolfe, Christopher M. Coley, and the Health Research Group, *Pills That Don't Work* (New York: Farrar, Straus and Giroux, 1981); Arthur S. Freese, *Managing Your Doctor: How to Get the Best Possible Health Care* (New York: Stein and Day, 1974); Arthur Levin, *Talk Back to Your Doctor: How to Demand and Recognize High Quality Health Care* (Garden City, N.Y.: Doubleday, 1975).

38. E.g., Lerner, *The Breast Cancer Wars*; Epstein, *Impure Science.*

39. Doris Zames Fleischer and Frieda Zames, *The Disability Rights Movement: From Charity to Confrontation* (Philadelphia: Temple University Press, 2001); Joseph P. Shapiro, *No Pity: People with Disabilities Forging a New Civil Rights Movement* (New York: Three Rivers Press, 1994); James I. Charlton, *Nothing about Us without Us: Disability Oppression and Empowerment* (Berkeley: University of California Press, 2000).

40. For a critique of the corporate capture of disease activism, see, e.g., Samantha King, *Pink Ribbons, Inc.: Breast Cancer and the Politics of Philanthropy* (Minneapolis: University of Minnesota Press, 2008).

41. James Morone, *The Democratic Wish: Popular Participation and the Limits of American Government* (New Haven: Yale University Press, 1998); Colleen M. Grogan and Michael K. Gusmano, *Healthy Voices, Unhealthy Silence: Advocacy and Health Policy for the Poor* (Washington, D.C.: Georgetown University Press, 2007).

42. Institute of Medicine, *Scientific Opportunities and Public Needs.*

43. Sandy Heierbacher, "Upgrading the Way We Do Politics," *Yes! Magazine*, August 21, 2009, http://www.yesmagazine.org/people-power/upgrading-the-way-we-do-politics, accessed May 30, 2010.

Part I

Voices of the Silent

The chapters in part 1 ask how health policies might take into account the perspectives of patients who are incapable of speaking for themselves or have special difficulties being heard when they do attempt to speak. Barriers to patient engagement are endemic. Here, these widespread impediments are illustrated by patients as diverse as those in a persistent vegetative state due to brain injury whose family members are reluctantly thrust into advocacy; low-income minority patients whose communication difficulties with physicians undermine their understanding of their diagnoses and treatments and thus inhibit their capacity for mobilization; women giving birth in the United States whose voices and preferences are mostly unknown or ignored in the creation of labor and delivery practices; and, finally, patients whose body tissues are taken and sold without their knowledge or consent for use in medical research. The chapters are organized into two pairs: the first focuses on constraints that limit activation by individual patients, their advocates, or both, the second on factors that inhibit collective mobilization.

Constraints on Individual Engagement

Most people in their first encounter with the American health care system are largely unprepared for its limitations. Numerous studies highlight patients' optimistic expectations for the outcomes of medical care and the ways in which they will be treated while obtaining that care.[1] It is most often only after they or their family members experience care that patients come to recognize the system's substantial failings, in what could be described a learning curve of shocked discovery about the limitations of medical knowledge and paucity of patient protections in American health care. It is an odyssey that people traverse at different rates, depending on their health problems, personal circumstances, familial and other resources, and the availability of allies to facilitate the learning process.[2] These factors also help determine whether patients will eventually give voice to their own medical experiences.

The process of patient activation is mediated in crucial ways by the involvement of other key actors, including the patient's family and friends and personal physician. Both family and clinicians have been shown to play a crucial role in advising patients about their health care choices and acting as their advocates.[3] Patients who lack these forms of support are at a clear disadvantage in both understanding their health care experiences and determining how best to respond to them.

The first two chapters in part 1 illustrate constraints on and pathways to patient engagement. What happens when patients *literally* cannot speak? In the case of victims of severe brain injury, authors Joseph Fins and Jennifer Hersh found that patients' family members were forced into reluctant advocacy as they confronted the medical system on behalf of their loved ones. Family members became policy actors first at the stage of acute care in the hospital, when they refused to accept a hopeless prognosis predicated on what the authors contend are outdated medical understandings of severe brain injury (Fins is a clinician, researcher, and ethicist who works with patients who are severely brain injured or minimally conscious). When patients with brain injury are released from the hospital, family members next must struggle with a fragmented and grossly underfunded system of long-term care. Although such families generally do not—and many cannot, given the burdens of their caregiving roles—join together in organized action, their individual advocacy still gives voice within the health care system to those least able to speak for themselves.

Patients can be silenced not only by their particular health condition, but also by social and economic constraints. In chapter 2, psychologist Robin DiMatteo and colleagues emphasize the importance of physician-patient communication in enabling low-income, racial minority, and non-English-speaking patients to be heard. The authors argue that in order for vulnerable patients to have an effective voice, greater education for patients will never be enough. What is also needed, as a matter of policy, is more extensive training of physicians about how to listen to and elicit patient voices.

Constraints on Collective Mobilization and Their Implications

Even when individuals are motivated to promote change in health care or health policies, their energies are most often focused on remediation of their personal circumstances.[4] The personal will be transformed into the political via the mobilization of patients only if individual patients can readily identify with others as a group, if this group has the capacity to collectively imagine how things might be different, and if the group finds the means to promote its goals.[5] Neither collective identification nor a strategic vision of patients' interests emerges readily, however, in a health care system that persistently frames patient experiences in individualized terms and treats them less as rights-based claims on collective resources and more as the result of informed consumer choice.[6] Under these circumstances, the collective representation of at least some patient interests may depend on the supportive engagement of other advocates—and certainly conditions are sometimes ripe for sustaining coalitions of patient and health professional interests promoting policy change. Yet it's equally crucial to recognize that the efforts of these other advocates can become diverted from authentic representations of patient voice.

The second pair of chapters in this cluster examines challenges to the mobilization of collective representation regarding silent patients' perspectives. The interdisciplinary team of Elizabeth Armstrong (a sociologist) and Eugene DeClercq (a political scientist) ask why we know so little about mothers' preferences in the delivery room, and why a group we might expect to be vocal is instead mostly silent on a policy level. Who has the authority to speak for patients whose collective voice is weak or muted? The authors argue that U.S. childbirth policies and practices reflect the goals of the obstetric profession and (occasionally) politicians, each claiming to represent patient interests but in ways that are not entirely legitimate or authentic. The concept of informed consent is central to patient empowerment. But how can patients involved in research give consent, speak, and be heard if they are not even aware that they are research subjects? In a powerful example of how uneven awareness and inadequate legal safeguards can constrain effective patient voice, legal scholars Lori Andrews and Julie Burger Chronis describe an emerging group of advocates: patients whose body tissues have been taken and used for research without their consent or knowledge. Some patients who find out that their tissues were used for unconsented research or for private profit are catapulted into awareness and activation and have taken physicians, researchers, and biotech companies to court. This chapter forces us to recognize that legal protections for patients and research subjects have lagged far behind rapidly changing technologies and shifting alliances between patients, clinicians, researchers, and the government and private sectors.

Notes

1. See, e.g., Larry A. Allen, Jonathan E. Yager, Michele Johnsson Funk, Wayne C. Levy, James A. Tulsky, Margaret T. Bowers, Gwen C. Dodson, Christopher M. O'Connor, and Michael Felker, "Discordance between Patient-Predicted and

Model-Predicted Life Expectancy among Ambulatory Patients with Heart Failure," *JAMA* 299, 21 (2008): 2533–2542; D. W. Barry, T. V. Melhado, K. M. Chacko, R. S. Lee, J. F. Steiner, and J. S. Kutner, "Patient and Physician Perceptions of Timely Access to Care," *Journal of General Internal Medicine* 21, 2 (2006): 130–133.

2. J. H. Hibbard, J. Greene, and M. Tusler, "Plan Design and Active Involvement of Consumers in Their Own Health and Healthcare," *American Journal of Managed Care* 14, 11 (2008): 729–736.

3. R. Antonelli and R. M. Turchi, "The Family-Centered Medical Home in Pediatrics," *Pediatric Annals* 38, 9 (2009): 472–474; M. L. Clayman, D. Roter, L. S. Wissow, and K. Bandeen-Roche, "Autonomy-Related Behaviors of Patient Companions and Their Effect on Decision-Making Activity in Geriatric Primary Care Visits," *Social Science and Medicine* 60, 7 (2005): 1583–1591; P. Reid Ponte and K. Peterson, "A Patient- and Family-Centered Care Model Paves the Way for a Culture of Quality and Safety," *Critical Care Nursing Clinics of North America* 20, 4 (2008): 451–464; M. Schlesinger, S. Mitchell, and B. Elbel, "Voices Unheard: Barriers to the Expression of Dissatisfaction with Health Plans," *Milbank Quarterly* 80, 4 (2002): 709–755.

4. R. D. Friele and E. M. Sluijs, "Patient Expectations of Fair Complaint Handling in Hospitals: Empirical Data." *BMC Health Services Research* 6 (2006): 106.

5. David Kirp, "Look Back in Anger: Hemophilia and AIDS Activism in the International Tainted-Blood Crisis," *Journal of Comparative Policy Analysis* 1 (1999): 177–202.

6. J. Donohue, "A History of Drug Advertising: The Evolving Roles of Consumers and Consumer Protection," *Milbank Quarterly* 84, 4 (2006): 659–699; David J. Rothman, "The Origins and Consequences of Patient Autonomy: A Twenty-Five-Year Retrospective," *Health Care Analysis* 9, 3 (2001): 255–264.

Solitary Advocates

The Severely Brain Injured and Their Surrogates

Some of society's most vulnerable members cannot speak for themselves and depend upon others to serve as their advocates. Infants and children who have yet to become self-determining, as well as infirm and elderly persons who may have lost their autonomy, rely upon the advocacy of others. For them, the notion of "patient as advocate" becomes something of an oxymoron. Theirs is an advocacy by proxy, by surrogate decision makers, who by dint of relationship or obligation step up and help the patient access appropriate care.

Under these circumstances advocacy is difficult, but it is especially challenging for surrogates of patients with severe brain injury causing disorders of consciousness. Emerging scientific findings about these disorders are calling into question prevailing clinical practices and perceptions about diagnosis and treatment, creating even more difficult challenges for advocates. In this chapter, we explore patient advocacy from the perspective of these surrogate decision makers. We trace their empowerment as advocates, starting with the onset of injury and continuing with the challenges of chronic care. Drawing upon in-depth interviews of family members of patients with severe brain injury, the experience of coauthor J. J. Fins as a clinical ethicist, and the growing genre of brain injury narratives, we describe the experiences of patients and surrogates.

When confronted by a family member with severe brain injury, many families decide to withdraw life-sustaining therapy in accord with the patient's prior wishes or based on their perception of the patient's prognosis. Other families, presented with the same medical facts, decide to pursue ongoing care for the patient in hopes of a favorable outcome. Our interviews are with families who chose the second course of action, and who have brought their injured family member to Weill Cornell Medical College to participate in a series of neuroimaging studies designed to elucidate mechanisms of recovery after severe brain injury. These families often confront a health care system well positioned to provide acute care but unable to meet chronic care needs. In their ongoing journey through the system, patient surrogates are transformed in their orientation toward it. Facing an often hostile and unprepared clinical context, these advocates morph from grateful and passive recipients of acute care that saves lives into increasingly informed advocates as the drama of emergent care fades and the struggle for ongoing care for their loved ones begins.

These surrogate advocates struggle alone quietly, consumed by the burden of care giving. Generally, they do not have time for public advocacy. They are just too busy learning about diagnostic and treatment options and managing, often micromanaging, the care of a child or a spouse trapped in clinical settings that may be plagued by medical ignorance and profound discontinuities between acute and chronic care. Societal biases about disability in general and brain injury in particular further complicate matters by distorting surrogates' expectations and falsely dichotomizing outcomes as either miraculous or catastrophic. These distortions make the achievement of realistic goals difficult and leave surrogates settling for pyrrhic victories and advocating for the barest minimum: a basic diagnosis and some information about prognosis and possible treatments.

We give voice to these voiceless surrogates, too often silenced by burdens of care that seem insurmountable. Their narratives tell us much about the challenge of severe brain injury and how structures of care might be reformed to ameliorate their burden. Beyond that, their stories expose the more generic challenges encountered by patients and advocates whose disease or injury straddles the acute and chronic care divide. Bridging that gap will benefit those patients whose unmet chronic care needs were created by a highly responsive acute care system capable of saving lives but incapable of sustaining them. Finally, their narratives speak to the resilience of surrogates and their ability to learn about brain injury and become more effective spokespersons for the patients who have been entrusted to their care. Their experiences, while not enviable, may be instructive to other surrogates entrusted with the care of others.

No one expects to become a surrogate decision maker, especially for a loved one who has sustained a sudden brain injury. Although brain injury is the leading cause of death and disability for young people in the United States, no one can be prepared for the complete transformation it brings.[1] This transformation occurs "in an instant," as the title of Lee and Bob Woodruff's memoir of his near-fatal brain injury in Iraq suggests.[2] In that moment, the world is changed, and the surrogate finds herself alone precisely when she would have reached out to her partner for guidance. Instead, he needs her.

It is a dramatic change in status. One moment your family is secure and safe. Then comes an urgent call from an emergency room or the police saying that there has been an accident, and that security and sense of well-being are disrupted. With brain injury, lives that had been thought shatterproof become broken, often irrevocably, without warning or preparation.

This lack of preparation is especially important for surrogates because, unlike sudden medical dramas with which the public is more familiar, brain injury is obscure and shrouded in mystery. This mystery is reflective not only of a biology we are only beginning to understand, but also of the confusing nomenclature that seeks to describe brain states. Physicians use terms like "coma," "brain death," and "persistent vegetative state" with surrogates— sometimes incorrectly and often prematurely—which betray the biases of practitioners in the acute care setting, and which may discount the possibility of recovery.

A mother describes how she heard about her son's accident and the dire prognosis that welcomed her upon her arrival in the Emergency Department. Her son had been in a car accident in the middle of the night—he had lost control and was projected out of the vehicle, landing unconscious in a pool of water. As she later learned, he was "knocked out, his nose was under the water and they estimated it was about eight minutes that he was under. I find that a little hard to believe—eight minutes is not so long to get all the rescue people there to get him out. But when he came out of, when he was pulled out of the car he was not breathing and they tried to resuscitate him on the ground and I believe I was told they finally got his heart going in the chopper on the way to the hospital."[3]

She was called to the hospital but not informed about the nature of her son's injury. Without any forewarning, she was immediately introduced to the prospect that her son might be brain dead: "I got the call from the hospital, all they said was that he was on life support and that I knew it was something very serious. That I didn't know until I got there and the neurosurgeon met us downstairs and proceeded to even not give him any hope that—first initially saying something to the effect that he had ordered some sort of blood-flow study to prove to us that he was brain dead, and that was the first time the brain was mentioned."[4]

Such discourse puts the stunned surrogate at a tremendous disadvantage, compelling her to understand the implications of what "brain death" might mean and how it might be different than conventional assessments of death.

Not only did the neurosurgeon immediately deprive her of hope or an opportunity to adjust to her new circumstance, he asked her to grapple with the challenging paradox of figuring out why proof is needed to determine that someone is dead.

In conventional parlance, one is either dead or alive. But brain death is a liminal state in which a patient retains a heartbeat and can be sustained on mechanical ventilation. It can be confusing to laypeople and evoke strong responses by professionals, who, as a recent survey of practice patterns revealed, may make errors in this diagnostic assessment.[5]

In this case, the flow study was meant to determine whether there was any arterial blood flow into the brain.[6] Although a clinical exam to determine brain death is employed in most circumstances, patients must be stable enough to withstand that evaluation, which involves removing them from a ventilator to see if respiration can be sustained independently. The young man was too unstable for this evaluation. These details were not shared with the mother, and she next heard of her son's status when she asked a nurse for an update. The neurosurgeon had vanished and no other doctor was available. It is unclear why no one was keeping her abreast of developments, but one hypothesis about why she had to initiate the line of questioning was that, unbeknownst to her, there had been a change in plans. She reports that the neurosurgeon had "disappeared and within—I think about six in the morning when we were finally able to see him and I questioned the nurse in trauma ICU had they done the tests and what were the results, and she at that time told me that those tests had been canceled and I asked why and they said that he, that his pupils had reacted and that meant that there was blood flow and he canceled the tests at that time."[7]

Just two hours earlier, the neurosurgeon had thought the patient to be brain dead. The mother's advocacy led to her being better informed but also revealed something that the clinical team may have perceived as a prognostic error.

Although it seems clinically appropriate to consider brain death testing in a patient who has sustained prolonged brain injury from trauma and prolonged anoxia (oxygen deprivation, here for a reported eight minutes), the patient's improvement exposed the fallibility of the neurosurgeon's judgment. Proposing brain death testing in this circumstance could have indicated good judgment and a desire to constrain unrealistic expectations. But neurosurgery is a culture that does not tolerate error, real or imagined, and the consequences of the neurosurgeon's prognostic miscalculation may have undermined the information flow between practitioner and advocate: "I actually had to constantly keep asking," the mother said, "because the, there was never any, I guess the severity of it, I guess they don't like to get your hopes up, there were never any words of hope or him coming out of this. Everything was grim and worse-case scenario."[8]

Within hours, confronted by a resistant system, the patient's mother had to begin advocating on her son's behalf, not to push an agenda and to obtain more or enriched information, but merely to protect and defend her child from preemptive brain death testing or other actions that might force a decision of which she was unaware. Here, the surrogate's stance toward care—and her emergent advocacy—is triggered by context in reaction to biases that might be embedded in that clinical setting.

The mother elaborated on how her feelings changed and how she began to view her responsibility to her son. Although she does not label her actions and decisions as advocacy, she quickly becomes more forceful in asserting her views and asking questions about diagnostic tests. Speaking of the neurosurgeon who had first discussed the flow study to determine whether her son was brain dead, she notes:

> It was like he was hell-bent on proving that P [the patient] was never, never, never gonna get any better. And when the blood study test didn't happen, his next step was he wanted to get him into an MRI machine. And he was trying to rush me into deciding to put him into an MRI machine. And he was so medically challenged that I kept asking him, "What's the rush for an MRI scan? Is the MRI machine gonna heal him?" And he says, "Well, no." So I say, "Then what is it going to tell me that I don't know already? What is the big rush?" Because behind me were some very caring nurses who were whispering in my ear, "Don't let him do the MRI, your son is not stable enough. If we remove him from the ventilator, we might lose him." And they have to switch ventilators to get him in the MRI machine. And the nurses weren't comfortable with that decision. They kept telling me, "Don't say that we told you, but don't let him put him in the MRI machine yet."[9]

Perhaps sensitized by her initial engagement over the flow study, the patient's mother is mobilized into a defensive stance, seeking to keep her son safe from medical mistakes. Her transition is importantly aided by the counsel of friendly, but hesitant nurses, who advise against the MRI because it would necessitate a switch of breathing machines, which could lead to complications. These nurses' advocacy—outside the usual chain of command—is appreciated by the patient's mother, who ascribes her analysis to their counsel. Tellingly, she notes that "behind me were some very caring nurses," suggesting that she was supported in her confrontation with the neurosurgeon by the nurses' help, which was invisible to him but felt by her.

Contrast this case with that of a mother whose twenty-two-year-old daughter had suffered a brain-stem stroke. Her dilemma initially was how best to represent her daughter's interests and preferences—not how to defend her from a potentially damaging clinical context but to make "right decisions" as a surrogate and eventually to defend her child's interests as her advocate.

The young woman was just weeks away from graduating college when her friends, after hearing strange noises, found her unconscious in her dorm room; the noises turned out to be signs of a seizure. Her mother rushed home from a vacation to find herself in the position of being her child's surrogate decision maker and eventual advocate.

As we will see in this vignette, surrogate decision makers, especially ones suddenly thrust into that role, do not start off as advocates. Instead, they begin as representatives of a patient unable to engage in self-representation because of decisional incapacity. In the initial impulse, the surrogate seeks to represent what the patient's wishes are, or might have been. In a bioethical or legal frame, this becomes a reliance upon "expressed wishes" when the explicit preferences of the patient are known or "substituted judgment" when these views must be inferred. When there are no antecedent wishes to guide deliberations, the surrogate decision maker falls back on a "best interests" standard of what a "generic" person might decide and do. This decision-making hierarchy is well ensconced in ethical norms, court rulings, and statutes.[10]

Although all good surrogates are at their core advocates for patients who are dependent upon them, surrogates seem unaware of this aspect of their pleadings at the outset. In the beginning, the focus is on representation and a desire not to veer too far from the wishes of the patient, if they are known. The goal is accuracy and fidelity to those wishes. If advocacy implies a degree of independence on the part of the surrogate, then the initial refrains of surrogacy are more muted. At least at the outset, the situation calls for close adherence to the score written by the patient when that individual was able to articulate preferences—a challenge when dealing with brain injury in young people who had never considered the prospect of disability and decisional incapacity.

One of us (J. J. Fins) conducted an empirical study of the moral obligations of patients and their surrogate decision makers designated through an advance directive such as a durable power of attorney or health care proxy.[11] In that analysis, surrogates were cautious in their representations, adhering to patient wishes. Although more discretionary or interpretative judgments could be made when the diagnosis and prognosis were clear, when there was uncertainty, surrogates tended toward conservatism and caution.

This conservatism is seen in this mother's initial effort to make a correct decision, not to engage in a broader vision of advocacy. Her caution was further compounded by the fact that her daughter—like most young people—had not completed an advance directive, depriving her mother as surrogate decision maker of both substantive guidance and moral authority to make life and death judgments. Speaking of her early encounters with medical providers, the mother said:

> I don't know that the word "advocate" is immediately used. You know, you start out and it's an emergency and so you just jump in to where you need to, but of course when you have the sort of emergency that relates to someone being in a coma, then obviously end-of-life issues come up immediately. And so since the person can't speak for themselves or perhaps like in my daughter's case she didn't have her own living will, or anything that said what she would have wanted, I had to decide what I thought she would want. So immediately you have to make decisions that have to do with being an advocate for this person. And say, "Well, I think this is what they want." And I actually was very pressed by a doctor immediately in P's treatment about "do you really think she would want you to keep her alive in this situation, when her chances of any sort of recovery are perhaps 5 percent or less?"
>
> So I actually had to, I sought out a paper that my daughter had written about something slightly related, which was euthanasia, because she was a veterinary student, and about her thinking about animals and when you would put someone down, an animal down versus when you would say, "Well, let's keep treating them." And so it really was so clear from that paper that she had an opinion about sort of quality of life and when you might say, "Now is time to have someone—to die."[12]

The patient's mother seeks to discern her daughter's prior wishes by inference from her past experience and her daughter's writings in college. Although not directly on point, they do help inform her stance as a surrogate and move her toward a prudent wait-and-see attitude that coheres with her daughter's views, as best as they can be discerned.

This faithfulness to her daughter's wishes leads to a degree of caution and makes the mother's advocacy something private between them. Its scope expands when the surrogate is called upon to respond to unanticipated challenges that will require a discretionary response. As in our first case vignette, this mother is, as she says, "put in a position" that compels public advocacy beyond the mere representation of the patient's wishes and an implicit or explicit pact between patient and surrogate. Her sense of responsibility changes when she is approached to see if her still living daughter might be considered an organ donor: "I guess after that then there were other times immediately as she, it became clear, someone came to me and said, 'Do you think your daughter would want to be an organ donor if she dies?' So that was another case where because she couldn't answer for herself I had to make a decision about that. And, not that it's hard, but it's something I had to decide on. So immediately you're put in the position of being an advocate."[13]

The way in which suspicion transforms a trusting representative-surrogate operating under a presumption of good faith into an advocate who needs to defend the prerogatives of a loved one is illustrated in the following exchange between a neurologist and the mother of a nineteen-year-old pedestrian who was struck by a drunk driver. Just days before her son's deployment to Iraq as a marine, he lay unresponsive after a severe brain injury. A neurologist told his mother that he did not even "have the reflexes of a frog."

> *Mother*: And actually I had a neurologist tell me, "Your son is basically just an organ donor now."
> *JJF*: And when did that happen?
> *Mother*: Within the first seventy-two hours. She said, "Well, he doesn't have the reflexes of a frog."
> *JJF*: He doesn't have the reflexes of a . . . ?
> *Mother*: Of a frog . . . She said, "You should really just consider him being an organ donor. That's the best thing you can do for your son." And I said, "I completely disagree with you. I'm not making him an organ donor. Go back in there and do the best you can."[14]

The three cases described here occurred in different regions of the country with families that were socioculturally distinct. Their experiences are reflective of a broader pattern of care that views the treatment of patients with severe brain injury as hopeless, even early on before a clear prognosis is evident. The broader institutional articulation of these attitudes is seen in a paper published in *Neurology*, the official journal of the American Academy of Neurology. The authors, critical care neurologists at the Mayo Clinic, counsel practitioners:

> Families should be given an explanation of the success rate and complexity associated with resuscitation, but the physician should avoid needless detail, . . . have an understanding of the accumulating costs of

intensive care if a major advancement of level of care is pursued. . . . The attending physician of a patient with a devastating neurologic illness will have to come to terms with the futility of care. . . . Those families who are unconvinced should be explicitly told they should have markedly diminished expectations for what intensive care can accomplish and that withdrawal of life support or abstaining from performing complex interventions is more commensurate with the neurologic status.[15]

This is not a value-neutral discourse but one with an agenda to engineer a specific outcome. In addition, it is scientifically inaccurate on several important counts. A coma is a self-limited, eyes-closed state of unconsciousness that typically lasts ten to fourteen days.[16] As we will see in the stories of our surrogate-advocates, brain states evolve, with a patient's prognosis becoming clearer over time. To put it plainly, it is premature to be so categorical about outcomes and goals of care with patients who are still in a comatose state because it is the first way station on the road to a potential recovery.

One surrogate, whose fifty-five-year-old wife suffered a ruptured anterior communicating artery aneurysm, tells of an exchange he had with a neurosurgeon just ten days after her injury. In years past his wife had made him her durable power of attorney for health care, with the authority to withdraw life-sustaining therapy. He felt it premature at that early juncture and decided to advocate for waiting, countering staff recommendations:

Husband: . . . We had both decided that . . . that we would, don't pull the plug too soon, make sure that you're right, but I don't want to be a burden to you and you don't want to be a burden to me, and we, we were in absolute synch as to what we wanted, but [pause] it, it, it's different in practice than in theory.

JJF: So when the neurosurgeon put his arm around you and said that letting her go would be an altruistic or kind thing to do, when was that exactly, how long into the course . . . ?

Husband: Before the end of July, probably within ten days.

JJF: She was in a coma?

Husband: Right.

JJF: How did you know it was in your gut of guts that it was too early to make that decision? . . . what was the internal clock telling you? How did you know?

Husband: Um, kinda silly. When I kissed her [starts crying], she kissed me back. And [pauses] the neurosurgeon minimalized that, saying it was . . . a primitive, instinctive reflex, and the longer she was at the hospital the more I was positive that she was, that her personality was still there [*crying*]. . . . And to further minimalize that which I felt, one of the nurses in the neuro-ICU said, "She's probably just kissing you goodbye." So everyone who I dealt with was negative. There was no one who said, "I think that there's hope. I think you should wait."[17]

Perhaps more than most cases, this one shows the wide range of outcomes that can attend a coma. Nearly three years later, at the time of this writing, the patient is learning how to talk again. This evolution suggests that the kiss was not a primitive reflex, but rather, as a song puts it, "just a kiss."

As time goes by, comas can lead to a wide range of outcomes, from death to complete recovery.[18] If consciousness is not recovered within two weeks, the patient will become vegetative. This state was first described by Bryan Jennett and Fred Plum in 1972 as a paradoxical one of "wakeful unresponsiveness" in which the eyes are open but there is no awareness of self or the environment.[19] There is the return of autonomic functions and a sleep-wake cycle marking the recovery of the most primitive part of the brain, the brain stem. This was the state that Karen Ann Quinlan was in when the New Jersey Superior Court reached its landmark 1976 right-to-die decision. The court justified the removal of Quinlan's ventilator based on the testimony of neurologist Fred Plum, who described the brain as a mix of higher-order sapient functions and more primitive vegetative ones.[20] Judge C. J. Hughes, writing for the court, noted the irretrievable loss of Karen Quinlan's cognitive, sapient state as the moral warrant for the removal of her ventilator. Confronted with such a dire prognosis and degree of medical futility, the court asserted:

We have no hesitancy in deciding . . . that no external compelling interest of the State should compel Karen to endure the unendurable, only to vegetate a few more measurable months with no realistic possibility of returning to any semblance of *cognitive or sapient life.* . . . Upon concurrence of the guardian and the family of Karen, should the responsible attending conclude that there is no reasonable possibility of Karen's ever emerging from her present comatose condition to a cognitive, sapient state and that the life-support apparatus . . . be discontinued, they shall consult with the hospital "Ethics Committee" or like body.[21]

We quote at length because of the importance of this decision and its reasoning to the emerging right-to-die movement. In *Quinlan*, the right to die began not as a global right but as a temperate one, limited to the state of profound futility characterized by the vegetative state.[22] Although the right-to-die would extend eventually to non-vegetative patients, its origins in *Quinlan* and link to the persistent vegetative state would long effect how patients with severe brain injury would be viewed.

The medical recommendations we heard from our participating family members reflect this historical legacy that equates severe brain injury with futility. This has led severe brain injury to be viewed with clinical nihilism, a sense that nothing can or should be done.[23] To pursue treatment in such "hopeless" cases is seen as ethically disproportionate, with burdens outweighing any foreseeable benefits.[24]

Practitioners suggesting that care be withheld or withdrawn reflect a thirty-year acculturation to patients' and surrogates' rights that have their origins in the nascent right to die embodied in the *Quinlan* decision. This professional acknowledgement of patients' self-determination or their delegated autonomy bequeathed to surrogates is well intentioned. It seeks to spare families the burden of caring for one forever destined to a non-sapient life, as Plum eloquently noted, and who can neither relate to the outside world nor speak, see, feel, sing, or think.

Since *Quinlan*, this professional concern has become something more. In fostering self-determination of patients and their surrogates, it has also become increasingly paternalistic and ideological, asserting a proper course of action when confronted by severe brain injury. Our participating surrogates report practitioners who, rather than respecting choices, engineer certain outcomes and obscure the choices. They conflate the diagnoses of different brain states that need to be disaggregated so that informed choices can be made to pursue additional treatment, engage in watchful waiting to see if the situation changes, or make a decision to withhold or withdraw life-sustaining therapy.[25] Perhaps most critically, linking the futility of the vegetative state to the right to die effectively compels patients with severe brain injury to be viewed indiscriminately, carrying an equally dire prognosis irrespective of etiology of injury or time course.[26] Here the right to die has overwhelmed the right to care.[27]

But we now appreciate that some vegetative states are transient and not permanent. There is a diagnostic sequence of events that is material to judgments about proportionate care. Temporally, when a vegetative state continues beyond thirty days, it is described as *persistent*. Prospects for the recovery of consciousness become grim when the vegetative state becomes *permanent*, three months after anoxic injury (without oxygen) and twelve months after traumatic injury.[28]

More critically, we now appreciate that consciousness can be regained in vegetative patients before that state becomes permanent. In the period between the persistent and permanent vegetative state, there is a window within which patients can progress to what has been described as the minimally conscious state (MCS).[29] Unlike vegetative patients, the minimally conscious demonstrate episodic but unequivocal evidence of awareness of self and the environment. They may say words or phrases and make gestures and may also show evidence of memory, attention, and intention. Patients are considered to have emerged from MCS when they can reliably and consistently communicate.

To put this technical digression into prognostic context, which is so important for well-founded surrogate advocacy, 77 percent of comas resulting from anoxic brain injury will result in death or the permanent vegetative state. This contrasts with 50 percent for those who have sustained a coma because of traumatic injury.[30] The remainder will span a continuum of brain states from MCS to full recovery. Although a patient's outcome may be grim, these data do not invariably equate with futility. Rather, they support the advocacy of the surrogates we have studied.[31]

Certain moments are transformative for a surrogate. The husband who had been kissed by his wife told us he felt isolated in his decisions, alone, confronted by medical facts with which he was unfamiliar. In those moments he became her champion, the one person who would advocate for her right to care. Like many whom we interviewed, he came to believe that he was a better gauge of his wife's progress than were those around him who urged a deescalation of care or were uninterested.

By virtue of their devotion to their loved ones—and long hours at the bedside—these surrogates may observe even the subtlest changes in patients' behaviors that may herald the return of consciousness and migration into MCS, which is marked by fluctuating signs of awareness of self, others, or the environment. Because these demonstrations of behavior are episodic and not readily reproducible, they are easily missed or dismissed, although this pattern is part and parcel of the biology of MCS and to be expected.[32]

Patients who are making this migration are incredibly vulnerable without the attention of a vigilant surrogate who will make observations and seek their clinical validation.[33] Absent informed and effective surrogacy, diagnostic errors can occur, labeling patients who have become minimally conscious as vegetative. Such is the now oft-told story of Terry Wallis, a thirty-nine-year-old Arkansan who resided in a nursing home for nineteen years under a false diagnosis.[34] Brain-imaging studies done nineteen years after his injury revealed axonal sprouting, or new connections between existing neurons, that investigators speculated might be related to his late recovery.[35] He now has emerged out of the minimally conscious state and has regained fluent speech; his case is starting to focus the attention of policy makers on the needs of this population and the need for systematic study.[36]

But until such study occurs, practice patterns will persist that turn a blind eye to the needs of this population and the observations of surrogates. Even after the worldwide front-page coverage of the Terry Wallis case, families are still struggling simply to obtain a credible diagnosis for their loved ones once they have left the acute care setting and entered chronic care. This is a difficult challenge.[37] Although brain states can and will change with time, patients who are moved to chronic care are often locked into a diagnostic frame supplied by the more acute institution from which they were transferred.

This was the case with a woman in her thirties who was in a motor vehicle accident. She presented very poor prognostic indicators, though she was eventually stabilized with highly aggressive neuroprotective surgery. After a rocky hospital course she was discharged to a skilled nursing facility with the diagnosis of being in a permanent vegetative state.

Like so many of those we interviewed, her mother had observed behaviors that would have put the patient functionally above the level of being vegetative. She struggled to have her daughter properly assessed:

> We were seeing improvements and changes but we couldn't get the staff. I was constantly trying to get a nurse or somebody in there to document what we were seeing because we had been told early on, whatever you see, have them document it. And so we tried desperately to have that happen and yet as a family member, I really and truly felt they were just patronizing me. . . . I just felt that people weren't really listening to what we were saying, and that why was it that we were seeing these changes and I couldn't get them there for her, and I couldn't get the staff to say she's making forward progress instead of not doing anything, but it just wasn't happening. So it was very, very frustrating and it was scary because I felt that she was going to be pigeonholed into a, into a spot that we would have a hard time getting out of.[38]

Despite her mother's advocacy, the patient was discharged with the diagnosis remaining vegetative.

> She was discharged with that diagnosis of PVS [persistent vegetative state], and I kept trying to get that changed because when she went to this new nursing care facility, the day that they got her they called me in and wanted to meet with me the very next morning. And so they had this big team of people—the speech therapist, occupational and

physical therapists, and the director of nursing—and they told me that the patient that they received the day before, my daughter, was not the patient that they were told they were going to get. They said she obviously isn't in PVS, you know, she's responding to her name, obviously when we talk to her she looks at us, she's tracking people across the room, she's moving her limbs, not a lot, but she's moving. This isn't a patient that apparently they told her was just basically going to have custodial care and be there to die. And I was upset when I found this out because here I thought that the professionals, the medical team at [a university hospital] thought that P was looking better and I'm thinking, "Ok, what's happening?"[39]

The diagnosis of a vegetative state facilitated this patient's transfer out of the university hospital and provided more options for placement.[40] It then limited the amount of rehabilitation to which the patient was entitled. The mother reported:

As time went on I realized that that [diagnosis] facilitated them having more nursing care facilities that would take her. If she's going to be laying there, not doing anything, then the nursing care facilities will take her, and they just wanted to get her out of the hospital. So they left her with that diagnosis; . . . one of my key things was to get her diagnosis changed. And one of the reasons was so I could get more therapy for her so that the insurance would pay for it and the therapists could start seeing her and she would hopefully move forward . . . [but] when she left that nursing care facility [she] still had the diagnosis of PVS.[41]

The misdiagnosis, which eased her placement out of the hospital, coupled with the nursing home's bureaucratic stasis resulted in limiting the amount of rehabilitation to which she was entitled. These lapses, which the mother viewed as ethical ones, reconfigured her advocacy into a mobilization of the institution's physical therapists. With an element of civil disobedience, she motivated physical therapists to provide necessary services in spite of the regulations and to do so on their own time. An alliance was struck with these therapists, most of whom were parents themselves. This dynamic, enjoining of a group of practitioners in the face of questionable administrative practice, was in direct response to the mother's rallying call:

So I said [to the therapists], "Well, are you gonna tell me that you can't take care of my daughter now that I've got her here?" And they said, "Oh no, no, we'll do whatever we can, we want P to get better here." It was

a battle. And there's where I say the therapists there took an interest in
P and they fought for her. And I have to say that they were very ethical,
the therapists were; the administrators, however, were not. And so it
was a constant battle for them to just be able to treat P, and they treated
her when they were not supposed to. They would stay after hours and
treat her and things like that. And I mean, that's the kind of care I know
people can't do it, they have busy lives and families and they have to go
home to their loved ones too. But I tell you that it was my hope, was in
my faith in the people who took an interest in her.[42]

Most surrogates are less successful in their advocacy when challenging
insurance constraints. The nature of these brain disorders makes it appear as
though patients are not benefiting from treatments or rehabilitation regimens.
Although an NIH consensus panel on brain injury stated that "persons with
TBI [traumatic brain injury] should have access to rehabilitation services
through the entire course of recovery, which may last for many years after the
injury," the patient's inability to demonstrate progress in a reliable fashion or
to meet medical necessity time frames makes it difficult to justify continued
interventions.[43]

The wife of a man who suffered a brain-stem stroke and is currently in a
locked-in state, like that of Jean-Dominique Bauby in *The Diving Bell and the Butterfly*, captured the difficulty of obtaining needed benefits in an interview with
us.[44] Her husband is entirely aware of his surroundings and is able to reliably
communicate. In much the same way that Bauby wrote his memoir, the patient
uses a letter board to spell out words by blinking his eyes or slightly nodding his
head. His wife's frustration and dire circumstances are evident in her comments:

I see some improvement. They stopped his physical therapy . . . I don't
understand their logic for not doing it. You know, they were saying . . .
he's not making an effort to roll or get to, try to get from the bed to a
chair, you know. . . . Now, I was like very upset over that. Because why
can't you do physical therapy forever? If the brain is so complex, what
he might not do today he might do three months from now. But if you
don't continue to do it with him, he's not gonna do it at all. . . . I don't
understand the logic to this. Not to mention the fact that it cost me my
insurance because they won't cover him now. . . . I have to become poor
in order for them to help him.[45]

The financial responsibilities of these surrogates is daunting, placing
tremendous pressure upon them and making it difficult for them to remain ever

vigilant for their loved ones. Many surrogates we interviewed had a defeatist attitude, feeling beaten down by the system. The husband of the patient who had suffered from an aneurysm—and who kissed him back—eloquently described this feeling of defeat. A lawyer and skilled advocate himself, he invoked the myth of Sisyphus to explain his circumstances and burdens:

> *Husband*: . . . In terms of how to deal with Medicaid issues, I'm kind of stuck. . . . They don't do any advocacy for us whatsoever. So if I want more assistance or anything like that, I don't know in any way how to go to Medicaid and ask for more assistance . . . or if I even can.
>
> *JH*: What sort of advocacy issues do you think this population is most . . . troubled by? What do they need the most? What do you need?
>
> *Husband*: What I need the most is money and services. I think, you know, help at home, caring for her, I've gotten three days paid for by Medicaid and I pay for three days myself. And it cost me about a little more than $120,000 out of my own pocket to have her home last year. Which leads me to believe that there aren't many people who can do that.[46]

For most of these surrogate-advocates, their cause is personal. It is corporeal and real, not abstract and policy driven. It is neither a task to be delegated to another nor a burden of their choosing. It is more a responsibility than a burden. As the mother of the young woman who had the seizure in her dorm room put it: "If I were to leave her advocacy to a social worker alone to answer the questions alone, I would feel neglectful. Because I know my daughter better. . . . I think if a social worker has a caseload of people . . . they have a job to do but their love or passion for that particular individual can never be the same as the family's passion and love; . . . no matter how loving and passionate they are about their work, it isn't the same thing. I think you just have to know how to use their knowledge but you can't expect them to do it for you."[47]

And yet, the assumption of this highly personal degree of responsibility extracts a hefty toll: financial hardship and exhaustion. One of the certainties of brain injury advocacy is that it does not draw upon a limitless fount. Studies have shown that depression in caregivers of patients with severe brain injury increases when the caregiver feels overwhelmed and perceives a lack of external support.[48]

The mother of the young man who was hit by the drunk driver reached out to her state's secretary of welfare in desperation, simply asserting: "I need your help. They're not helping me. I need your help. People in power need to help." She perhaps described the burdens surrounding cost of care and insurance coverage best when she said: "It's like having an extra job just doing this."[49] She and her fellow surrogate-advocates are not pleading for a cause but for loved ones for whom they care deeply. This is not a political act, a march for some sort of cure, that one can choose to attend or not. Instead it is an obligation that strikes at the core of love and family.

Like most of these surrogates, her battle is a solitary one, ill-fitting with the advocacy groups that purport to help. In her view:

> *Mother*: A lot of times these groups are so, like, fragmented. And especially for brain injury groups. There's not a lot of—people who don't vote, I don't think there are a lot of groups out there to help them. I mean, even if you're paralyzed you can still vote, hopefully. But when you're brain injured, you don't . . . there's no power there, none; . . . and it is sad to find out like all these groups, . . . they tell you there's nothing they can do for you, . . . nothing fits his needs, . . . if you have AIDS, they have a Medicaid waiver for that, if you're paralyzed, there's a waiver for that. But brain injury, no.
>
> *JH*: So you think it's a very marginalized population?
>
> *Mother*: Extremely marginalized, that's the exact word! They don't think, there's no hope for them getting better. You can tell when you're talking to someone, they don't have the respect for his being. Much less, you know, how's he doing. They don't see them as a value to society in any way. I'm shocked by what I saw.[50]

Her eloquence gives proper voice to the challenges confronted by this marginalized population and by the diligent surrogate-advocates who defend them one by one, as she continues: "You're not seeing people who are brain injured . . . on the street. They're not going to baseball games, they're unseen and unheard. And that's the problem. People in wheelchairs, they're out and about. They have jobs . . . you kind of can't mess with . . . people who are aware of their surroundings; . . . when do you see people like P except in an institutional environment? . . . They're the unseen and unheard . . . and even the people who were supposed to help him really didn't want to help him."[51]

This mother's poignant words encapsulate the many challenges that patients and families touched by severe brain injury encounter. Patients are placed in facilities unsuited to their needs and isolated from society, sequestered out of sight. Their surrogate advocates struggle with individuals and institutions, from neurologists to nursing homes, but have remained silent as policy actors.

We hope that this biopsy of their concerns gives voice to their advocacy and points to the need to reform the untenable context of care that presently exists. Although one story is merely an anecdote, the collective narratives of many patients and families reveal recurring patterns of care that is deficient.

Like many stories, these narratives are also a collective parable, stories with a moral lesson: we must become aware of the shortcomings of the current system in order to remedy them. The challenge is clear: the tragedy of young people residing in nursing homes designed for what is euphemistically described as "custodial care" distanced from academic medical centers where scientific innovation might ameliorate their conditions.

This discordance of clinical need and policy response is a public health challenge that needs to be rectified by a reconfiguration of institutional care structures. If we are to meet the needs of these patients—as articulated so cogently by their surrogate-advocates—we need to better integrate acute care venues with their chronic care counterparts and decrease the abrupt discontinuities of care that place patients in low-tech facilities unable to promote clinical innovation or sustain vanguard research that might ultimately make a difference in their diagnosis and treatment. This effort will be capital intensive and require the collaboration of the neurological, neurosurgical, and rehabilitative medicine communities and a transformation of the built environment.[52]

Until this longer-term objective is realized, the more immediate pragmatic challenge is to make the care environment more hospitable to the needs of these patients and their surrogates. These narratives tell us that one of the ways this happens is through the formation of alliances. If surrogates hope to become advocates, they will need to engage with others. Advocates need interlocutors and even willing adversaries who will engage them—physicians, nurses, social workers, and administrators—and take their requests seriously. But as these tales of woe indicate, surrogates are often met with disinterest from the medical community. This neglect can in turn extinguish advocacy and replace it with complacency and frustration. Laudable exceptions to this trajectory are noteworthy because they illustrate alternative patient-centered responses that might be prompted, if not institutionalized.

Bringing this degree of humanity to the bedside of those with severe brain injury will not be simple because the object of surrogates' advocacy, the local clinical establishment, has also historically been where patients and families obtain credible information. Local clinicians' ignorance of scientific advances, be it from errors of omission (lack of continuing medical education) or commission (cultural priming: believing that all brain injuries are catastrophic and it is best to let these patients die), compounds the problem because they misinform families or do not engage in empowering community-based education.

This is further complicated by the inherent conservatism in medical practice, outside of isolated research and academic settings. Physicians are often uncomfortable questioning the diagnostic frameworks under which they were trained, preferring older nosologies with which they are comfortable. Like scientists clinging to an old Kuhnian paradigm, physicians will remain defensively confident in frameworks that are increasingly revealed as imperfect when challenged.

Yet for advocates to have any sway with physicians, doctors need a requisite amount of humility about their pronouncements and a willingness to acknowledge gaps in their knowledge. Previously, one of us (J. J. Fins) suggested that physicians separate their diagnoses into "time-delimited" elements recognizing their contingency and potential inaccuracy as recovery ensues and new diagnostic tools, such as neuroimaging, are brought into the assessment process.[53] In these circumstances, diagnostic imprecision can have an overwhelming impact on prognostic possibilities and patient outcomes.

Properly empowered surrogate-advocates can help clinicians achieve diagnostic temperance by being informed and asking good questions. Clinicians should acknowledge their reciprocal obligation to give surrogates the information they need to ask good questions and participate in the decision-making process. Removed from the bedside of individual patients, clinicians should develop educational materials that are both accessible and accurate.[54] Although knowledge is power, education in isolation may not be powerful enough to break reified practice patterns. Substantive knowledge needs to be met with procedural reform. For this reason, it is especially critical that care structures seek to institutionalize ways to give surrogate-advocates *access to those in power.* Organizations should sanction regularly scheduled interdisciplinary meetings or forums that provide many points of contact for surrogate-advocates to initiate alliances with members of the clinical team. These meetings should be nonhierarchical and held as group sessions so that surrogate-advocates can overcome their solitary efforts and collectively alter the status quo.

Writing of the extremes of partisanship during the French Revolution, Samuel Taylor Coleridge famously noted: "The first duty of a wise advocate is to convince his opponents that he understands their arguments, and sympathizes with their just feelings."[55] We hope that our proposals give surrogates the wisdom they need and the forum they deserve to serve those who are dependent upon their care.

Acknowledgments

J. J. Fins is the recipient of an Investigator Award in Health Policy Research ("Minds Apart: Severe Brain Injury and Health Policy") from the Robert Wood Johnson Foundation. He also gratefully acknowledges grant support from the Charles A. Dana Foundation ("Mending the Brain, Minding our Ethics II") as well as the Buster Foundation ("Neuroethics and Disorders of Consciousness") and the Richard Lounsbery Foundation ("Sustaining and Building Research Infrastructure for the Study of Disorders of Consciousness at Weill Cornell Medical College and Rockefeller University"), which have also funded Jennifer Hersh's research.

We thank the family members who have shared their stories with such generosity of spirit and Dr. Nicholas D. Schiff for his collaboration and counsel.

Notes

1. "NIH Consensus Development Panel on Rehabilitation of Persons with Traumatic Brain Injury," *JAMA* 282 (1999): 974–983.
2. J. J. Fins, review of *In an Instant: A Family's Journey of Love and Healing*, by Lee and Bob Woodruff, *JAMA* 297, 23 (2007): 2642–2643.
3. Interview IN301M. All interviews are taken from J. Fins and J. Hersh, "Neuroethics and Disorders of Consciousness: A Qualitative and Quantitative Assessment of Clinical Practice and Healthcare System Epidemiology/Barriers to Care," Institutional Review Board–approved research study in progress, January 2007 to the present. Interviews are identified by an internal code to protect subject anonymity. In all interview excerpts, the patient is referred to as "P."
4. Ibid.
5. D. M. Greer, P. N. Varelas, S. Haque, and E. F. Wijdicks, "Variability of Brain Death Determination Guidelines in Leading US Neurologic Institutions," *Neurology* 70, 4 (2008): 284–289; S. Laureys and J. J. Fins, "Are We Equal in Death? Avoiding Diagnostic Error in Brain Death," *Neurology* 70, 4 (2008): 14–15.
6. J. Posner, C. B. Saper, N. D. Schiff, and F. Plum, *Plum and Posner's Diagnosis of Stupor and Coma*, 4th ed. (New York: Oxford University Press, 2007).
7. IN301M.
8. Ibid.
9. Ibid.
10. J. J. Fins, *A Palliative Ethic of Care: Clinical Wisdom at Life's End* (Sudbury, Mass.: Jones and Bartlett, 2006).
11. J. J. Fins, B. S. Maltby, E. Friedmann, M. G. Greene, K. Norris, R. Adelman, and I. Byock, "Contracts, Covenants, and Advance Care Planning: An Empirical Study of the Moral Obligations of Patient and Proxy," *Journal of Pain and Symptom Management* 29 (2005): 55–68.
12. IN316W.
13. Ibid.
14. IN314W.
15. E.F.M. Wijdicks and A. A. Rabinstein, "The Family Conference: End-of-Life Guidelines at Work for Comatose Patients," *Neurology* 68 (2007): 1092–1093.

16. Posner et al., *Diagnosis of Stupor and Coma.*

17. IN300E.

18. J. J. Fins, "Rethinking Disorders of Consciousness: New Research and Its Implications," *Hastings Center Report* 35, 2 (2005): 22–24.

19. B. Jennett and F. Plum, "Persistent Vegetative State after Brain Damage: A Syndrome in Search of a Name," *Lancet* 1, 7753 (1972): 734–737.

20. *In the Matter of Karen Quinlan, an Alleged Incompetent*, 70 N.J. 10, 355 A.2d 677 (1976).

21. Ibid.

22. Fins, *A Palliative Ethic of Care.*

23. J. J. Fins, "Constructing an Ethical Stereotaxy for Severe Brain Injury: Balancing Risks, Benefits, and Access," *Nature Reviews Neuroscience* 4 (2003): 323–327.

24. H. K. Beecher, "Ethical Problems Caused by the Hopelessly Unconscious Patient," *New England Journal of Medicine* 278, 26 (1968): 1425–1430; H. K. Beecher, "After the 'Definition of Irreversible Coma,'" *New England Journal of Medicine* 281, 19 (1969): 1070–1071.

25. J. J. Fins, "Rethinking Disorders of Consciousness," 22–24; J. J. Fins and F. Plum, "Neurological Diagnosis Is More Than a State of Mind: Diagnostic Clarity and Impaired Consciousness," *Archives of Neurology* 61, 9 (2004): 1354–1355.

26. Ibid.

27. J. J. Fins, "Affirming the Right to Care, Preserving the Right to Die: Disorders of Consciousness and Neuroethics after Schiavo," *Supportive and Palliative Care* 4, 2 (2006): 169–178.

28. "Medical Aspects of the Persistent Vegetative State (1 and 2): The Multi-Society Task Force on PVS," *New England Journal of Medicine* 330, 21 (1994): 1499–1508, and 22 (1994): 1572–1579.

29. J. T. Giacino, S. Ashwal, N. Childs, R. Cranford, B. Jennett, D. I. Katz, J. P. Kelly, J. H. Rosenberg, J. Whyte, R. D. Zafonte, and N. D. Zasler, "The Minimally Conscious State: Definition and Diagnostic Criteria," *Neurology* 58, 3 (2002): 349–353.

30. Posner et al, *Diagnosis of Stupor and Coma.*

31. Fins, "Constructing an Ethical Stereotaxy," 323–327.

32. J. J. Fins, "Clinical Pragmatism and the Care of Brain Injured Patients: Towards a Palliative Neuroethics for Disorders of Consciousness," *Progress in Brain Research* 150 (2005): 565–582.

33. J. J. Fins, "Border Zones of Consciousness: Another Immigration Debate?" *American Journal of Bioethics* 7, 1 (2007): 51–54.

34. N. D. Schiff and J. J. Fins, "Hope for 'Comatose' Patients," *Cerebrum* 5, 4 (2003): 7–24.

35. H. U. Voss, A. M. Uluc, J. P. Dyke, R. Watts, E. J. Kobylarz, B. D. McCandliss, L. A. Heier, B. J. Beattie, K. A. Hamacher, S. Vallabhajosula, et al., "Possible Axonal Regrowth in Late Recovery from Minimally Conscious State," *Journal of Clinical Investigation* 116 (2006): 2005–2011.

36. J. J. Fins, N. D. Schiff, and K. M. Foley, "Late Recovery from the Minimally Conscious State: Ethical and Policy Implications," *Neurology* 68 (2007): 304–307.

37. J. J. Fins, M. G. Master, L. M. Gerber, and J. T. Giacino, "The Minimally Conscious State: A Diagnosis in Search of an Epidemiology," *Archives of Neurology* 64, 10 (2007): 1400–1405.

38. T-x. Quotes in the text attributed in the notes to Tx are drawn from a transcript of a taped public talk given by the patient's mother and are used with her permission.

39. Ibid.
40. Had the misdiagnosis been deliberate (as the patient's mother believed in this case), it would have been in startling contrast with the more common scenario of physician manipulation of reimbursement rules to help patients obtain care. See M. K. Wynia, D. S. Cummins, J. B. VanGeest, and I. B. Wilson, "Physician Manipulation of Reimbursement Rules for Patients: Between a Rock and a Hard Place," *JAMA* 283, 14 (2000): 1858–1865.
41. T-x.
42. Ibid.
43. "NIH Consensus Development Panel on Rehabilitation of Persons with Traumatic Brain Injury," *JAMA* 282, 10 (1999): 974–983.
44. Jean-Dominique Bauby, *The Diving Bell and the Butterfly* (New York: Vintage, 1998).
45. IN321D.
46. IN300E.
47. IN316W.
48. J. K. Harris, H. P. Godfrey, F. M. Partridge, and R. G. Knight, "Caregiver Depression Following Traumatic Brain Injury (TBI): A Consequence of Adverse Effects on Family Members?" *Brain Injury* 15, 3 (2001): 223–238.
49. IN314W.
50. Ibid.
51. Ibid.
52. J. Berube, J. J. Fins, J. T. Giacino, D. Katz, J. Lanlois, J. Whyte, and G. A. Zitnay, *The Mohonk Report: A Report to Congress Improving Outcomes for Individuals with Disorders of Consciousness* (Charlottesville, Va.: National Brain Injury Research, Treatment, and Training Foundation, 2006).
53. J. J. Fins, "Ethics of Clinical Decision Making and Communication with Surrogates," in Fins, *Diagnosis of Stupor and Coma*; J. J. Fins, J. Illes, J. L. Bernat, J. Hirsch, S. Laureys, E. Murphy, and Participants of the Working Meeting on Ethics, Neuroimaging, and Limited States of Consciousness, "Neuroimaging and Disorders of Consciousness: Envisioning an Ethical Research Agenda," *American Journal of Bioethics* 8, 9 (2008): 3–12; J. J. Fins, "Neuroethics and Neuroimaging: Moving towards Transparency," *American Journal of Bioethics* 8, 9 (2008): 46–52.
54. J. Illes, P. W. Lau, and J. T. Giacino, "Neuroimaging, Impaired States of Consciousness, and Public Outreach," *Nature Clinical Practice Neurology* 4, 10 (2008): 542–543; J. J. Fins, "Brain Injury: The Vegetative and Minimally Conscious States," in *From Birth to Death and Bench to Clinic: The Hastings Center Briefing Book for Journalists, Policymakers, and Campaigns*, ed. M. Crowley (Garrison, N.Y.: Hastings Center, 2008), 15–19.
55. S. T. Coleridge, *The Friend: A Series of Essays in Three Volumes to Aid in the Formation of Fixed Principles in Politics, Morals, and Religion, with Literary Amusements Interspersed*, vol. 2 (London: Rest Fenner, Paternoster-Row, 1818), 23.

Chapter 2

M. Robin DiMatteo, Kelly B. Haskard-Zolnierek,
Summer L. Williams, and Desiree Despues

Physician-Patient Communication in the Care of Vulnerable Populations

The Patient's Voice in Interpersonal Policy

Effective communication with their providers is an essential element of health care for all patients. To accept and adhere to prescriptions and treatment recommendations, patients need clear information about their conditions, attention to their questions and concerns, informative explanations about treatment options, support to make the medical decisions that are right for them, and preservation of their dignity and emotional well-being in dealing with the challenges of illness. Unfortunately, in the United States today, these important aspects of care are often denied to economically and socially vulnerable patients—specifically those of low income, ethnic minority status, low education, or low health literacy. Vulnerable patients receive less effective medical care and have less optimal health outcomes than do patients with greater economic resources and greater social advantage, even when controlling for access to medical services.[1]

One important element at the root of these health disparities is inequality in provider-patient communication. Socioeconomically vulnerable patients receive less positive communication, less information, fewer treatment options, and overall less effective care compared with more advantaged patients. Communication disparities challenge patients' ability to adhere to preventive and treatment recommendations, reducing the quality of their health outcomes. More broadly, these communication difficulties differentially privilege and empower patients' voices at institutional, community, and national levels; patients of higher education and income are often heard, and patients of low income, education, or health literacy are often silenced. Empowerment and provider-patient communication are thus essential targets for policy intervention to reduce disparities in health and health care.

The Silent Voices of Vulnerable Patients

Effective physician-patient communication is essential to a multitude of health care outcomes, including patient satisfaction, adherence, and treatment response.[2] When physician-patient communication is effective, physicians are more likely to address patients' treatment expectations, and there are fewer misunderstandings.[3] Shared, participatory decision-making gives patients a greater sense of control over their medical care and allows them to take greater personal responsibility for their treatment adherence, resulting in earlier detection of treatable problems, better health care outcomes, and lower treatment costs.[4] When provider-patient communication is effective, patients are less likely to delay reporting their symptoms and they provide more accurate medical histories, facilitating better treatment outcomes.[5] Physicians who work to build therapeutic partnerships tend to have more active patients who ask questions, express concerns, and are assertive in relaying their needs.[6]

Patient involvement, participation, and partnership in the medical visit—when they occur—allow patients to have a broad experience of empowerment in their health care. They learn about their disease conditions, come prepared for their medical visits, and discuss with their providers various options for medications, screening tests, and interventions. They expect to have alternatives available to them, and to choose among these as a matter of policy. Without information and the power of decision making, participation, and involvement, patients cannot advocate on the individual level for themselves or their family members. Without a sense of empowerment in the medical visit, individuals also cannot advocate on a broader scale for all patients by affecting health policy at the organizational, community, and national levels.

To examine the subtle role of physician communication in silencing a vulnerable patient, consider the interaction between this physician and a low-income patient (with identifying information and verbal disfluencies removed):

Patient: So, what does hyperventilation involve?

Doctor: Lotta stuff . . . has to do with anxiety. They used to say 'breathe into a paper bag.' Do that. . . . Um, [medication #1] will help you. M'kay?

P: But I, I can't take [medication #1] anymore—

D: [*Interrupts*] Just try taking one. Do you have some at home?

P: Because I hallucinate.

D: M'kay. Do you have some still at home?

P: What?

D: Do you still have some at home?

P: Yeah but I . . . put it away.

D: Okay. Just take one.

P: But what if I hallucinate?

D: It'll go away. It's only temporary. Okay?

P: I can take it . . . [patient is *panting*], but that hallucination comes.

D: Okay. Okay. I just want you to calm down and rest assured that it's not serious, okay?

P: So [medication #1] is the only thing that . . .

D: No, [medication #2] . . . let's increase [medication #2].

P: [Medication #2] pill?

D: [Medication #2], correct. I want you to take more than just a quarter . . . half of a half.

P: Yeah. [*panting, coughing*] So when the, when the . . .

D: You have to learn to relax.

P: Huh?

D: You have to learn to relax . . .

P: How do you do that?[7]

In this dialogue, the physician dominates the conversation with a vulnerable patient who cannot assert her concerns. He fails to listen to her clear distress about a medication that has caused problematic side effects. Despite briefly attempting to reassure her about the medication, the physician fails to address the patient's anxiety and reduces the patient's sense of control by persisting with his directive to take the medication. Communication about dosage of the second medication is also unclear, and there is no explanation of the reason for adding it. The physician fails to explain "hyperventilation" to the patient after being questioned directly about it. The physician also seems to subtly blame the patient for experiencing anxiety, suggesting that she should control it and "relax." Ineffective communication such as this is common in medical care when patients are of lower income or ethnic minority status or have limited health literacy; poor health outcomes can be the direct result. This patient is unlikely to be empowered to complain about, or try to improve, her care; she is surely unlikely to advocate for better communication for all patients. She has been left feeling helpless and anxious by her physician, and as an economically vulnerable patient, she is not alone.

Consider the next interaction, in which a physician gives directives to a patient who has limited education. The physician does not recognize this patient's low health literacy as the cause of considerable difficulty in the

patient's understanding and processing the information the doctor is providing. Reluctant to question the physician, this patient remains passive.

> *Doctor*: Okay um . . . what I'll do is this. I'm gonna prescribe a nasal spray
> in addition, okay? . . . Nasal sprays—have you used one of those
> before?
>
> *Patient*: No.
>
> *D*: No, okay. It's um—it's an inhaled steroid. . . . It helps reduce the inflam-
> mation and congestion . . . in the nasal area. . . . The full effect comes
> up, you know, after three to five days, okay?
>
> *P*: Oh.
>
> *D*: So, use it about a week or so, and use one two weeks, and see how you
> do with this, okay? Get some, it will help . . . makes your sinus allergy
> down—symptoms down. And—and um-um you know you can also
> take some Tylenol for that discomfort that you have. I'm gonna go
> ahead and give you some medicine, that antibiotic. First to treat this—
> I think you may have ah, you know, perhaps, you know, some signs of
> sinus congestion and sinus infection.
>
> *P*: I got it all!
>
> *D*: So I'm gonna give you treatment. And—and, ah, at least your blood
> pressure today is um . . . um . . . I would probably recommend that we
> get you scheduled for a full physical.
>
> *P*: Yeah . . .
>
> *D*: And—and um, we evaluate your blood pressure again. And at that time,
> ah, we may put you back on, ah, the medicines you were taking.
> You're not taking it anymore so . . .
>
> *P*: Uh, uh.
>
> *D*: It's just, ah, we're gonna recheck the blood pressure and see how you
> do—could be also pain that will cause it to come back again, . . . just
> to make sure your blood pressure is okay, make it next visit . . . okay?
>
> *P*: Okay.
>
> *D*: Any questions for me?
>
> *P*: No.
>
> *D*: Any allergies to medication?
>
> *P*: Not that I know of,
>
> *D*: Now, what is your wife's name?[8]

At several places in the conversation (almost a physician monologue), the
physician's statements are not clear. Medical terms are used and not explained
(e.g., "inhaled steroid"); some directives don't make complete sense (e.g., "use

it about a week or so, and use one two weeks, and see how you do with this, okay?"). It would not be surprising if this patient has little idea of what is supposed to be done. The patient is passive, expresses no concerns, asks no questions. The physician appears to accept an utter lack of patient involvement, thus risking communication errors and nonadherence to treatment.

In contrast, the next interaction is with an affluent and highly educated patient; it is characterized by the physician's engagement with the patient, and by the patient's active involvement in care.

Patient: M' kay, so this is what? This is a cough syrup?

Doctor: First one is—Yeah. Cough syrup; one or two teaspoons every four to six hours as needed for cough. And the *[antibiotic #1]*.

P: The last time you gave me *[antibiotic #2]*.

D: [Antibiotic #2]? You don't need [antibiotic #2] right now.

P: You sure? Okay.

D: No, I'm sure.

P: Last time was good.

D: Yeah? Worked for you? Well, you know the other thing is that if it doesn't work for you, yes, I may need to switch your antibiotic. But, let's try with something that's good and it's always proven to be effective, okay?

P: Okay. Okay.

D: Take care, but get a lot of rest an' drink a lot of fluids.

P: Okay, thank you.[9]

Here the physician is not at all defensive and allows the patient to challenge the treatment plan. The medication choice is clearly explained, and a plan is offered to revisit the issue if the initial antibiotic is ineffective. The physician responds to the patient's concerns with respect. In this interaction, the patient's higher health literacy and social status allows a partnership between physician and patient.

Communication and Involvement in Care among Vulnerable Patients

As seen in the examples of poor communication given here, the voices of socially and economically vulnerable patients are often not heard. When patients and their physicians are separated by significant differences in income, education, health literacy, and social class, status differences that exist in the wider society influence their patterns of verbal and nonverbal behavior.[10]

Interpersonal behaviors that reflect differences in social power are more likely to occur when physicians communicate with socially and economically vulnerable patients than with those who are more affluent and better educated. The latter receive more information about their health care and more detailed explanations from their physicians, and greater social distance between physicians and their lower income/education patients brings about subtle difficulties in communication, empathy, and affective behavior.[11] Physicians offer their low-income patients less responsiveness and fewer expressions of positive affect; they are less friendly, less concerned, and less interpersonally engaged. They are more likely to ignore the comments of their minority patients, and to give them less information, nonverbal attention, courtesy, and empathy. They spend less time answering their questions and providing health information, and they are more verbally dominant and negative in emotional tone.[12] Among patients with depression, the disparities are even greater; African American patients experience less discussion of their distress, and their physicians make less of an effort to build a relationship with them and to offer them depression treatments.[13] In the oncology setting, physicians spend more time communicating with white, affluent, and educated patients than with those who are less advantaged.[14]

Socioeconomically vulnerable patients are less likely to achieve patient agency; they are less apt to ask for, understand, and manage health information and to guide decision making about their own care in the medical visit.[15] Low-income patients are less likely to present their ideas to and disagree with their physicians; they ask fewer questions, are less emotionally expressive, and participate less in medical decisions; their physicians are consequently less informative.[16] This is true despite reports from these patients that they want more information than their physicians realize, express a strong desire for relational communication with their physicians, and aspire for control in decision making.[17]

Overt interpersonal behavior such as the expression of disrespect toward minority patients occurs often, resulting in less trust in the physician-patient relationship and in the health care system.[18] Patients who are more affluent have more choices and options in their care, and they are better liked by their physicians than are poorer patients.[19] Patients with greater means receive more help with disease prevention efforts, more health behavior counseling, greater continuity of care, and more chances to have discussions of ways to improve their treatment adherence.[20]

Health behavior counseling is essential to achieving beneficial patient outcomes, but poor, uninsured, and minority ethnicity patients tend to receive fewer preventive care recommendations and less screening, and they are consequently diagnosed later with progressive diseases.[21] African American breast cancer patients want information about health behavior changes that might reduce their risk of recurrence, but more than 90 percent of such patients in one study did not receive *any* counseling about lifestyle changes.[22] When counseling is provided, more vulnerable patients tend to be prevented from asking questions, voicing their concerns, expressing their preferences, and negotiating treatment regimens; thus, their efforts to follow preventive health care regimens can be ineffective and contribute to poor health care outcomes.[23]

Training for Better Communication

Although some physicians and health care professionals are naturally gifted at communicating with their patients, many would benefit from training in crucial communication skills. Furthermore, training patients to be more active and involved in their health care can have positive effects on their health outcomes. Recent experimental research conducted by the authors and their colleagues provides an example of what can be done to train physicians and patients in communication skills and the effects such training can have. This study involved randomly assigning 156 physicians and 2,196 of their patients either to a control group or to one of three treatment conditions (physician, patient, or both trained). It was conducted at a university medical center, a staff-model HMO, and a veteran's medical center on the West Coast. The physician-training program was intensive, involving 18 hours of workshops as well as approximately 1.5 hours of coaching sessions covering a variety of communication concepts. Trained patients received a twenty-minute previsit intervention in which they listened to a brief audiotape and followed along with a guidebook that provided them with strategies to be more involved and active in their care.[24]

Results of this research showed that communication training for physicians improved patients' satisfaction with the explanations and information their physicians gave them, and increased physicians' use of health-behavior counseling. Training also improved physicians' satisfaction with aspects of the visit. According to third-party raters, the physicians were more connected with and sensitive to their patients after the physician training. Training patients to participate in their care influenced physician satisfaction with the medical visit: physicians felt they received better information from trained patients and were better able to understand them.

This was the first study to train both physicians and their patients in communication skills; of interest were possible synergistic effects of training both groups. Not surprisingly, the results of training both physicians and patients were complex. One important result is that physicians experienced more stress and less satisfaction when only one member of the dyad was trained, suggesting that it was overall better to train *both* physician and patient in communication than to train only one of them. When only one member of the medical visit dyad is trained to focus on better communication, conflict with the other member may ensue.

Policy Implications and Recommendations

Changes in policy at the levels of health care education and delivery may help to remedy the inequities in the health care visit that socially and economically vulnerable patients experience. These changes ideally would involve efforts to inform, activate, and support patients to participate in their medical care, and to facilitate physician-patient communication by enhancing physicians' communication skills. Patient empowerment and physician acceptance of that empowerment are critically important, not only for care at the individual visit level, but also for patient activation at the level of system change. The voices of vulnerable patients are comparatively silent at all levels, and diminished health care outcomes for the socially and economically disadvantaged in our society can be traced to, among other things, disparities in communication and the interpersonal process of their medical care. Vulnerable patients have worse health outcomes than do those with greater social and economic resources partly because, at the microsocial level, they feel limited both in their degree of empowerment and in their physicians' acceptance of that empowerment and effective communication with them. Limited empowerment at the individual level limits activation and empowerment at the levels of health care organization, community, and social policy.

No established health policy guarantees all patients effective interpersonal interactions. Angeles and Somers argue that disparities in care for socially and economically vulnerable patients are so severe that states should investigate the possibility that they are paying for inadequate services delivered to their Medicaid beneficiaries.[25] Policies should seek to eliminate disparities by *requiring* interventions and training in communication for contracting health care organizations and their providers, and by offering education and support to patients. Evidence cited here suggests that such training can be effective.

Recommendations for Provider Communication Training

All health professionals should be taught, and consistently reminded of, the importance of effective communication and empathy in the care of all their patients. Research findings demonstrate that interventions to improve communication behaviors for physicians have positive outcomes.[26] Survey data suggest that medical residents typically do not believe they are ready to provide culturally sensitive health care to their patients. As many as half the residents surveyed received no training in cross-cultural care beyond medical school, and as many as 83 percent in some specialties received no such training at all.[27] Managed care organizations paid on a capitated basis have business incentives to implement quality initiatives to eliminate health disparities, including emphasis on effective communication with patients. Such rewards as special teaching status could be granted to those who demonstrate the greatest ability to treat vulnerable patients, and health professionals should be recruited and trained from the ranks of those who have a demonstrated commitment to the care of the socially and economically vulnerable. There is growing evidence that communication goals might best be achieved with racial/ethnic concordance of physician and patient, which results in longer, more participatory, partnership-oriented communication, and higher patient satisfaction, greater patient trust in and access to the physician, greater trust in the health care system, and greater respect and listening in the process of communication and medical care.[28]

Recommendations for Patient Communication Training and Feedback

Opportunities to improve patient care require patients' feedback about their care experiences to their providers and health care organizations at all levels. Survey questionnaires and follow-up telephone calls can accomplish this aim, protecting patient confidentiality. Surveys should always be translated into the most common local languages in addition to English. For instance, the Interpersonal Processes of Care survey was translated from English to Spanish using items that focus groups revealed would be relevant for both languages and for Latino, white, and African American groups.[29] Other surveys such as the Spanish version of Consumer Assessments of the Health Care Providers and Systems Hospital Survey (CAHPS) have been shown to be comparable to the English version, and to provide reliable and valid feedback from patients.[30] Illustrated versions of such patient surveys have been developed, providing opportunities for clearer and more accurate questioning; these surveys can also be administered in an interview format, allowing for further clarification and patient elaboration.[31]

Feedback can be offered at the level of organizations, such as having participants provide comments to their HMOs (as discussed in later chapters in this book), and at the level of public programs, such as nonprofit groups assisting seniors in navigating the Medicare program (e.g., the Medicare Rights Center and the Center for Medicare Advocacy). Employer-based health insurance programs should offer expert liaison between employees and health insurers to improve service and give patients a voice in their care.

Patients' social power often limits their opportunity to provide feedback and evaluation, and the very factors that inhibit patients' negotiation and participation in the medical visit may inhibit their ability and willingness to complain about suboptimal care. Health care organizations therefore should have strict policies about reliability, validity, equal opportunity, and confidentiality in assessing consumer satisfaction, and should respond to these assessments with appropriate systemic change. The experiences of vulnerable patients are not often assessed; compared to more advantaged groups, nonwhite, non-English-speaking patients tend to be clustered into managed care plans with lower consumer ratings.[32] Greater effort should be focused on surveying perceptions of care via culturally and linguistically appropriate surveys.

The improvement of patients' agency requires concerted efforts to increase knowledge of health and health care among patients who are less educated, less health literate, and less economically advantaged, and among those for whom English is not the primary language. Beyond the health care interaction, access to health education for vulnerable populations is essential to the improvement of communication in the health care visit, to patient adherence to medical treatment, to individual health care outcomes, and to efforts at change on the broader levels of institution and social policy. At every level, individuals should have ready access to the Internet and reliable sources of health information so that they can ask questions of their health professionals, make decisions for themselves, and actively engage at the broader policy level to offer better health care to all.[33] Balanced, independent health information should be available in print or multimedia formats at libraries, health maintenance organizations, and public clinics, encouraging patients to be informed, collaborative participants in their own care.[34]

Translation and interpretation needs of all patients should be accommodated at every health care interaction (including with new systems for interpreting, such as the Remote Simultaneous Medical Interpreting System in which an off-site interpreter assists with the medical interaction). Patients report satisfaction with the quality and privacy of remote interpreting.[35] Web sites and other informational content for patients should offer culturally specific materials at the appropriate reading level (adapting existing materials as needed).[36] Interactive computer-based educational modules directed at specific illnesses and proper medication use could provide helpful information to patients in their primary language.[37] Free Internet services for patients at hospitals, primary health care clinics, outpatient centers, and community clinics should include help for patients to navigate these sources, and health education assistance to identify concerns and questions before the visit. Prepared patients tend to be more involved in the medical visit, and more verbally active and interpersonally engaged; they elicit more information from their doctors, have higher rates of appointment keeping and adherence, and may be more actively involved in bringing their knowledge and skills to their communities at large.[38]

Long-term disease self-management, and support groups composed of patients with similar illnesses within a medical practice, health care organization, or community, should be available to all chronic disease patients who need them. Organized and run by a trained health professional, these groups could help educate patients, provide critical social support for patient adherence, and serve as a platform for voicing concerns about providers, health care insurers, and institutions, laying the groundwork for community-based policy endeavors. Information could be provided to the schools, churches, cultural groups, radio stations, and local businesses that serve more vulnerable populations. Lay health workers could assist in the creation of culturally and linguistically appropriate groups that target specific health challenges in various vulnerable populations.[39] Health advocates in the community should be of the same ethnicity and speak the same language as the patients they serve, helping patients to have their voices heard about the care they wish to receive from their health professionals.[40]

Communication training can help patients—including patient populations that are primarily minority or non–English speaking—participate more actively in their care, with resultant improvements in health outcomes, patient communication, and adherence to treatment.[41] Specific interventions to improve patients' voice have focused, for example, on providing patients with a wallet-sized personal medication list and examining how this affects their knowledge and sense of responsibility or on giving patients with terminal cancer a "question prompt list," which has been found to improve the communication process about difficult end-of-life issues.[42] A Canadian program, It's Safe to Ask, provides posters and brochures in multiple languages, which are posted in physicians' offices and give patients a list of important questions to ask and suggestions on how to ask questions as well as room to write down the answers.[43]

Researchers have studied communication between providers and patients since the 1950s. This research has uncovered areas where the communication process can be improved and has spurred more recent scholarship on interventions to improve communication. New interventions conducted by researchers have encouraged changes in the training and education of health care providers. Some of the examples cited here represent more recent techniques for improving communication, many of which rely on advances in technology. The scope of interest in communication in medical care has increased in recent years due to several factors, including attempts to understand how communication may play a role in disparities in health care.

Additional research must explore the particular needs of underserved patients, who are most in need of guidance and instruction about how to communicate effectively with their health care providers. Research is also needed on the degree to which patients activated to participate in their personal medical encounters go on to become involved with improving care in their health care organizations and communities, and in efforts to improve health care policy. In addition, studies are needed on how training physicians to effectively work with trained and activated patients affects health outcomes.[44] Some studies currently in progress will provide valuable information on how culturally focused communication interventions can affect outcomes for vulnerable patients.[45]

Conclusion

Social power differentials in health care interactions are intimidating and difficult to traverse. Patients should not be prevented, overtly or more subtly (through unsupportive interpersonal communication), from deriving essential task-oriented and socioemotional support from those who provide their medical care. All patients, regardless of income, ethnicity, or education, should be sustained in their efforts to ask necessary questions, participate in and challenge medical decisions, and gain the information and support necessary to initiate and maintain personal responsibility for their health. Medical care, including interpersonal care, should be delivered in such a way that every patient has the opportunity to derive the most benefit from their health care and to enjoy the best possible health care outcomes.

Whether and how potential policy solutions are implemented will depend upon the values of the individuals who ultimately shape health policy. Disparities in the interpersonal communicative aspects of health care do not happen in a vacuum; they reflect wider societal issues of power and inequality. In the United States, health care remains a commodity; those with greater means purchase care of higher quality and tend to be vocal in insisting on its interpersonal quality. Those with fewer economic resources are often silenced and unable to insist upon interpersonally supportive, informed, and collaborative treatment at the individual level, leaving them powerless at the broader organizational and policy levels as well.

Societal values drive the microlevel and the macrolevel forces that silence socially and economically vulnerable medical patients. These forces are pervasive, and changing them requires a significant shift in values regarding the rights of all individuals to receive effective health care. Provider-patient communication is an essential prerequisite for effective, equitable care, and a critically important target for policy intervention.

Notes

1. Steven A. Schroeder. "We Can Do Better," *New England Journal of Medicine*, 357, 12 (2007): 1221–1228; Bruce G. Link and Jo C. Phelan, "Fundamental Sources of Health Inequalities," in *Policy Challenges in Modern Health Care*, ed. D. Mechanic, L. B. Rogut, D. C. Colby, and J. R. Knickman (New Brunswick, N.J.: Rutgers University Press, 2005), 71–84.

2. Lucille M. Ong, Johanna C. de Haes, Aloysia M. Hoos, and Frits B. Lammes, "Doctor-Patient Communication: A Review of the Literature," *Social Science and Medicine* 40, 7 (1995): 903–918; M. Robin DiMatteo, Lawrence S. Linn, Betty L. Chang, and Dennis W. Cope, "Affect and Neutrality in Physician Behavior: A Study of Patients' Values and Satisfaction," *Journal of Behavioral Medicine* 8, 4 (1985): 397–409; Loretto M. Comstock, Elizabeth M. Hooper, Jean M. Goodwin, and James S. Goodwin, "Physician Behaviors That Correlate with Patient Satisfaction," *Journal of Medical Education* 57, 2 (1982): 105–112.

3. M. Robin DiMatteo, "The Physician-Patient Relationship: Effects on the Quality of Health Care," *Clinical Obstetrics and Gynecology* 37, 1 (1994): 149–161.

4. On participatory decision making, see Sherrie H. Kaplan, Barbara Gandek, Sheldon Greenfield, William Rogers, and John E. Ware, "Patient and Visit Characteristics Related to Physicians' Participatory Decision-Making Style," *Medical Care* 33, 12 (1995): 1176–1187. On results of greater patient responsibility for treatment adherence, see Carol M. Ashton, Paul Haidet, Debora A. Paterniti, Tracie C. Collins, Howard S. Gordon, Kimberly O'Malley, Laura A. Petersen et al., "Racial and Ethnic Disparities in the Use of Health Services: Bias, Preferences, or Poor Communication?" *Journal of General Internal Medicine* 18, 2 (2003): 146–152; M. Robin DiMatteo, "The Role of the Physician in the Emerging Health Care Environment," *Western Journal of Medicine* 168, 5 (1998): 328–333.

5. Rainer S. Beck, Rebecca Daughtridge, and Philip D. Sloane, "Physician-Patient Communication in the Primary Care Office: A Systematic Review," *Journal of the American Board of Family Practice* 15, 1 (2002): 25–38.

6. Richard L. Street Jr., Edward Krupat, Robert A. Bell, Richard L. Kravitz, and Paul Haidet, "Beliefs about Control in the Physician-Patient Relationship," *Journal of General Internal Medicine* 18, 8 (2003): 609–616.

7. John Heritage and M. Robin DiMatteo, "Communication and Satisfaction with Primary Care Teams Study," 2003 (transcribed from unpublished raw data). For all transcripts quoted, details have been changed to protect privacy, and linguistic disfluencies and simultaneous speech have been removed or clarified.

8. Ibid.

9. Ibid.

10. Ana I. Balsa and Thomas G. McGuire, "Prejudice, Clinical Uncertainty, and Stereotyping as Sources of Health Disparities," *Journal of Health Economics* 22, 1 (2003): 89–116.

11. Howard Waitzkin, "Doctor-Patient Communication: Clinical Implications of Social Scientific Research," *Journal of the American Medical Association* 252, 17 (1984): 2441–2446; Mary Boulton, David Tuckett, Coral Olson, and Anthony Williams, "Social Class and the General Practice Consultation," *Sociology of Health and Illness* 8 (1986): 325–350.

12. Elizabeth M. Hooper, Loretto M. Comstock, Jean M. Goodwin, and James S. Goodwin, "Patient Characteristics That Influence Physician Behavior," *Medical Care* 20, 6 (1982): 630–638; Joke C. van Wieringen, Johannes A. Harmsen, and Marc A. Bruijnzeels, "Intercultural Communication in General Practice," *European Journal of Public Health* 12, 1 (2002): 63–68; Lisa A. Cooper, Debra L. Roter, Rachel L. Johnson, Daniel E. Ford, Donald M. Steinwachs, and Neil R. Powe, "Patient-Centered Communication, Ratings of Care, and Concordance of Patient and Physician Race," *Annals of Internal Medicine* 139, 11 (2003): 907–915; Rachel L. Johnson, Debra Roter, Neil R. Powe, and Lisa A. Cooper, "Patient Race/Ethnicity and Quality of Patient-Physician Communication during Medical Visits," *American Journal of Public Health* 94, 12 (2004): 2084–2090; Debra L. Roter, Moira Stewart, Samuel M. Putnam, Mack Lipkin Jr., William Stiles, and Thomas S. Inui, "Communication Patterns of Primary Care Physicians," *Journal of the American Medical Association* 277, 4 (1997): 350–356; Bri K. Ghods, Debra Roter, Daniel E. Ford, Susan Larson, Jose J. Arbelaez, and Lisa A. Cooper, "Patient-Physician Communication in the Primary Care Visits of African Americans and Whites with Depression," *Journal of General Internal Medicine* 23, 5 (2008): 600–606.

13. Julie A. Wagner, Denise W. Perkins, John D. Piette, Bonnie Lipton, and James E. Aikens, "Racial Differences in the Discussion and Treatment of Depressive Symptoms Accompanying Type 2 Diabetes," *Diabetes Research and Clinical Practice* 86, 2 (2009): 111–116; Laura A. Siminoff, Gregory C. Graham, and Nahida H. Gordon, "Cancer Communication Patterns and the Influence of Patient Characteristics: Disparities in Information-Giving and Affective Behaviors," *Patient Education and Counseling* 62, 3 (2006): 355–360.

14. Sharon W. Williams, Laura C. Hanson, Carlton Boyd, Melissa Green, Moses Goldmon, Gratia Wright, and Giselle Corbie-Smith, "Communication, Decision Making, and Cancer: What African Americans Want Physicians to Know," *Journal of Palliative Medicine* 11, 9 (2008): 1221–1226.

15. Elizabeth Murray, Lance Pollack, Martha White, and Bernard Lo, "Clinical Decision-Making: Patients' Preferences and Experiences," *Patient Education and Counseling* 65, 2 (2007): 189–196; David W. Baker, Ruth M. Parker, Mark V. Williams, Kathryn Pitkin, Nina S. Parikh, Wendy Coates, and Mwalimu Imara, "The Health Care Experience of Patients with Low Literacy," *Archives of Family Medicine* 5, 6 (1996): 329–334.

16. Boulton et al., "Social Class"; Dean Schillinger, Andrew Bindman, Frances Wang, Anita Stewart, and John Piette, "Functional Health Literacy and the Quality of Physician-Patient Communication among Diabetes Patients," *Patient Education and Counseling* 52, 3 (2004): 315–323.

17. Heritage and DiMatteo, "Communication and Satisfaction"; Mark P. Doescher, Barry G. Saver, Peter Franks, and Kevin Fiscella, "Racial and Ethnic Disparities in Perceptions of Physician Style and Trust," *Archives of Family Medicine* 9, 10 (2000): 1156–1163; L. Ebony Boulware, Lisa A. Cooper, Lloyd E. Ratner, Thomas A. LaVeist, and Neil R. Powe, "Race and Trust in the Health Care System," *Public Health Reports* 118, 4 (2003): 358–365. Sarah T. Hawley, Nancy K. Janz, Ann Hamilton, Jennifer J. Griggs, Amy K. Alderman, Mahasin Mujahid, and Steven J. Katz, "Latina

Patient Perspectives about Informed Treatment Decision Making for Breast Cancer," *Patient Education and Counseling* 73, 2 (2008): 363–370.

18. Doescher et al., "Racial and Ethnic Disparities"; Boulware et al., "Race and Trust"; Judith A. Hall, Arnold M. Epstein, Mary Lou DeCiantis, and Barbara J. McNeil, "Physicians' Liking for Their Patients: More Evidence for the Role of Affect in Medical Care," *Health Psychology* 12, 2 (1993): 140–146.

19. Judith A. Hall, Terrence G. Horgan, Terry S. Stein, and Debra L. Roter, "Liking in the Physician-Patient Relationship," *Patient Education and Counseling* 48, 1 (2002): 69–77; Michelle van Ryn and Jane Burke, "The Effect of Patient Race and Socio-Economic Status on Physicians' Perceptions of Patients," *Social Science and Medicine* 50, 6 (2000): 813–828; Valerie E. Stone, "Physician Contributions to Disparities in HIV/AIDS Care: The Role of Provider Perceptions Regarding Adherence," *Current HIV/AIDS Report* 2, 4 (2005): 189–193.

20. Johnson et al., "Patient Race/Ethnicity"; Sarah S. Casagrande, Tiffany L. Gary, Thomas A. LaVeist, Darrell J. Gaskin, and Lisa A. Cooper, "Perceived Discrimination and Adherence to Medical Care in a Racially Integrated Community," *Journal of General Internal Medicine* 22, 3 (2007): 389–395.

21. Pamela C. Heaton and Stacey M. Frede, "Patients' Need for More Counseling on Diet, Exercise, and Smoking Cessation: Results from the National Ambulatory Medical Care Survey." *Journal of the American Pharmacology Association* 46, 3 (2006): 364–369; Peter Franks, Kevin Fiscella, and Sean Meldrum, "Racial Disparities in the Content of Primary Care Office Visits." *Journal of General Internal Medicine* 20, 7 (2005): 599–603; Jun Ma, Guido G. Urizar Jr., Tseday Alehegn, and Randall S. Stafford, "Diet and Physical Activity Counseling during Ambulatory Care Visits in the United States," *Preventative Medicine* 39, 4 (2004): 815–822; Elizabeth J. Jackson, Mark P. Doescher, Barry G. Saver, and L. Gary Hart, "Trends in Professional Advice to Lose Weight among Obese Adults, 1994 to 2000," *Journal of General Internal Medicine* 20, 9 (2005): 814–818.

22. David R. Evans and Shahe S. Kazarian, "Health Promotion, Disease Prevention, and Quality of Life," in *Handbook of Cultural Health Psychology*, ed. D. R. Evans and D. R. Kazarian, 86–114 (San Diego: Academic Press, 2001).

23. Elisabeth Arborelius and Stefan Bremberg, "Prevention in Practice: How Do General Practitioners Discuss Life-Style Issues with Their Patients?" *Patient Education and Counseling* 23, 1 (1994): 23–31; M. Robin DiMatteo, Patrick J. Giordani, Heidi S. Lepper, and Thomas W. Croghan, "Patient Adherence and Medical Treatment Outcomes: A Meta-Analysis," *Medical Care* 40, 9 (2002): 794–811.

24. Kelly B. Haskard, Summer L. Williams, M. Robin DiMatteo, Robert Rosenthal, Maysel K. White, and Michael G. Goldstein, "Physician and Patient Communication Training in Primary Care: Effects on Participation and Satisfaction," *Health Psychology* 27, 5 (2008): 513–522.

25. January Angeles and Stephen A. Somers, "From Policy to Action: Addressing Racial and Ethnic Disparities at the Ground Level," *Issue Brief, Center for Health Care Strategies* (Hamilton, N.J.: Center for Health Care Strategies, 2007).

26. Ibid.; Jaya K. Rao, Lynda A. Anderson, Thomas S. Inui, and Richard M. Frankel, "Communication Interventions Make a Difference in Conversations between Physicians and Patients: A Systematic Review of the Evidence," *Medical Care* 45, 4 (2007): 340–349.

27. Joel S. Weissman, Joseph Betancourt, Eric G. Campbell, Elyse R. Park, Minah Kim, Brian Clarridge, David Blumenthal, Karen C. Lee, and Angela W. Maina, "Resident

Physicians' Preparedness to Provide Cross-Cultural Care," *Journal of the American Medical Association* 294, 9 (2005): 1058–1067.

28. Cooper et al., "Patient Centered Communication"; Lisa Cooper-Patrick, Joseph J. Gallo, Junius J. Gonzales, Hong T. Vu, Neil R. Powe, Christine Nelson, and Daniel E. Ford, "Race, Gender, and Partnership in the Patient-Physician Relationship," *JAMA* 282, 6 (1999): 583–589; Saha et al., "Patient-Physician Racial Concordance"; Nancy Lynn Sohler, Lisa K. Fitzpatrick, Rebecca G. Lindsay, Kathryn Anastos, and Chinazo O. Cunningham, "Does Patient-Provider Racial/Ethnic Concordance Influence Ratings of Trust in People with HIV Infection?" *AIDS Behavior* 11, 6 (2007): 884–896.

29. Anita L. Stewart, Anna M. Napoles-Springer, Steven E. Gregorich, and Jasmine Santoyo-Olsson, "Interpersonal Processes of Care Survey: Patient-Reported Measures for Diverse Groups," *Health Services Research* 42, 3, part 1 (2007): 1235–1256.

30. Margarita P. Hurtado, January Angeles, Steven A. Blahut, and Ron D. Hays, "Assessment of the Equivalence of the Spanish and English Versions of the CAHPS Hospital Survey on the Quality of Inpatient Care," *Health Services Research* 40, 6, part 2 (2005): 2140–2161.

31. Judy A. Shea, Abigail C. Aguirre, John Sabatini, Janet Weiner, Michael Schaffer, and David A. Asch, "Developing an Illustrated Version of the Consumer Assessment of Health Plans (CAHPS)," *Joint Commission Journal on Quality and Patient Satisfaction* 31, 1 (2005): 32–42; Janet Weiner, Abigail Aguirre, Karina Ravenell, Kim Kovath, Lindsay McDevit, Joan Murphy, David A. Asch, and Judy A. Shea, "Designing an Illustrated Patient Satisfaction Instrument for Low-Literacy Populations," *American Journal of Managed Care* 10, 11, part 2 (2004): 853–860.

32. Robert Weech-Maldonado, Marc N. Elliott, Leo S. Morales, Karen Spritzer, Grant N. Marshall, and Ron D. Hays, "Health Plan Effects on Patient Assessments of Medicaid Managed Care among Racial/Ethnic Minorities," *Journal of General Internal Medicine* 19, 2 (2004): 136–145.

33. Jean A. Gilmour, "Reducing Disparities in the Access and Use of Internet Health Information," *International Journal of Nursing Studies* 44, 7 (2007): 1270–1278.

34. Michael C. Gibbons, "A Historical Overview of Health Disparities and the Potential of eHealth Solutions," *Journal of Medical Internet Research* 7, 5 (2005): e50.

35. Francesca Gany, Jennifer Leng, Ephraim Shapiro, David Abramson, Ivette Motola, David C. Shield, and Jyotsana Changrani, "Patient Satisfaction with Different Interpreting Methods: A Randomized Controlled Trial," *Journal of General Internal Medicine* 22, supp. 2 (2007): 312–318.

36. Feleta L. Wilson, Eric Racine, Virginia Tekieli, and Barbara Williams, "Literacy, Readability, and Cultural Barriers: Critical Factors to Consider When Educating Older African Americans about Anticoagulation Therapy," *Journal of Clinical Nursing* 12, 2 (2003): 275–282.

37. Bonnie A. Leeman-Castillo, Kitty K. Corbett, Eva M. Aagaard, Judith H. Maselli, Ralph Gonzales, and Thomas D. Mackenzie, "Acceptability of a Bilingual Interactive Computerized Educational Module in a Poor, Medically Underserved Patient Population," *Journal of Health Communication* 12, 1 (2007): 77–94.

38. Sheldon Greenfield, Sherrie Kaplan, and John E. Ware Jr., "Expanding Patient Involvement in Care: Effects on Patient Outcomes," *Annals of Internal Medicine* 102, 4 (1985): 520–528; Debra L. Roter, Judith A. Hall, and Nancy R. Katz, "Patient-Physician Communication: A Descriptive Summary of the Literature," *Patient Education and Counseling* 12 (1988): 99–119.

39. Cheryl Rucker-Whitaker, Sanjib Basu, Glenda Kravitz, Marlease K. Bushnell, and Carlos F. de Leon, "A Pilot Study of Self-Management in African Americans with Common Chronic Conditions," *Ethnic Disparities* 17, 4 (2007): 611–616; Linda Larkey, "Las Mujeres Saludables: Reaching Latinas for Breast, Cervical, and Colorectal Cancer Prevention and Screening," *Journal of Community Health* 31, 1 (2006): 69–77.

40. Beverly J. McElmurry, Chang G. Park, and Aaron G. Buseh, "The Nurse-Community Health Advocate Team for Urban Immigrant Primary Health Care," *Journal of Nursing Scholarship* 35, 3 (2003): 275–281.

41. Douglas M. Post, Donald J. Cegala, and William F. Miser, "The Other Half of the Whole: Teaching Patients to Communicate with Physicians," *Family Medicine* 34, 5 (2002): 344–352; Debra L. Roter, "Patient Participation in the Patient-Provider Interaction: The Effects of Patient Question Asking on the Quality of Interaction, Satisfaction, and Compliance," *Health Education Monograph* 5, 4 (1977): 281–315; Lynda A. Anderson, Brenda M. DeVellis, and Robert F. DeVellis, "Effects of Modeling on Patient Communication, Satisfaction, and Knowledge," *Medical Care* 25, 11 (1987): 1044–1056.

42. Sung Yu Chae, Mark H. Chae, Nicole Isaacson, and Tarika S. James, "The Patient Medication List: Can We Get Patients More Involved in Their Medical Care?" *Journal of the American Board of Family Medicine* 22, 6 (2009): 677–685; Josephine M. Clayton, Phyllis N. Butow, Martin H. Tattersall, Rhonda J. Devine, Judy M. Simpson, Ghauri Aggarwal, Katherine J. Clark et al., "Randomized Controlled Trial of a Prompt List to Help Advanced Cancer Patients and Their Caregivers to Ask Questions about Prognosis and End-of-Life Care," *Journal of Clinical Oncology* 25, 6 (2007): 715–723.

43. Jan Byrd and Laurie Thompson, "'It's Safe to Ask': Promoting Patient Safety through Health Literacy," *Healthcare Quarterly* 11, 3 (2008): 91–94.

44. Haskard et al., "Physician and Patient Communication Training."

45. Lisa A. Cooper, Debra L. Roter, Lee R. Bone, Susan M. Larson, Edgar R. Miller, Michael Barr, Kathryn A. Carson, and David M. Levine. "A Randomized Controlled Trial of Interventions to Enhance Patient-Physician Partnership, Patient Adherence, and High Blood Pressure Control among Ethnic Minorities and Poor Persons: Study Protocol Nct00123045," *Implementation Science* 4 (2009): 7.

Is It Time to Push Yet?

The Challenges to Advocacy in U.S. Childbirth

Women in New Jersey in 2007 demonstrated outside the Underwood-Memorial Hospital in Woodbury. They demanded to know why two women had died in childbirth following cesarean sections at this hospital within a fifteen-day period.[1] They sought, at a minimum, the publication of hospital and obstetrician cesarean rates; their efforts garnered regional media coverage and resulted in—very little. The hospital expressed its regret but did not begin publishing its cesarean rates. Ironically, several months after the protest the hospital received a national award for its childbirth services.[2] The limited impact of the protest was characteristic of the difficulties faced by those trying to change the nature of childbirth in the United States and serves as a reminder of the challenges faced by patient advocates when the elements needed for successful advocacy are not present.

Traditional interest group theory suggests preconditions for interest group development and involvement in the political system: a sense of felt need among individuals resulting from a shared focus on a common problem. To be successful in political advocacy, such groups need to join or develop an organizational structure that provides the institutional support critical to the long-term commitment necessary for success. Consensus on an identifiable and, ideally, a simple solution to the problem of concern, and a clear place (bureaucratic entity, legislative branch) to target advocates' efforts, will greatly enhance their venture. As is often the case for childbirth advocates, almost none of these characteristics were part of the New Jersey demonstration. Activists had no leverage over the local hospital they were trying to influence and no connection whatever with the local obstetricians. Government officials were able to view this matter as simply a private tragedy. The case exemplifies childbirth's paradoxical dual status as at once a public and a private issue.

Steven Epstein's chapter in this volume describes the various types of success patients have achieved in shaping the conceptualization of disease, research agendas, attitudes of professionals, and government policy. One can find examples of attempts at each of these in the case of childbirth, only they almost invariably fail. Efforts to humanize childbirth were largely co-opted by hospitals' adoption of the form but not the substance of change with the development of birthing centers and childbirth classes.[3] Officials met with disdain attempts by activists to shift the National Institutes of Health (NIH) research agenda away from cesarean delivery on maternal request. A successful major effort at state reform of hospital practices—extending postpartum stays—was led not by consumers but by groups representing clinicians. Throughout the debates about childbirth policies and practices, the voices of women themselves have mostly remained silent.

The Challenges to Advocacy: Why Is Childbirth Different?

As feminists and advocates for less medical intervention in childbirth have been arguing for decades, pregnant, parturient, and postpartum women are not ill. To what extent, then, are they patients? Ought we to consider advocacy around childbirth an instance of "patients as policy actors"? This question actually taps into a much broader (and heavily value-laden) debate about the experience of childbirth and how we conceptualize it. The midwifery or normal birth model posits that labor and delivery are normal, physiological processes that women's bodies evolved to accomplish; only in cases where something goes wrong is it appropriate or helpful to intervene in this process. In contrast, the medical model (the dominant paradigm in the United States) views every birth as potentially (if not definitely) pathological and thus insists that births are safe only in hospitals, where a full armamentarium of technologies is accessible at a moment's notice. Whereas midwifery insists that birth is a normal process, an obstetrical axiom holds that "birth is normal only in retrospect." The first complication in our thinking about patient advocacy around childbirth is the simple matter of whether pregnant and parturient women are patients at all. Indeed, to the extent that they look like or act like patients in the traditional sense, it is mostly because they have been put in this position by the process of medicalization that modern obstetrics insists on.

The second complication around the very notion of patient advocacy regarding childbirth is the vexed question within maternity care of just who *is* the patient: the pregnant woman or the fetus or both? Are there two patients or one? Arguably, for most of its history, obstetrics regarded the pregnant woman as the patient, but increasingly obstetrics has embraced the "fetal patient," and many obstetricians speak explicitly about "the two-patient model" of obstetrics.[4] Although in many respects this is a false dichotomy (maternal health and well-being remain the best guarantors of fetal health and well-being), this two-patient model further confounds the notion of patient advocacy in maternity care. Not only are the goals of advocacy unclear, but even the beneficiary is uncertain.

In fact, the supposed benefits for fetal well-being are among the primary justifications for many of the medical interventions during pregnancy, labor, and delivery. Among the more than 4 million women in the United States who give birth every year, the vast majority do so under the medical model—in the hospital, under the direct care of an obstetrician. Less than 1 percent of U.S. births occur outside the hospital. Interventions are routine: 34 percent of labors are induced, three-fourths of laboring women receive epidural anesthesia, nine out of ten are subject to continuous electronic fetal monitoring, one in four giving birth vaginally have an episiotomy, and three out of ten deliveries in the United States are cesareans.[5] The ubiquity of these interventions means that "normal birth" is decidedly not the norm among women in the United States, a fact with important consequences for childbirth advocacy.

In the face of these blunt facts, there is a small, organized advocacy community fighting to maintain what they call "normal birth" but which is more widely known as "natural childbirth."[6] Notably, many of the principal actors in the normal birth community are professional associations like the American College of Nurse-Midwives, Doulas of North America, Midwives of North America, the Coalition for Improving Maternity Services, and Lamaze International, which certifies childbirth educators. Consumer-led groups like Citizens for Midwifery remain more marginal, though the grassroots group International Cesarean Awareness Network, founded in 1982, has been growing in numbers, savvy, and impact recently, in part as the number of women who have experienced a cesarean section (and been radicalized by that often unwanted experience) has skyrocketed. Lamaze International, for example, maintains an Institute for Normal Birth and works to promote what it calls the "six care practices that support normal birth." These are: labor that begins on its own, freedom of movement throughout labor, continuous labor support, no routine interventions, nonsupine positions for birth, and no separation of mother and baby after birth, with unlimited opportunity for breastfeeding. Based on these standards, which notably do not limit mothers' use of pain medications, fewer than 2 percent of mothers experienced a normal physiological birth, according to a 2006 national survey.[7]

There are additional aspects of childbirth that are inimical to the conditions of grassroots advocacy. Like illness, it is an experience that people devote very little attention to until it is upon them—almost no one reads pregnancy or childbirth books until she is pregnant or trying to conceive. Like illness, childbirth is an all-consuming experience. And parenting a newborn affords little time or energy for anything else. Thus, at the most basic level, the natural constituency for maternity care reform—pregnant women and the parents of newborns—is a challenging group to mobilize.

Moreover, throughout pregnancy, labor and delivery, and early mothering, U.S. culture and medicine pointedly focus on first the fetus, then the newborn, often to the exclusion of the mother. This focus on the infant emphasizes outcome while eliding process. It is hard to argue with a good outcome—that is, a healthy baby—in order to draw attention to the process by which that outcome is achieved. This focus also reflects the two-patient perspective, while highlighting that one patient seems to count more than the other. This focus on birth outcomes happens at both the individual level and the societal one. Many parents subject to a cascade of medical interventions around birth (e.g., induction of labor, leading to the need for pain medications, leading to stalled labor, leading to efforts to accelerate labor, culminating in an eventual cesarean delivery) end up grateful to the doctors and nurses who "saved" their baby by virtue of technology. It is difficult for parents to feel aggrieved about unnecessary medical care in the midst of such gratitude.

Consumer-driven childbirth advocacy first emerged in the United States in the late 1950s, when women began to protest publicly the often harsh and impersonal maternity care delivered in hospitals, most notably in hundreds of letters on the subject of "cruelty in maternity wards" sent to *Ladies' Home Journal* in 1957 and 1958.[8] Direct consumer involvement with the organization and delivery of maternity care has its roots in the movement to bring the Lamaze method of childbirth to the United States in the late 1950s. Originally, the Lamaze method consisted of childbirth education classes for expectant parents, relaxation and breathing techniques, and continuous emotional support of the expectant mother from the expectant father and a specially trained nurse. Dr. Fernand Lamaze first developed the method in France in the 1950s, based on pain-management practices he had observed in Russia. *Thank You, Dr. Lamaze*, published in 1959 by U.S. expatriate Marjorie Karmel, recounted her childbirth experience with the techniques Lamaze developed in Paris.[9] The Lamaze method—and with it a sea change in attitudes toward childbirth—took off in the United States when Karmel and Elisabeth Bing founded what they called the American Society for Psychoprophylaxis in Obstetrics (later renamed Lamaze International) in 1960. Bing began teaching classes for expectant parents in her New York City apartment; as the Lamaze approach spread, couples began to make new demands on hospitals—most significantly, to have male partners present throughout labor and delivery.[10]

Throughout the 1970s, the vogue for natural—that is, demedicalized—childbirth grew and midwifery enjoyed a brief renaissance.[11] The women's health movement as well contributed to demands to humanize obstetrics by ceasing such routine interventions as pubic shaving, enemas, and episiotomy that offered no real benefit to women or babies and by establishing freestanding birth centers. Hospitals responded to the consumer push for natural birth by creating birthing suites that cleverly concealed medical equipment behind quilts and other accoutrements meant to invoke the comforts of home. During the 1980s and 1990s, women and their partners eagerly embraced these amenities, even as obstetrics embraced new technologies like electronic fetal monitoring that pushed maternity care back in the direction of medicalization. This trend is apparent most vividly in the rapidly rising cesarean section rate over the last three decades, from 5.5 percent in 1975 to 32 percent in 2007.[12] Thus, despite the efforts of childbirth educators, midwives, and other proponents of natural birth, maternity care remains an especially technology-intensive arena of medicine.

What Do Women Want?

In the context of patient advocacy around childbirth, there are two ways to think about the question of what women want. The first is to note that in contrast to most other patient advocacy movements, what childbirth advocates want is less, not more—less medical intervention during labor and delivery, less medical technology, less medicalization of birth. Those seeking more technological interventions related to maternity care—for example, advocates for assisted reproductive technologies—have invariably fared better. Advocating to lose services rather than to gain access to services goes against the grain of most U.S. citizen movements. This difference may also be a function of how patient interests coincide with those of professional groups and manufacturers who use patient advocates to legitimize their own advocacy efforts. One is not likely to engage industry support from manufacturers of electronic fetal monitors or pharmaceutical companies producing the drugs used in epidurals when the goal is to reduce interventions in childbirth.

The second way to think about this question in the context of maternity care reform today is to understand that the organized advocates may be profoundly out of sync with the consumers. Consider that fewer than 8 percent of births are attended by a midwife and fewer than 1 percent of U.S. births take place outside the hospital.[13] "Why do women go along with this stuff?" was the plaintive topic of extended debate among normal birth advocates in two recent issues of *Birth*, one of the major academic journals devoted to childbirth.[14] Why, indeed. Many women seem to want hospital births, to seek out epidurals, to feel reassured by electronic fetal monitoring, unnecessary IVs, and the whole armamentarium of modern medicalized birth. This leaves advocates of normal birth contemplating an uncomfortable gap between what they think women ought to want, expect, and demand, and what women themselves seem to want and expect during childbirth. Thus, much childbirth advocacy takes the form of educating the public about nonmedical models of birth in an attempt to induce demand for alternative modes of birth.

Pain presents another conundrum for childbirth advocacy. Of particular note here is the prevalence of epidural anesthesia during labor. Unlike earlier forms of pharmacological labor-pain relief (chloroform, ether, scopolamine), epidurals leave women conscious during birth. They are a magic bullet, in that they make relatively painless labor and delivery possible. Most women in the United States seem to regard an epidural as a valuable and desirable part of the birth regimen. Take, for example, the common linguistic habit among women of referring to "my epidural," as in, "I want my epidural now." One Internet site sells a t-shirt that reads, "Biggie size my epidural!"[15] Maternity care providers share this linguistic habit. In contrast, surgery patients do not talk about "my general anesthesia." And many labor and delivery nurses as well as obstetricians regard epidurals positively because they make laboring women easier to manage clinically. In addition, a powerful medical subspecialization—obstetrical anesthesiology—has developed largely around the administration of epidurals. In the face of epidurals, advocacy for nonmedicalized modes of childbirth is often interpreted as sentencing women to unnecessary suffering during labor and delivery, though in fact these modes of childbirth do not preclude pain relief.

Thus, the goals of policy action around childbirth are not only diffuse but also unclear. Do women want epidurals or not? If they knew better, would they still want epidurals? If the health care system took seriously nonpharmacological means of pain relief, would women still want epidurals? It has been well documented that much of what happens to modern American women during labor and delivery is done for the convenience and ease of providers, rather than for the woman's benefit.[16] Thus, efforts to reconfigure the delivery of maternity care run inevitably into opposition from the institutions who benefit from and are professionally committed to the status quo.

Moreover, the target of policy reform efforts is unclear. Is it the American College of Obstetricians and Gynecologists? Hospitals? Insurance companies? Policy makers? Consumers themselves? Whose hearts, minds, and practices are childbirth advocates aiming to change? Early consumer-driven efforts at childbirth advocacy in the 1960s and 1970s focused on hospitals, particularly the policies of banning partners (at that point, husbands) from labor and delivery rooms and of not allowing mothers to keep their babies in their room while in the hospital.[17] Once successful with these efforts, the focus of advocacy (e.g., to reduce cesarean rates) became unclear because the causes were more diffuse. In the case studies that follow, we explore recent reform efforts aimed at various target groups.

What Do Women Know?

In trying to address the goals of a patient advocacy effort related to childbirth, we will utilize an examination of what women know and think about the childbirth process. *Listening to Mothers II* was a 2006 national survey of 1,573 women who had given birth in 2005, only the second national survey to explore mothers' experiences in pregnancy, labor, birth, and postpartum.[18] It also asked mothers about their views on several matters central to a discussion of advocacy—their perception of their rights, their information needs, and the decision-making process in childbirth. Table 3.1 presents mothers' attitudes in two areas—their knowledge of their rights and what they felt they needed to know about side effects of three common interventions—by key demographic characteristics. Overall, about three-fourths of mothers felt they fully understood two key rights: the right to full explanations concerning any procedure done to them, and the right to accept or refuse any procedure, drug, or test.

Mothers were also asked about the extent to which they should be informed about possible side effects associated with labor induction, epidural anesthesia, and cesarean birth. Roughly three-fourths thought they should be informed of *every* possible side effect. Education had the strongest relationship to these attitudes, with less-educated mothers most likely to want to learn about every side effect and college graduates least likely to feel such a need. What is of interest here in assessing the potential for mothers to act as advocates is the degree to which mothers expected more information on side effects than is ever provided, but at the same time generally asserted that they fully understood all their rights.

Mothers were also given some options concerning decision making during labor and childbirth; these results are summarized in Table 3.2. When asked to describe who should be making decisions in cases where there were no medical

Table 3.1 Maternal Perspectives on Rights and Knowledge Needed in Childbirth, by Demographic Characteristics

	Full and clear explanations[a] (n = 1,370)	Accept/ refuse care[b] (n = 1,370)	Labor induction side effects[c] (n = 525)	Cesarean side effects[d] (n = 493)	Epidural side effects[e] (n = 549)
	% I fully understood		% Patient should know all		
All respondents (n = 1,370)	75	78	78	81	79
Race/ethnicity					
White non-Hispanic	*76	77	76	*79	*75
Black non-Hispanic	65	72	91	90	94
Hispanic	81	85	87	88	84
Parity					
Parity = 1	*66	*73	75	76	*70
Parity = 2+	79	81	80	84	85
Age					
18–24	72	74	75	89	*85
25–34	75	77	79	77	80
35+	80	84	82	80	71
Education					
High school or less	72	77	*86	*92	*89
Some college	78	79	81	81	83
College grad+	78	79	63	69	63
Income					
<$35,000	74	73	82	*91	*92
$35,000–$74,999	76	81	81	81	85
$75,000+	77	79	71	66	65
Paid for maternity care					
Private insurer	75	79	75	*75	*75
Public insurer	74	78	86	92	89

Source: Adapted from data collected for Eugene R. Declercq, Carol Sakala, Maureen Corry, and Sandy Applebaum, *Listening to Mothers II: Report of the Second National U.S. Survey of Women's Childbearing Experiences* (New York: Childbirth Connection, 2006).

[a]While pregnant and giving birth, a woman has the legal right to receive clear and full explanations of any procedure/drug/test offered to her. During the time you were pregnant and giving birth, did you *fully* understand that you *had* a right to accept or refuse? % represents those who agreed, "I fully understood."

[b]While pregnant and giving birth, a woman has the legal right to *accept or refuse* any procedure, drug, or test offered to her. During the time you were pregnant and giving birth, did you *fully* understand that you *had* a right to accept or refuse? % represents those who agreed, "I fully understood."

[c]Quite a few women experience labor induction while giving birth. Before consenting to labor induction, how important is it to learn about possible side effects of labor induction? % represents those who agreed, "It is necessary to know *every* complication."

[d]Quite a few women experience cesarean section while giving birth. Before consenting to cesarean section, how important is it to learn about possible side effects of cesarean section? % represents those who agreed, "It is necessary to know *every* complication."

[e]Quite a few women experience an epidural while giving birth. Before consenting to an epidural, how important is it to learn about possible side effects of an epidural % represents those who agreed, "It is necessary to know *every* complication."

*p < .01

Table 3.2 **Maternal Attitudes on Who Should Control Decision Making in Childbirth**

	Primary elective cesarean[a]	Vaginal birth[b]	VBAC[c]	I should make labor/birth decisions[d]
				% Agree
	% Agree should be patient's choice (n = 1,370)			(n = 1,370)
All respondents (n = 1,370)	46	93	85	73
Race/ethnicity				
White non-Hispanic	*45	*94	*87	73
Black non-Hispanic	52	96	81	75
Hispanic	41	86	77	74
Parity				
Parity = 1	*55	92	85	69
Parity = 2+	41	93	85	75
Age				
18–24	*54	*88	81	69
25–34	42	97	87	73
35+	45	89	85	78
Education				
High school or less	46	91	*81	75
Some college	44	93	89	76
College grad+	47	94	88	69
Income				
<$35,000	47	*91	83	*77
$35,000–$74,999	48	95	86	75
$75,000+	43	94	88	70
Paid for maternity care				
Private insurer	45	*95	87	74
Public insurer	46	90	83	72

Source: Adapted from data collected for Eugene R. Declercq, Carol Sakala, Maureen Corry, and Sandy Applebaum, *Listening to Mothers II: Report of the Second National U.S. Survey of Women's Childbearing Experiences* (New York: Childbirth Connection, 2006).

[a] If a woman who has never had a cesarean wants to have a cesarean, she should be able to do so. % represents those who agreed.

[b] If a woman who has never had a cesarean wants to have a vaginal birth, she should have the opportunity to do so. % represents those who agreed.

[c] If a woman who had a previous cesarean wants to have a vaginal birth after cesarean [VBAC], she should have the opportunity to do so. % represents those who agreed.

[d] Assuming there are no medical complications, who should make most decisions about your labor and birth experience? % represents those who agreed, "I should make decisions after considering the advice of my caregivers."

*p < .01

complications, 73 percent of mothers stated that they should, after considering the advice of their maternity care providers. Mothers were also asked about their right to choose the method of delivery given three scenarios: a woman wanting an elective primary cesarean; a woman wanting a vaginal birth; and a woman seeking a vaginal birth after cesarean (VBAC). Mothers were generally supportive of a woman's autonomy in all cases, particularly in the case of vaginal birth and VBAC. Mothers were more evenly split over the right to choose an elective cesarean.

The findings presented in Tables 3.1 and 3.2 raise two general questions. First, is it heartening or disappointing that three out of four women feel they fully understand their rights related to maternity care? Should we expect universal awareness? Likewise, is the 46 percent support for a mother's right to choose an elective cesarean a call for more widespread use of cesareans or a testimony to a desire to protect maternal autonomy? The latter might be the correct interpretation, based on even higher levels of support for vaginal birth and VBAC, but at the NIH meeting we discuss later, expert panel members cited the former interpretation as justification to explore expanding the options for additional cesareans. It is important to note the juxtaposition between maternal responses that advocated having knowledge of every possible side effect of procedures, and their desire for control of key decisions about labor and birth and for autonomy in choosing method of delivery, in the context of advocates' argument that mothers have been passive players (or worse, dupes) in accepting the increasing medicalization of birth.

Case Studies of Policy Reform around Childbirth

In the sections that follow, we present two cases of organized, visible advocacy around childbirth. By "visible" we mean that in each instance the activity around childbirth made it onto the mainstream public agenda—it commanded mass media attention, it generated controversy and conflict, and it resulted in legislative or regulatory action or both—in other words, it resulted in policy change. These examples of "successful" childbirth advocacy are also distinguished by the relative lack of participation of the very groups we might consider typical childbirth advocates: the normal birth community and mothers themselves. In the first case discussed, drive-through deliveries, it was physicians, not mothers, who primarily demanded additional private insurance coverage for a longer postpartum hospital stay. In the second, the NIH meeting on maternal request cesareans was sought not by women or their advocates, but by obstetricians. That these interventions in maternal care did result in policy change suggests that nonpatient advocates claiming to speak for mothers have been more successful at capturing the attention of policy makers than has the organized childbirth movement. The rest of this chapter thus explores the mechanisms by which other stakeholders attempt to speak for patients and how they are able to claim authenticity and win policy success without relying on actual patient voices or support.

A Consumer Protection Campaign that Didn't
Involve Consumers: Drive-through Deliveries

It was with great fanfare that President Bill Clinton signed the Newborns' and Mothers' Health Protection Act of 1996. Its most notable provision required insurers that provided medical benefits for maternity to "ensure that coverage is provided with respect to a mother . . . and her newborn child for a minimum of 48 hours of inpatient length of stay following a normal vaginal delivery, and a minimum of 96 hours of inpatient length of stay following a cesarean section."[19] This law followed the passage of similar legislation in more than half the states.[20] The national bill (S.969) proposing minimum stays had been submitted only fifteen months earlier. and its swift passage with generally bipartisan support was seen as a victory for consumer interests. However, consumers played a largely passive role in the initiation, development, or passage of these laws at the national or state levels. There were few consumer groups involved in lobbying for passage of the legislation, with the March of Dimes a member of the coalition supporting the legislation and a small group, the Center for Patient Advocacy (now defunct), using the issue to foster its own growth.

What and who, then, were behind the legislation? Three factors seemed to be crucial. The legislation was in essence an unfunded mandate on private insurers to pay for an extra hospital day, thereby avoiding substantial additional costs to the government (and hence opposition from conservatives). This was guaranteed when the federal law dropped a provision requiring Medicaid plans to provide the additional days in the hospital for mothers and babies. A provision to support postpartum home visiting was also dropped in the final legislation. If this legislation was about improving health outcomes, why explicitly exclude those mothers and babies presumably at greatest risk? The answer was political. In 1996, Republicans, having recently taken control of the House with a pledge to the states to eliminate unfunded mandates, were not likely to impose such a cost on Medicaid systems. Of course, Congress could have provided federal support to state Medicaid systems, but that would have required finding an offset to keep the legislation budget neutral. Given that Medicaid pays for about a third of all births in the United States, this provision in the legislation made a substantial dent in what it could be said to have achieved.

A second factor was the legislation's timing and symbolic nature. In the heat of the 1996 election season, it served as a way for legislators, as well as President Clinton, to identify their commitment to mothers and babies shortly after they had passed controversial welfare reform legislation. In responding to criticisms of their actions in the latter case, they could cite their support for the Newborns' and Mothers' Health Protection Act. The media was also strongly attracted to an issue that could be so powerfully personalized. Multiple stories appeared in both print and broadcast outlets, usually focusing on a tragic outcome associated with a mother or baby who had been discharged "too early." State and national legislative hearings focused on similar tragedies. This coverage did get consumers involved, at least to the extent that they would respond to such things as a *Good Housekeeping* article that included a coupon to mail to Senator Bill Bradley's office (65,000 cards and letters) or an advertisement titled "Your Baby's Life Is in Danger" in *Parents* posted by a small advocacy group (a reported 30,000 cards were sent to the group). However, the lack of more direct consumer involvement is evident in another compromise made in the legislation—the dropping of what was termed the "mother's veto." A provision in some states and in earlier versions of the national bill gave mothers the right to determine whether they felt they needed to stay longer than the forty-eight or ninety-six hours required by the law. At the insistence of Senator Bill Frist, who feared the precedent this provision would establish, the final bill gave the decision on an extended stay to "attending providers in consultation with the mother." If this legislation were about consumer empowerment, the mother's veto would seem a basic component.

The third factor moving the legislation forward at both the state and national levels was active interest group involvement, but from provider groups rather than consumer groups. Lobbyists for the American Medical Association, American College of Obstetrics and Gynecology, and the American Academy of Pediatrics worked on the issue at both the state and national level. Their motives for involvement appeared to involve a concern with clinical outcomes—though the research on the health consequences of early discharge has never been conclusive—combined with ongoing dissatisfaction with the increased intrusion of insurance companies into their clinical domains.[21] Senator Frist, as a physician, perfectly captures this perspective with his insistence that the mother's veto be dropped and that discharge decisions be the domain of doctors without interference from insurers.

Subsequent research shows the same kind of mixed impacts that were apparent in the research reported before the law's enactment. While postpartum length of stay undoubtedly increased, the studies examining whether or not longer stays were associated with better infant health outcomes continued to show mixed results.[22] From a simple political perspective, the policies were an unqualified success since elected officials, when discussing consumer protection in maternal and child health, could now cite these legislative efforts as an example of their commitment to mothers and children.[23] Yet consumers played little role in getting this issue on state or national agendas and only a secondary role in policy formation or adoption.[24] Moreover, rather than empowering women as consumers of maternity care, the drive-through delivery laws in effect drove the medicalization of childbirth by increasing physician control and reinforcing cultural beliefs about the hospital being the only safe place for a mother and newborn.

Cesarean Delivery on Maternal Request: The Missing Consumer Redux

In our next case, expert elites again drive the policy agenda, given a veneer of authenticity by mass media reports of women—most typically celebrities—who had opted for elective primary cesarean deliveries. Cesarean delivery was performed sparingly for most of the twentieth century. Beginning in the 1970s, however, the rate of cesarean births began to rise. Increasing sharply in the 1980s, cesareans accounted for 22.7 percent of all births by 1990. After a small decline to 20.7 percent in 1996, the rate continued to rise, reaching 32 percent in 2007, the highest rate ever reported in the United States.[25] These increases provoked widespread social concern and policy initiatives from the 1980s onward to lower the cesarean rate.[26] Yet concern about the rising cesarean delivery rate is now mixed with discussion of whether cesarean delivery on maternal request (CDMR) may be a mode of birth that some women do, or would if fully informed, genuinely prefer to vaginal delivery. Some investigators, for instance, have suggested that, after accounting for changes in medical practice and the characteristics of women giving birth (i.e., increasing age, obesity, gestational diabetes), maternal request may be a driving force behind the increase in the primary cesarean rate.[27] Further, with the growth of the discipline of urogynecology, increased attention to the purported potential pelvic floor sequelae of vaginal delivery has raised the question of whether cesarean delivery might be appropriately preferred by some women.[28]

Discussion about the medical appropriateness of CDMR heightened in the United States in 2000, when newly elected American College of Obstetricians and Gynecologists (ACOG) president Benson Harer wondered in a widely discussed editorial whether "the deciding factor [for route of delivery] should simply be the mother's preference for how her baby is to be delivered." He recast the issue as one of women's rights, calling physician refusal to grant elective cesarean "a major example of . . . physician paternalism," and listing free choice of delivery route among women's civil and reproductive rights, along with property holding, education, voting, contraception, and abortion.[29] Following Harer's statement, an ACOG position statement, as well as many commentators, argued that offering women a choice of primary elective cesarean section and providing cesarean when requested may indeed be ethical, underscoring the principle of autonomy.[30]

Some physicians and advocates raised concerns about making CDMR available, including worries that pregnant women may face cultural pressures to choose cesarean delivery;[31] that women may choose cesareans without adequate appreciation for the burdens of abdominal surgery or the implications for future deliveries;[32] that demand for repeat cesareans may be driven less by patients and more by restrictions on vaginal birth after cesarean (VBAC), or by providers who may prefer scheduled cesareans over waiting for labor and natural birth, or because providers have lost the skills necessary to manage a complicated vaginal birth;[33] or as a way of avoiding the perceived risks of medical malpractice associated with vaginal delivery.[34] Surveys of care providers regarding patient-requested cesarean delivery have reported divergent findings. Some studies indicate broad-based support for CDMR; others document considerable reluctance on the part of obstetricians to perform cesarean deliveries without medical indications.[35] Opinions among physicians appear to vary by specialty as well, with urogynecologists indicating more support for CDMR.[36]

Popular media accounts of women who were "too posh too push" began appearing in 1999 in England.[37] The U.S. media quickly jumped on the bandwagon and began reporting on the phenomenon here, particularly in the context of celebrity births. Britney Spears, Kate Hudson, Christina Aguilera, Madonna, Gwyneth Paltrow, and Catherine Zeta-Jones have all elected cesarean surgery for nonmedical reasons. In the popular media, journalists portrayed women alternately as exerting unreasonable, selfish demands for choice during birth, or as exercising a legitimate but hitherto-ignored interest in determining the mode of childbirth for themselves.[38] To the surprise and consternation of many, in 2005 the National Institutes of Health announced a State of the Science conference to assess the evidence around what it called "cesarean delivery on maternal request" (CDMR). The Agency for Healthcare Research and Quality commissioned a technical evidence report to evaluate existing data on maternal and fetal outcomes, comparing planned vaginal and planned cesarean deliveries. NIH assembled a panel of experts, including a lone patient representative, to evaluate the evidence and make recommendations to the institute. Mary D'Alton, an obstetrician-gynecologist at Columbia University, was appointed to lead the panel. As per NIH guidelines, the composition of the expert panel had to consist of professionals who had never published on the matter of CDMR.

The NIH meeting itself, in March 2006, was a highly ritualized staging of professional dominance, as reflected in my field notes. The expert panel sat above the audience on a stage. The chair of the panel, Mary D'Alton, carefully addressed her fellow physicians with the formal title "doctor." When a Ph.D. epidemiologist was called to present evidence, D'Alton introduced her by her first name only, Meera. Given this staging, it was hardly surprising when the interactions between the panel and the audience members, who were invited to address questions and comments to the panelists, turned antagonistic. It is necessarily an adversarial process when one group is elevated to expert status and another group, which cares passionately about the issue, is relegated to crashing the gates. This disparity was characterized by the editor of *Obstetrics and Gynecology*, the official journal of the American College of Obstetricians and Gynecologists, who referred to the "impartial panel of experts" and deemed the comments from the audience "personal, biased, and anecdotal."[39] In this case, the gate-crashing contingent was composed mainly of the normal-birth community, a loose confederation of midwives, childbirth educators, doulas, family practice doctors, public health researchers, and citizen advocates who regard birth as a normal, nonpathological process that requires minimal medical intervention. In other words, there was a large gulf between the assumptions of the expert panel that vaginal birth might be an inherently risky endeavor that even a woman deemed low risk might quite reasonably seek to avoid and those of the audience that cesarean delivery in a low-risk woman represented unnecessary medicalization and threatened severe adverse consequences for mother and baby alike. As one of the physician presenters acknowledged early on the first day (after being asked "Have you no shame, sir?" by a birth advocate in the audience): "This certainly is an emotional topic."

And what of the social construction of knowledge around this "emotional topic"? At the center of the consensus development process as envisioned by NIH is "the evidence." In this case, there is none. First, we do not know how many women request cesarean delivery; one maternal-fetal medicine specialist in the audience said that she got more requests from the media than from pregnant women. The only population-based survey to ask women their preferences directly, the *Listening to Mothers* survey, found 1 woman out of 252 who reported that she had requested a primary cesarean delivery.[40] Second, we do not know the consequences for women or newborns. As the Agency for

Healthcare Research and Quality evidence report put it: "Virtually no studies exist on CDMR, so the knowledge base rests chiefly on indirect evidence from proxies possessing unique and significant limitations. . . . The evidence is significantly limited by its minimal relevance to primary CDMR."[41] By narrowly constructing the key question around outcomes associated with a phenomenon that did not really exist, the organizers all but ensured they would find no relevant research. In fact, "we just don't know" ought to have been the mantra of the conference. However, the matter of what we know and what we don't was often blurred and confounded. And it turns out (again not surprisingly), there is wide disagreement about what evidence should even be looked at. The panel was charged, narrowly, with examining the medical aspects of birth—which slanted its deliberations strongly in the direction of morbidity and mortality, excluding any measure of optimal outcomes or any consideration of the social, cultural, and personal meanings and significance of birth. Note again the emphasis on the outcomes of birth while the process of birth receives scant consideration or weight.

The phrase "cesarean delivery on maternal request" would appear on its surface to describe a consumer movement. However, that it does not is characteristic of advocacy in the area of childbirth, because the movement, such as it is, appears to be more a media phenomenon based on a few celebrity cases and supported by some clinicians than a truly consumer-led effort. Even if it were led by consumers, they would have no target at which to direct their efforts in today's fragmented maternity care system. While maternity care is viewed as a matter for policy makers in some countries, notably England, it continues to be seen in the United States as a private matter between a mother and her doctor rather than an issue of public concern.[42] Indeed, during the 2009 efforts of President Barack Obama and his administration to achieve health care reform, U.S. Senator John Kyl argued against mandating that insurers provide coverage for maternity care, asserting, "I don't need maternity care," to which fellow senator Debbie Stabenow retorted, "I think your mom probably did." Despite this snappy rejoinder, Kyl's dismissal of maternity care as an essential benefit reflects a longstanding indifference to childbirth as a policy concern among U.S. policy makers.

Conclusions

As a matter of public policy, childbirth is virtually invisible. This is curious, since it involves some of the elements one would expect to draw policy makers' interest—with more than four millions births every year in the United States, large numbers of people are affected, resulting in increased health care costs as cesarean deliveries have become the most common major surgical procedure in the United States. There is also the enormous symbolic power of birth in our society. The issue is literally about motherhood (if not apple pie). From a patient perspective, it also seems to have the potential to engage large numbers of consumers (perhaps at least eight million parents a year). Birth is a major life event and a transformative experience for many. These would seem powerful preconditions for a consumer movement. Despite all these reasons, childbirth remains far below the political radar.

Why do so few care? We might resort to a gender explanation: childbirth happens to women, so who cares? But several of the other cases described in this book (e.g., breast cancer) show how issues can move from the personal to the policy level quickly and powerfully. Childbirth, however, is unique in one respect compared to these other cases—it involves two health outcomes, and the cultural model of childbirth, drawing on centuries of experience, emphasizes the singular importance of a healthy baby. This perspective is so ingrained that any questions raised by mothers challenging the medical model are deemed self-centered; mothers are asked why they would do anything (that did not involve medical intervention) that put their babies at risk. Alternatively, if they choose to take a step such as avoiding pain medications, they are asked why they seek to suffer.

As a result, those advocating for normal birth face several major barriers. First, many mothers may not be supportive of normal birth efforts since they too have accepted the premise of the medical model and the almost patriotic claim that the United States has the best maternity care system in the world (despite poor outcomes relative to other countries). Second, there is a general feeling that if the baby is healthy, a mother does not have the right to complain about her care. With a substantial majority of babies being born healthy, there is an implicit assumption that the system must be working. Third, there is the increasing specialization of obstetrics, with more provider groups (obstetrical anesthesiologists; urogynecologists; maternal-fetal medicine specialists) building their practices on greater intervention. Fourth, a legal climate exists that also rewards action over patience, encouraging clinicians to intervene in the myriad gray areas of clinical decision making—a problem that has not been resolved by the growing evidence-based medicine movement.[43] Finally, the structure of the U.S. maternity care system is based on a fragmented, privatized model of care that does not lend itself to the kinds of organized advocacy efforts described elsewhere in this book.

And yet we seem to be in the midst of a cultural moment in which there is at least the promise of change in advocacy around childbirth. It is always risky to forecast the trajectory of social change as it is happening; nonetheless, we cannot end this chapter without noting briefly some of the new developments on the horizon. Birth *is* on the agenda for a new generation; some young women seem to be searching for alternative models of birth, and discussion of birth is flourishing in popular culture and media. Discussion of childbirth is proliferating in the blogosphere and in new social media like Facebook and Twitter.

Three characteristics of recent advocacy warrant mention. First, greater numbers of younger women are involved. In particular, the emerging profession of doula is drawing women in their twenties and thirties to childbirth advocacy. Second, in an increasingly celebrity-oriented culture, celebrities are drawing attention to birth. It is true that the "too posh to push" phenomenon involved celebrities like Britney Spears and Posh Spice, but other celebrities like Ricki Lake, Julia Roberts, and Salma Hayek have prompted public discussion of natural childbirth and breastfeeding. Third, new forms of media—particularly the Internet—are playing a role by providing venues for discussions of childbirth. These three features of recent childbirth advocacy are synergistic.

Several documentary films that came out in 2008 are being widely distributed, including *The Business of Being Born* and *Orgasmic Birth*. Perhaps even more importantly, each of these films has attracted mainstream media attention. Deborah Pascali-Bonaro's *Orgasmic Birth* was featured on *20/20*. Ricki Lake's film, *The Business of Being Born*, shows footage of Lake's home birth; since its release Lake and director Abby Epstein have attracted regular media attention, culminating in an American Medical Association resolution condemning home birth in summer 2008. The AMA action became the target of outrage among birth advocates.

At the policy level, there are indications that institutions are at last paying greater attention to birth in a more systematic way as well. In March 2010 the NIH convened a consensus conference on vaginal birth after cesarean—a topic that advocates at the 2006 conference on CDMR had insisted deserved attention. In early 2010, the Joint Commission on Accreditation of Healthcare Organizations added a measure of hospitals' cesarean rate among low-risk (nulliparous, vertex presentation) women to its core measures of health care performance, a move that will force hospitals to pay closer attention to the rising rate of cesareans. Likewise, the National Quality Forum is developing a set of perinatal measures to assess the quality of maternity care services and women's satisfaction with care. These policy initiatives suggest that birth is making its way onto the health policy agenda in a way it never has before.

It is too early to determine the future of childbirth advocacy, but it may be in the process of being reborn; women's voices are perhaps less silent than before. The escalating cesarean rate, the malpractice crisis, lack of access to VBAC, stubbornly high preterm birth and infant mortality rates, and increasing maternal mortality have not escaped the notice of individual consumers or policy makers. New social media are providing forums for consumer organization and consciousness raising that overcome some of the traditional barriers to mobilizing new parents. At the same time, attention to issues of quality and to comparative effectiveness of care generally has provided childbirth advocates with new opportunities to advance the cause of maternity care reform.

Notes

1. Marie McCullough, "Teachers Joined in Birth, Death," *Philadelphia Inquirer*, May 10, 2007.

2. Valerie Levesque, "Award for N.J. Hospital Draws Anger," CBS3 New Jersey, January 2, 2008.

3. On birthing centers, see Raymond DeVries, "The Alternative Birth Center: Option or Cooptation," *Women and Health* (1980): 5; on childbirth classes, see Eugene R. Declercq, "The Politics of Co-Optation: Strategies for Childbirth Educators," *Birth* 10, 3 (1983): 167–172.

4. Frank Chervenak and Laurence B. McCullough, "The Fetus as a Patient: An Essential Concept for Maternal-Fetal Medicine," *Journal of Maternal-Fetal Medicine* 5, 3 (1996): 115–119; Susan S. Mattingly, "The Maternal-Fetal Dyad: Exploring the Two-Patient Obstetric Model," *Hastings Center Report* 22, 1 (1992): 13–18; Thomas H. Murray, "Moral Obligation to the Not-Yet Born: The Fetus as Patient," *Clinics in Perinatology* 142 (1987): 329–343; James David, "Fetal Medicine," *British Medical Journal* 316, 7144 (1988): 1580–1583.

5. Eugene R. Declercq, Carol Sakala, Maureen Corry, and Sandy Applebaum, *Listening to Mothers II: Report of the Second National U.S. Survey of Women's Childbearing Experiences* (New York: Childbirth Connection, 2006).

6. Birth advocates began using the term "normal birth" to signal a belief that birth is a normal, nonpathological process, in contradistinction to the medical model of birth as inherently risky. However, many people outside the so-called normal birth community find this term confusing, or disconcerting and off-putting. Thus, advocates are now turning to language about "physiologic" birth (as employed by Childbirth Connection) and "natural, safe, and healthy birth" (as employed by Lamaze International). In this chapter, we use the terms "normal birth" and "physiologic birth" interchangeably.

7. Eugene R. Declercq, Carol Sakala, Maureen Corry, and Sandy Applebaum, *Listening to Mothers: Report of the First National U.S. Survey of Women's Childbearing Experiences* (New York: Maternity Care Association, 2002).

8. Richard W. Wertz and Dorothy Wertz, *Lying-In: A History of Childbirth in America* (New Haven: Yale University Press, 1989).

9. Marjorie Karmel, *Thank You, Dr. Lamaze: A Mother's Experiences in Painless Childbirth* (Philadelphia: J. B. Lippincott, 1959).

10. Judith W. Leavitt, *Make Room for Daddy: The Journey from Waiting Room to Birthing Room* (Chapel Hill: University of North Carolina Press, 2009).

11. Ina May Gaskin, *Spiritual Midwifery* (Summertown, Tenn.: Book Publishing Company, 1975).

12. For 1975, see "Rates of Cesarean Delivery—United States, 1991," *Morbidity and Mortality Weekly Report* 42, 15 (1993): 285–289; for 2007, see Fay Menacker and Brady E. Hamilton, "Recent Trends in Cesarean Delivery in the United States," *NCHS Data Brief* 35 (2010): 1–8.

13. Marian F. MacDorman, Fay Menacker, and Eugene Declercq, "Trends and Characteristics of Home and Other Out-of-Hospital Births in the United States, 1990–2006," *National Vital Statistics Reports* 58, 11 (2010).

14. Sheila Kitzinger, Josephine M. Green, Beverly Chalmers, Marc J.N.C. Keirse, Kathleen Lindstrom, and Elina Hemminki, "Why Do Women Go Along with This Stuff? Roundtable Discussion Part 1," *Birth: Issues in Perinatal Care* 33, 2 (2006): 154–158; Michael C. Klein, Carol Sakala, Penny Simkin, Robbie Davis-Floyd, Judith P. Rooks, and Jane Pincus, "Why Do Women Go Along with This Stuff? Roundtable Discussion Part 2," *Birth: Issues in Perinatal Care* 33, 3 (2006): 245–250.

15. Zazzle Web site, http://www.zazzle.com/biggie_size_my_epidural_tshirt-235572969030373467, accessed March 17, 2010.

16. Elizabeth M. Armstrong, "Lessons in Control: Prenatal Education in the Hospital," *Social Problems* 47, 4 (2000): 583–605; William R. Arney, *Power and the Profession of Obstetrics* (Chicago: University of Chicago Press, 1982); Barbara K. Rothman, *In Labor: Women and Power in the Birthplace* (New York: W. W. Norton, 1983).

17. Leavitt, *Make Room for Daddy*.

18. Declercq et al., *Listening to Mothers II*; the first survey was Declercq et al., *Listening to Mothers*, published in 2002, four years earlier.

19. "Newborns' and Mothers' Health Protection Act of 1966," Senate of the United States, 104th Congress, 2nd session, amendment to H.R. 3666, 2.

20. Eugene Declercq and Diana Simmes, "The Politics of Drive-Through Deliveries: Putting Early Postpartum Discharge on the Legislative Agenda," *Milbank Quarterly* 75, 2 (1997): 175–202.

21. On concern about clinical outcomes, see Arthur Eidelman, "Early Discharge—Early Trouble," *Journal of Perinatology* 12, 2 (1992): 101–102; on applicable research, see Susan Egerter, Paula Braveman, and Kristen Marchi, "Follow-up of Newborns and Their Mothers after Early Hospital Discharge," *Clinics in Perinatology* 25, 2 (1998): 471–481.

22. Elizabeth J. Bragg, Barak M. Rosen, Jane Khoury, Menachem Miodovnik, and Tariq A. Siddiqi, "The Effect of Early Discharge after Vaginal Delivery on Neonatal Readmission Rates," *Obstetrics and Gynecology* 89, 6 (1997): 930–933; Kenneth E. Grullon and David A. Grimes, "The Safety of Early Postpartum Discharge: A Review and Critique," *Obstetrics and Gynecology* 90, 5 (1997): 860–865; David M. Mosen, Steven L. Clark, Michael B. Mundorff, Diane M. Tracy, Elizabeth C. McKnight, and Mary B. Zollo, "The Medical and Economic Impact of the Newborns' and Mothers' Health Protection Act," *Obstetrics and Gynecology* 99, 1 (2002): 116–124.

23. Eugene Declercq, "Making U.S. Maternal and Child Health Policy: From 'Early Discharge' to 'Drive Through Deliveries,' to a National Law," *Maternal and Child Health Journal* 3, 1 (1999): 5–17; Eugene Declercq and Judith Norsigian, "Mothers Aren't behind Vogue for Caesareans," *Boston Globe*, April 3, 2006.

24. Declercq and Simmes, "Politics of Drive-Through Deliveries."

25. Fay Menacker, "Trends in Cesarean Rates for First Births and Repeat Cesarean Rates for Low-Risk Women: United States, 1990–2003," *National Vital Statistics Reports*

54, 4 (2005); Fay Menacker and Sally C. Curtin, "Trends in Cesarean Birth and Vaginal Birth after Previous Cesarean, 1991–99," *National Vital Statistics Reports* 49, 13 (2001); Brady E. Hamilton, Joyce A. Martin, and Stephanie J. Ventura, "Births: Preliminary Data for 2007," *National Vital Statistics Reports* 57, 12 (2009).

26. Diony Young, "A New Push to Reduce Cesareans in the United States," *Birth: Issues in Perinatal Care* 24, 1 (1997): 1–3.

27. "National Institutes of Health [NIH] State-of-the-Science Conference Statement: Cesarean Delivery on Maternal Request," *Obstetrics and Gynecology* 107, 6 (2006): 1386–1397; Ginger L. Gossman, Jutta M. Joesch, and Koray Tanfer, "Trends in Maternal Request Cesarean Delivery from 1991 to 2004," *Obstetrics and Gynecology* 108, 6 (2006): 1506–1516; Susan F. Meikle, Cladia A. Steiner, Jun Zhang, and William L. Lawrence, "A National Estimate of the Elective Primary Cesarean Delivery Rate," *Obstetrics and Gynecology* 105, 4 (2005): 751–756.

28. Richard C. Bump, "Advising Prospective Mothers about the Maternal Morbidity of Vaginal Childbirth," *American Journal of Obstetrics and Gynecology* 187, 4 (2002): 823; W. Benson Harer Jr., "Elective Cesarean: An Option for Primiparas?" *Ob/Gyn Management* 14, 5 (2002): 38–44; Howard Minkoff, "The Ethics of Cesarean Section by Choice," *Seminars in Perinatology* 30, 5 (2006): 309–312; Howard Minkoff and Frank A. Chervenak, "Elective Primary Cesarean Delivery," *New England Journal of Medicine* 348, 10 (2003): 946–950; Ingrid Nygaard and Dwight P. Cruikshank, "Should All Women Be Offered Elective Cesarean Delivery?" *Obstetrics and Gynecology* 102, 2 (2003): 217–219; Amy L. O'Boyle, Gary D. Davis, and Byron C. Calhoun, "Informed Consent and Birth: Protecting the Pelvic Floor and Ourselves," *American Journal of Obstetrics and Gynecology* 187, 4 (2002): 981–983; Jennifer M. Wu, Andrew F. Hundley, and Anthony G. Visco, "Elective Primary Cesarean Delivery: Attitudes of Urogynecology and Maternal-Fetal Medicine Specialists," *Obstetrics and Gynecology* 105, 2 (2005): 301–306.

29. W. Benson Harer Jr., "Patient Choice Cesarean," *ACOG Clinical Review* 5, 2 (2000): 1–16.

30. ACOG Committee Opinion 289, November 2003, "Surgery and Patient Choice: The Ethics of Decision Making," *Obstetrics and Gynecology* 102, 5 (2003): 1101–1106. Also see Minkoff, "Ethics of Cesarean Section by Choice"; Minkoff and Chervenak, "Elective Primary Cesarean Delivery"; Frank A. Chervenak and Laurence B. McCullough, "An Ethically Justified Algorithm for Offering, Recommending, and Performing Cesarean Delivery and Its Application in Managed Care Practice," *Obstetrics and Gynecology* 87, 2 (1996): 302–305; Lisa H. Harris, "Counselling Women about Choice: Balliere's Best Practice and Research," *Clinical Obstetrics and Gynecology* 15, 1 (2001): 93–97; Anne D. Lyerly and Peter Schwartz, "Is the Patient Always Right?" *Hastings Center Report* 34, 2 (2004): 13–14; Barbara L. McFarlin, "Elective Cesarean Birth: Issues and Ethics of an Informed Decision," *Journal of Midwifery and Women's Health* 49, 5 (2004): 421–429; Howard Minkoff, "Ethical Dimensions of Elective Primary Cesarean Delivery," *Obstetrics and Gynecology* 103, 2 (2004): 387–392; Geeta Sharma, F. A. Chervenak, L. B. McCullough, and H. Minkoff, "Ethical Considerations in Elective Cesarean Delivery," *Clinical Obstetrics and Gynecology* 47, 2 (2004): 404–408; Andrea L. Tranquilli and Guiseppe G. Garzetti, "A New Ethical and Clinical Dilemma in Obstetric Practice: Cesarean Section 'On Maternal Request,'" *American Journal of Obstetrics and Gynecology* 177, 1 (1997): 245–246.

31. For physician concerns, see Susan Bewley and Jayne Cockburn, "The Unfacts of 'Request' Caesarean Section," *BJOG: An International Journal of Obstetrics and Gynaecology* 109, 6 (2002): 597–605.

32. On abdominal surgery burdens, see Declercq and Norsigian, "Mothers Aren't behind Vogue for Cesareans"; on effects on future deliveries, see "NIH State-of-the-Science Conference Statement on Cesarean Delivery on Maternal Request," *NIH Consensus and State-of-the-Science Statements* 23, 1 (2005): 1–29.

33. Atul Gawande, "The Score: How Childbirth Went Industrial," *New Yorker*, October 9, 2006, 58–67.

34. McFarlin, "Elective Cesarean Birth"; A. C. Angeja, A. E. Washington, J. E. Vargas, R. Gomez, I. Rojas, and A. B. Caughey, "Chilean Women's Preferences Regarding Mode of Delivery," *BJOG: An International Journal of Obstetrics and Gynaecology* 113, 11 (2006): 1253–1258; Dominique Behague, Cesar G. Victora, and Fernando C. Barros, "Consumer Demand for Caesarean Sections in Brazil," *BMJ* 324, 7343 (2002): 942–945; Susan Bewley and Jayne Cockburn, "The Unethics of 'Request' Caesarean Section," *BJOG: An International Journal of Obstetrics and Gynaecology* 109, 6 (2002): 593–596; Denise Grady, "Trying to Avoid 2nd Cesarean, Many Find Choice Isn't Theirs," *New York Times*, November 29, 2004; I. Hildingsson, I. Rådestad, C. Rubertsson, and U. Waldenström, "Few Women Wish to Be Delivered by Caesarean Section," *BJOG: An International Journal of Obstetrics and Gynaecology* 109, 6 (2002): 618–623; Michael C. Klein, "Elective Cesarean Section," *Canadian Medical Association Journal* 171, 1 (2004): 14–15, and author reply, 15–16; Michael C. Klein, "Obstetricians' Fear of Childbirth: How Did It Happen?" *Birth* 32, 3 (2005): 207–209; Michael C. Klein, "Quick Fix Culture: The Cesarean-Section-on-Demand Debate," *Birth* 31, 3 (2004): 161–164; Zosia Kmietowicz, "NICE Advises against Caesarean Section on Demand," *BMJ* 328, 7447 (2004): 1031; L. Penna and S. Arulkumaran, "Cesarean Section for Non-medical Reasons," *International Journal of Gynaecology and Obstetrics* 82, 3 (2003): 399–409; J. E. Potter, E. Berquó, I. H. Perpétuo, O. F. Leal, K. Hopkins, M. R. Souza, and M. C. Formiga, "Unwanted Caesarean Sections among Public and Private Patients in Brazil," *BMJ* 323, 7322 (2001): 1155–1158; Cecilia Souza, "Caesarean-Sections as Ideal Births: The Cultural Construction of Beneficence and Patients' Rights in Brazil," *Cambridge Quarterly of Healthcare Ethics* 3, 3 (1994): 358–366; Diony Young, "'Cesarean Delivery on Maternal Request': Was the NIH Conference Based on a Faulty Premise?" *Birth* 33, 3 (2006): 171–174; Diony Young, "The Push against Vaginal Birth," *Birth* 30, 3 (2003): 149–152; Mary Ellen Schneider, "Insurers Set Criteria for VBAC Coverage," *OB GYN News*, 40, 3 (2005): 1–2; Susan P. Walker, Elizabeth A. McCarthy, Antony Ugoni, Anna Lee, Sharon Lim, and Michael Permezel, "Cesarean Delivery or Vaginal Birth," *Obstetrics and Gynecology* 109, 1 (2007): 67–72.

35. On support for CDMR, see Christina S. Cotzias, Sara Paterson-Brown, and Nicholas M. Fisk. "Obstetricians Say Yes to Maternal Request for Elective Caesarean Section: A Survey of Current Opinion," *European Journal of Obstetrics, Gynecology, and Reproductive Biology* 97, 1 (2001): 15–16. On obstetricians' reluctance, see Barbara A. Bettes, Victoria H. Coleman, Stanley Zinberg, Catherine Y. Spong, Barry Portnoy, Emily DeVoto, and Jay Schulkin, "Cesarean Delivery on Maternal Request: Obstetricians-Gynecologists' Knowledge, Perception, and Practice." *Obstetrics and Gynecology* 109, 1 (2007): 57–66.

36. Wu, Hundley, and Visco, "Elective Primary Cesarean Delivery"; Bettes et al., "Cesarean Delivery on Maternal Request"; K. Kenton, C. Brincat, M. Motone, and

L. Brubaker, "Repeat Cesarean Section and Primary Elective Cesarean Section: Recently Trained Obstetrician-Gynecologist Practice Patterns and Opinions," *American Journal of Obstetrics and Gynecology* 192, 6 (2005): 1872–1875; discussion on 1875–1876.

37. Joanna Moorhead. "Are You Too Posh to Push? The Way You Give Birth Has Become the Status Symbol of Our Times," *London Daily Mail*, January 26, 1999; Marie McCullough, "C-Section Trend Emerges," *Philadelphia Inquirer*, March 25, 2001.

38. Moorhead, "Are You Too Posh to Push?"; Karen Springen, "The Right to Choose," *Newsweek*, December 4, 2000, http://www.newsweek.com/2000/12/03/the-right-to-choose.html, accessed November 10, 2010; Sora Song, Andrew Downie, Helen Gibson, Kristin Kloberdanz, and Jeanne McDowell, "As More Pregnant Women Schedule C-Sections, Doctors Warn That the Procedure Is Not Risk-Free," *Time*, April 19, 2004, http://www.time.com/time/magazine/article/0,9171,993857,00.html, accessed November 10, 2010.

39. James R. Scott, "Cesarean Delivery on Request: Where Do We Go From Here?" *Obstetrics and Gynecology* 107, 6 (2006): 1222–1223.

40. DeClercq et al., "Listening to Mothers II."

41. M. Viswanathan, A. G. Visco, K. Hartmann, M. E. Wechter, G. Gartlehner, J. M. Wu, R. Palmieri, M. J. Funk, L. J. Lux, T. Swinson et al., "Cesarean Delivery on Maternal Request," Evidence Report/Technology Assessment No. 133 (Rockville, Md: Agency for Healthcare Research and Quality, 2006), v.

42. Eugene Declercq, "Changing Childbirth in England: Lessons for US Health Reform," *Journal of Health Politics, Policy, and Law* 23, 5 (1998): 833–859.

43. The malpractice climate greatly affects childbirth practices in the United States, an issue beyond the scope of this chapter.

A Pound of Flesh

Patient Legal Action for Human Research Protections in the Biotech Age

Daniel and Debbie Greenberg's son Jonathan seemed healthy at birth, but six months later he was still functioning at a newborn's level. After many medical missteps, he was diagnosed as having Canavan disease, a fatal genetic disorder. Following the devastating diagnosis, his parents began to mobilize other parents to fund and participate in research to create a genetic test to allow Canavan screening and prenatal testing for the disease.

In 1987, the Greenbergs convinced geneticist Dr. Reuben Matalon to try to develop a prenatal test for Canavan disease. For years, the Greenbergs provided Matalon with tissue samples from themselves, their children, and other families and raised money for Matalon's research. When Jonathan died, they provided pieces of his brain for research. Throughout, the families and Matalon thought of the enterprise as a partnership whose goal was to create an accessible genetic test for carrier and prenatal screening.

When Matalon discovered the Canavan disease gene in 1993, the families felt that their prolonged efforts had paid off. The Canavan Foundation, which had been founded to support the research, launched a free testing program at major university centers in four states. Unbeknownst to the families or the foundation, though, Matalon and his hospital patented the Canavan gene. In 1998, the hospital began to charge royalties and limit the availability of testing, decreasing access and potentially impeding research. The patent holder stopped the free testing program.

"We gave our samples to be used for the public good," says Judith Tsipis, the mother of a child with Canavan disease and a genetic counselor. "Had they told us they wanted to patent the gene, we probably would have found another researcher who had the same goals as we did."[1]

As a result of the constraints put on research and clinical testing by the patenting of the gene, the Greenbergs and the other families joined a growing group of research subjects who have sued research institutions to enforce their rights as human subjects. The suits indicate a paradigm shift in the type of policy work patients and their families have undertaken with respect to human research.

When the AIDS epidemic began, activism by patients led to numerous policy changes—increased funding for research, fast-tracking of drugs at the FDA, laws forbidding HIV testing without consent, and legal policies protecting HIV seropositive individuals from discrimination.[2] Breast cancer patients followed a similar strategy, leading to increased funding for research on the disease and state laws aimed at preventing insurance discrimination against people with genetic predispositions to disease, including those with mutations in their breast cancer genes.[3] The success of those efforts may have been due to the combination of grassroots lobbying and public support from noted researchers. With the patients, providers, and researchers all on the same side, policy change may have been inevitable.

New policy struggles involving patients are taking a much different turn. In the current conflicts, the patients generally do not have the bond of a common disease as a rallying point. And they often do not have the support of the scientific community for their efforts to change the law. This new generation of disputes, in fact, pits patients against doctors and researchers. In court cases and legislative initiatives, patients are fighting for the right to be informed about and have control over what type of research is done on their blood and tissue and over who should gain the commercial fruits of that research. They seek a buffer against the most extreme market in medicine, in which patients provide, often unwittingly, the raw material for products. The advocacy goal in this arena is to move toward more democratic participation, allowing patients and research subjects to have greater control over what is done with their tissue.[4]

The First Wave of Human Research Laws

The backdrop for the current conflicts over the protection of patients in research studies is a set of regulations adopted in the 1970s to govern federally funded research. The adoption of those regulations did not come about because of the political activism of patients. Instead, the atrocities committed in the name of research by Nazi doctors—and the subsequent revelation of unethical research in the United States in an influential 1966 study by Henry Beecher in the *New*

England Journal of Medicine—prompted an effort by a federal commission of doctors, lawyers, and philosophers to implement guidelines for researchers.[5]

The trial of the Nazi doctors led to the promulgation of the Nuremberg Code, the first principle of which is that "voluntary consent of the human subject is absolutely essential."[6] Similarly, the federal research regulations enacted in 1974 emphasize the need to ensure that participation in research is voluntary and that people receive adequate information in advance of their decision about whether to be part of a research study.[7] The regulations also assure people that they are free to withdraw from research at any time.[8] The federal regulations created a mechanism—the local Institutional Review Board (IRB)— to review federally funded research proposals to assure that the benefits to the subjects outweigh the risks.[9]

The nature of the research enterprise in the United States has changed vastly since the federal research regulations were adopted in the 1970s, especially with respect to the "expanded commercialization of the research enterprise."[10] Today, federally funded university researchers are more likely to have a commercial interest that conflicts with the needs of their patient/ subjects. The regulations were adopted before the enactment of the federal technology transfer laws that allow university researchers and government researchers using federal funds to personally benefit financially from the research, such as by patenting a gene they have identified in a patient's tissue.[11]

With the advent of biotechnology research and the chance to profit personally from research projects, some physicians began to view their patients as sources of raw materials for biotech research. Today, hospitals make deals with biotech companies to sell pathology samples from patients. Doctors contact preeminent genetic researchers and say something like, "I'll sell you my families"—offering to provide the researchers with tissue samples from, for example, all their patients with asthma or diabetes. Some medical school researchers report that when they seek tissue samples within their hospitals for nonprofit research, they find that the samples have already been sold.[12]

In addition to a change in the financial incentives for research, the type of research being undertaken has changed profoundly. The 1970s federal regulations were geared toward protecting people against the physical risks inherent in, for example, human experimentation involving new drugs. When subjects signed up as part of a research project, they usually knew what disease they had and were volunteering for a test of a new diagnostic or treatment. But genetics research has shifted the paradigm. People's tissue often is used without their consent for research that may reveal information unknown to the research subject, such as increased risk of illness or predisposition to a stigmatizing behavior—information they might not want others to know or may not want to know themselves. People's confidential health records, phenotypic data (such as blood pressure, weight, and psychiatric information), exposure information (such as drug use and environmental factors), and pedigree information (including sensitive information about familial relationships) are linked to their tissue samples or their genomes in large-scale, genomewide association studies; such studies compare the genomes, medical histories, and social histories of thousands of people to locate genetic differences between people with specific illnesses and people without those illnesses.

The federal research regulations were not specifically designed to address the situations of research in which the physical intervention might be minor (such as a blood draw) or nonexistent (such as the use of a previously collected tissue sample) but other risks loom. As research into AIDS, genetics, embryo stem cells, and human cloning makes clear, people have interests in what happens to their tissue even when the research presents no physical risks to them. Research on tissue—whether it is performed with identifiable or anonymized tissue samples—may violate people's personal or religious beliefs or lead to stigmatization or discrimination against them as individuals or members of a group.

The possible risks to genetic research subjects are numerous. For example, studies done on identifiable tissue samples could lead to discrimination against the tissues' owners in insurance or employment. In one such case, a participant in a study of predisposition to colon cancer lost his health insurance.[13] Relatives of people with Huntington's and Alzheimer's disease have been denied admission to school, been fired or denied employment, and lost insurance coverage.[14] Psychological risks exist when patients find out they do (or do not) have a genetic propensity to develop a certain disease.

A federal law passed on May 21, 2008, provides a starting point to address some of these concerns.[15] The Genetic Information Nondiscrimination Act (GINA) prohibits employers from using genetic information to make decisions about the hiring, firing, promotion, and compensation of employees.[16] Although employers are also forbidden from collecting genetic information, there are exceptions, such as allowing employers to purchase the information from publicly available sources or "inadvertently" request a family history, so long as they do not discriminate against those individuals because they have a genetic predisposition to disease.[17] Yet, it would be difficult to prove that an employer discriminated on the basis of that genetic information and not for some other reason.

Even research undertaken on an anonymized tissue sample is generally reported according to demographic categories, which could lead to discrimination against people of an ethnic group, race, or Native American tribe.[18] In 2006, for example, a researcher made the controversial claim that he had discovered a "warrior" gene in the Maori that makes them more aggressive, more violent, and more likely to be criminals.[19] The Maori and others protested this claim as stigmatizing and scientifically questionable.

Research on tissue from people from certain ethnic or religious groups may cause distress to other members of that group, including relatives of the people whose tissues were used for research. In the Orthodox Jewish community, for instance, unauthorized use of body tissue violates religious beliefs which require that the body be buried whole.[20] If a living person's leg is amputated during his or her life, arrangements are made to store that body part for burial with the individual after death.[21] Similar issues were raised by research on Native Americans, when graves of their ancestors were disturbed to acquire bones for research. Research that results in gene patents may be opposed by those, like some Baptists, who believe the genetic code should not be owned.[22]

The growth of private-sector research—with studies being undertaken by biotech firms, pharmaceutical companies, and in private doctors' offices—highlights another glaring problem with the federal research regulations. Unlike most industrialized countries, whose regulations cover both government-funded research and privately funded research, the federal research regulations in the United States do not apply to research conducted using private funds.[23] Yet a substantial amount of biomedical research is privately funded. Industry support from pharmaceutical, biotechnology, and medical device firms accounts for 57 percent of funding for biomedical research.[24]

Patients as Policy Actors in Research Disputes

Patients—as individuals and, on occasion, in groups—have begun to protest against the way physicians and other researchers are using their tissue. Three types of disputes have come before courts and legislatures, involving: (1) the researcher's use of patients' tissue without consent; (2) the researcher's use of tissue provided for one type of research for a different type of research to which the patient has not given consent; and (3) the researcher's commercialization through patents of the tissue or its genetic information in a way that could disadvantage patients as a whole.

Conflicts about Research Conducted on Tissue without Consent

In the United States, research is not a matter of conscription. People are free to refuse to participate. Yet despite the fact that the federal research regulations and all medical and research codes of ethics stress the importance of informed consent, patients' tissue is often used for research without their consent. Patients rarely find out about this unless a whistleblower within an institution discloses the research, or the researchers inadvertently disclose something that leads to suspicion.

In 1951, a thirty-one-year-old African American woman, Henrietta Lacks, died of ovarian cancer. Without the knowledge or consent of Lacks or her family, her tissue was taken and made into a cell line that has been extremely valuable for research and is still sold today. Her family became aware of the use of Henrietta's tissue only when, years later, the researchers began to call family members and ask for their tissue too. In an interview in 1994, her husband said: "As far as them selling my wife's cells without my knowledge and making a profit—I do not like that at all. They are exploiting both of us."[25] In the years since, however, researchers have even more incentive to use people's tissue.

Patients seeking to change the policy in this area have turned to lawyers. But the law is not well developed with respect to the use of tissue without consent and therefore has provided some, but not sufficient, protection to patients. The main legal challenges have involved claims of violation of a right to informed consent and claims about conversion of the patient's property.

Actions in court about research conducted without consent

John Moore felt something was amiss in the early 1980s when his physician, David Golde, kept asking him to fly back to Los Angeles from his home in Seattle to provide samples of blood and other tissues. Moore had been diagnosed several years earlier with hairy cell leukemia, underwent a splenectomy at U.C.L.A., and was cured. So it seemed strange that his doctor was insisting that he keep coming back for tests and telling him that those tests could not be done by a doctor in Seattle.

The situation was disturbing enough that Moore contacted a lawyer to explore whether he had been a victim of medical malpractice. The lawyer went online to read about the doctor's scientific publications and found a staggering admission. Golde had created a special cell line from Moore's blood, patented it, and named it the Mo cell line.[26] He had then sold rights to the cell line to a biotechnology firm.

Moore at first reacted with disbelief. Then, as he thought more about what had happened, he felt "violated for dollars," "invaded," "raped." His body had been appropriated without his knowledge or consent. He asked his lawyer to sue his doctor for theft.[27]

The case was so unusual that the trial court judge quickly threw it out of court. But on appeal, the California Court of Appeals ruled that Moore had indeed been wronged. The decision underscored the growth of the market: "Until recently, the physical human body, as distinguished from the mental and spiritual, was believed to have little value, other than as a source of labor. In recent history, we have seen the human body assume astonishing aspects of value." The appeals court reviewed cases involving celebrities like Bela Lugosi, who was held to have a property interest in his own likeness that prevented other people from marketing photos of him. "If the courts have found a sufficient proprietary interest in one's persona, how could one not have a right in one's own genetic material, something far more profoundly the essence of one's humanity than a name or a face?" On a practical note, the court wrote: "If this science has become science for profit, then we fail to see any justification for excluding the patient from participation in those profits."[28]

The appellate decision was not the last word on the matter. In 1988 the doctor and biotechnology company appealed to the California Supreme Court. The justices were deeply divided. Each wrote eloquently about the meaning of the body, some describing it as a sacred temple, others as a biomedical factory. An acrimonious dispute surfaced in four opinions about whether Moore could claim that his tissue was his property. A majority of the justices, for differing reasons, rejected the idea that Moore could claim a property interest in his body. Even though the law in many ways was on his side, the justices seemed swayed by the heady promise of biotechnology. They did not want to slow down research by universities or by the nation's biotechnology companies. They described researchers as "innocent parties" engaged in socially useful activities who have no reason to believe that their use of a particular cell sample may be against a donor's wishes. They were concerned that giving Moore a property right to his tissue would "destroy the economic incentive to conduct important medical research."[29]

Several justices dissented to the *Moore* decision, pointing to its ironies. Justice Allen Broussard wrote: "Far from elevating these biological materials above the marketplace, the majority's holding simply bars *plaintiff* [Moore], the source of the cells, from obtaining the benefit of the cells' value, but permits *defendants*, who allegedly obtained the cells from plaintiff by improper means, to retain and exploit the full economic value of their ill-gotten gains free of their ordinary common law liability for conversion."[30] Justice Stanley Mosk also dissented, suggesting the paradox in the view that the patient could not own his tissue while the doctor could.[31]

Although the California Supreme Court justices refused to recognize Moore's property right under these circumstances, they did recognize his right to sue his doctor for lack of informed consent and for breach of what is known as the doctor's "fiduciary duty"—his responsibility to put the patient's interest first. They held that a physician must tell his patient if he has a personal interest unrelated to the patient's health that might affect his judgment, whether that interest is scientific or commercial.

Using the fiduciary duty approach protects patients from physicians who collect the tissue, but it does not protect patients from other researchers and other institutions that may be collecting or testing tissue samples without patients' knowledge or consent. In an even larger loophole, it does not protect the patient who is sick—as Moore was—and who probably would have consented to the operation, no matter what the doctors were planning to do with his tissue.

Although Moore filed suit as an individual, the largest patient advocacy group in the United States, the People's Medical Society, filed an amicus brief in the *Moore* case on behalf of its 85,000 members. The People's Medical Society, a patient/consumer empowerment group founded in 1983, argued that the possibility of commercialization touched more aspects of medical care than in the past. It noted that Arnold Relman, then editor of the *New England Journal of Medicine*, had expressed concern that physicians' growing commercial desire weakened their professional ethics. Similarly, Leon Rosenberg, then dean of the Yale University School of Medicine, acknowledged that "the goals of some scientists—clinical or basic—are different than in the past. . . . The biotechnology revolution has moved us, literally or figuratively, from the class room to the board room and from the *New England Journal* to the *Wall Street Journal.*"[32]

The *Moore* court specifically noted that it did not need to give the patient/research subject a property right because his interests were thought to be adequately protected by the causes of action for lack of informed consent and breach of fiduciary duty.[33] But the court stated that "we do not purport to hold that excised cells can never be property for any purpose whatsoever."[34] Indeed, a subsequent California case ended in a different result than the *Moore* case and found that a person had a property interest in his tissue where a contract existed that showed that the person providing the tissue had an "expectation he would in fact retain control."[35]

In fact, since the 1980 decision in *Moore*, numerous courts have held that human tissue outside the body can be considered the property of an individual or the next of kin.[36] For example, in *Mansaw v. Midwest Organ Bank*, a Missouri federal court held that a father had a property interest in his son's dead body and that the "property interest" covered the right to control the removal of tissue and organs from the body.[37] Because *Moore* was a California case, interpreting California law, it does not have legal precedence in other states. Yet researchers and research institutions continue to use the case to claim that they can own patients' tissue, while simultaneously arguing that patients cannot own their own tissue.

Legislative and professional actions about unauthorized research

Patient groups such as the National Breast Cancer Coalition have also gone to legislators to fight for control over what is done with patient tissues in research. One umbrella consumer lobbying group, People with Genes, points out that since we all have genes, we all need to be protected against discrimination. Their lobbying led ultimately to the passage of the federal Genetic Information Nondiscrimination Act. Some states have responded by adopting statutes asserting patients' right to consent in the use of their tissues. In Florida, for example, a person's genetic material may not be tested without consent, even for important research purposes.[38]

Today, various professional organizations, and even some biotechnology companies, require that, when the tissue is first extracted, people be given information about potential research and commercial uses of their tissue and a chance to refuse to allow the use of their tissue for such purposes.[39] The American Medical Association's Code of Ethics provides that "[p]otential commercial applications must be disclosed to the patient before a profit is realized on products developed from biological materials" and that "[h]uman tissue and its products may not be used for commercial purposes without the informed consent of the patient who provided the original cellular material."[40]

With respect to the initial decision of patients about whether their tissue will be used in research, there is previous case law and statutory law in some instances that requires advance consent. This is particularly true when the researcher is a physician. But the law does not spell out what information is required to be disclosed. Should it be sufficient if researchers ask for consent for all future research purposes, or should researchers have to disclose the nature, risks, and problems particular to the research studies they are proposing, including the risks of group stigmatization? If they are supposed to inform prospective subjects about commercialization, is it sufficient to have a sentence (as is customarily done) that tells participants that if there is financial gain they will not receive a portion, or should the participants be told that they could participate in the same sort of study (such as research identifying genes) by another researcher, who will not commercialize the scientific information but will instead share it with others?

Conflicts about Research on Tissue That Goes
Beyond What the Patient Consented To

Because research on tissue presents risks, a committee of the National Academy of Sciences on genetic research noted, "it is not ethically or legally acceptable to ask research participants to 'consent' to future yet unknown uses of their identifiable DNA samples."[41] Yet researchers now commonly make secondary use of blood samples that patients have provided for another purpose without getting additional consent. Again, this has led to legal cases brought by individual patients and groups of patients.

In the early 1980s, William Catalona, an internationally known prostate cancer surgeon, began asking his patients if they were willing to let him use the tissue removed during their surgery, their blood, and other tissue for prostate cancer research. Patients were told they could withdraw consent to research on their tissue sample at any time in the future. Under these terms, Catalona amassed tissue samples from more than thirty thousand people.

But Catalona's institution, Washington University, began to see the tissue samples not solely as a resource for prostate cancer research advances, but additionally as a capital resource for the university. As the conflicts between research protections and financial interests escalated, Catalona decided to leave Washington University for a new position at Northwestern University medical school. He wrote to his patients, telling them that he was transferring to a new institution and asking whether they were willing to transfer their samples to Northwestern. Six thousand of his patients wrote that they wanted their samples to move with him.

Washington University refused to transfer the samples and sued Catalona to have the tissue samples declared the university's property and thus to prevent him from moving them. In its lawsuit, Washington University requested a declaratory judgment that it owned the tissue samples, which it said were worth more than $1 million, and asserted that it had the right to use them as it wished "in its sole discretion."[42]

A group of patients sued to intervene in the case and were eventually added by the judge as necessary parties because he found that the outcome of the case could affect their interests. In their arguments to the court, the patients pointed out that they had not turned over their property—their tissue—to the university for its unconditional use and that they wanted to exercise their federally guaranteed right to withdraw from the study by withdrawing their samples. They argued that transferring the samples to Northwestern would effectuate their original intent of having a specific researcher, Catalona, undertake a specific kind of research, prostate cancer research, on their tissue samples.

Washington University argued that the patients had no ownership rights to their tissue since it was a gift—a donation—to the university. Its lawyers argued that the patients' right to withdraw from the study did not include the right to withdraw the sample and that the university should be able to make the samples anonymous and do whatever research it pleased with them.

In April 2005, a federal district court judge held a hearing solely to answer the question, who owns these tissue samples? All patients who testified indicated that they chose to participate because of the type of research Catalona was performing and because Catalona would be the one leading the studies. "I [can't] think of anybody that I would have more faith in to do the kind of research that might help my grandsons on my samples, my tissues, my body parts, than Doctor Catalona," testified one of the patients, James Ellis.[43] The patients also testified that they interpreted the right to withdraw from the study as evidence that they had retained some control over their tissues.

The patients' arguments were consistent with the federal regulations, which prohibit research subjects from waiving their legal rights to their tissue. Section 46.116 of Title 45 of the Code of Federal Regulations provides: "No informed consent, whether oral or written, may include any exculpatory language through which the subject or the representative is made to waive or appear to waive any of the subject's legal rights, or releases or appears to release the investigator, the sponsor, the institution or its agents from liability for negligence." This regulation prohibits the very action the research institution sought in the case: requiring research participants to give up rights to their tissue.

In the *Catalona* case, the patients argued that if Washington University prevailed, research in this country would be threatened. Patients would be unlikely to allow the use of their tissue if they had no control over how their tissue was used, because their own tissue might be used for a type of research that violated their religious beliefs, such as embryonic stem cell research.[44] Or it could be sold to a biotech company for research for sheer commercial gain.[45]

The Association of American Medical Colleges (AAMC) filed an amicus curiae brief with the trial court in support of Washington University, arguing that allowing the research participants to own their tissue would seriously impede medical research and "threaten the integrity and utility of all biorepositories, and the progress of biomedical research."[46] The AAMC pointed to the enormous archive of human tissue samples in hospitals and medical centers around the country that might be used in research unimaginable at the time of the collection of the samples.

Judge Stephen Limbaugh, the trial court judge, relied heavily on the AAMC brief in his ruling that the patients had made a gift of their tissue to Washington University, finding that the AAMC's doomsday prediction "succinctly mirrors the Court's concerns."[47] The judge also ruled that the university was not bound by what it had provided patients in the informed consent form, stating that "informed consent was inconsequential."[48]

The case was appealed. The AAMC filed another amicus brief at the appellate level on behalf of itself and universities, including Cornell, Duke, Emory, and Johns Hopkins. The AAMC described research using human tissue as a "national imperative" and said that overturning the lower court would threaten research, "to the detriment of mankind."[49]

Yet, as argued by the patients, this language—suggesting that people can be forced into having their tissue used in studies to which they object—conflicts with the legal and ethical principle that informed consent is the cornerstone of research. Research institutions have successfully conducted research for years using exactly the system the patients in the case were fighting for. The patients were asking nothing more than that the court enforce their already-existing rights under the federal research regulations, including their right to withdraw their tissue from research.

Various organizations purporting to be patients' groups filed briefs in the case. Yet, the groups with clear research interests weighed in, not surprisingly, on the side of researchers. The American Cancer Society (ACS), the largest source of cancer research funding other than the government, has established biorepositories and undertakes its own research. The ACS filed a brief supporting Washington University, arguing that a ruling allowing the patients to own their tissue and decide who could perform research on it would cause devastating results: "ongoing and future research would suffer, jeopardizing discovery of desperately needed new disease detection tools, treatments, and cures."[50]

In contrast, a prostate cancer survivors' group, Us Too, filed an amicus brief in support of the patients. Us Too, which encourages members to participate in research protocols, financially supports research but does not conduct research on its own. The group argued for enforcing the individual rights of research participants, including enforcing the patient's decision about whether to continue participating. As in the *Moore* case, the People's Medical Society (a patients' advocacy group which does not undertake research or fund it) filed a brief in the *Catalona* case. The organization argued that if courts fail to recognize people's rights to control the research undertaken on their tissue, the public will lose trust in medical research. They pointed out that, "taking this one step further, it is even possible that people will not seek out medical care if they cannot trust that their tissue will not be taken and used in medical research against their will. This is especially a concern for minority individuals, who have been shown to be less likely to seek medical care for existing conditions due to apprehension about what an institution will do with their tissue."[51]

In 2007 an appellate court affirmed the decision of the lower court, ruling that excised tissue is property of the patients that can be given as a gift, thus transferring ownership rights from a patient to a research institution if the facts of the case demonstrate that is the intent of the patient.[52] The court, however, recognized that research participants have a continuing interest in their tissue, including the right to require that the tissue no longer be used for research.[53] Nevertheless, attorneys now advise their research institution clients to look at their state's gift law to ensure that the language in their informed consent documents will suffice to make patients give up their rights to their tissue.

The problems of doing research that goes beyond initial consent are raised by another lawsuit brought by research participants. In 2004, the Havasupai tribe of Arizona filed a $50 million lawsuit claiming that four hundred samples provided to local universities for diabetes research were used for studies on inbreeding, schizophrenia, and ancient human population migrations to North America. The tribe asserted they were stigmatized by the schizophrenia and inbreeding research and would not have consented to the origins studies because the theories directly conflicted with the tribe's religious beliefs. The National Congress of American Indians (NCAI), the largest national organization of American Indian and Alaska Native tribal governments, and the Navajo Nation expressed their support for the Havasupai legal action. NCAI issued a resolution "support[ing] the effort of the Havasupai Indian Tribe to protect against unauthorized genetic research on its Members and other indigenous populations."[54]

A federal district court found that the Havasupai had asserted valid claims for intentional infliction of emotional distress, negligent infliction of emotional distress, civil rights violations, negligence, and gross negligence, but had not stated claims for an informed consent violation.[55] The federal court ruled against the tribe on its claim that its property had been taken fraudulently.[56] The plaintiffs then voluntarily dismissed the federal claims and are litigating the case in state court.

In negating even the simple protection of informed consent that the *Moore* court had recognized, the *Catalona* and *Havasupai* courts were responding in part to pressure from medical researchers who have both a professional and a financial stake in access to patients' tissue. Subsequently, however, the *Havasupai* case was settled.

In other health policy arenas, such as health care financing, the interests of patients as a group might conflict with that of individual patients. With respect to policy on tissue, however, the existing law is clear that the rights of patients as individuals should predominate. The idea that individuals can choose whether to participate in research—and cannot be conscripted to participate in research, no matter what the social benefits of participation—is a cornerstone of human research law and ethics. Research does go forward under just these conditions, which are embodied in the federal research regulations and university practice.[57]

Conflicts about the Commercialization of Patients' Tissue

Another set of conflicts has arisen in which patients have actually consented to the particular type of tissue research but not to the commercialization of their tissue. Much of the current focus of genetic research is on the identification—and subsequent patenting—of genes and segments of DNA that might be useful in diagnostic testing, gene therapy, and drug development. With a single gene patent potentially worth over a billion dollars a year to the patent holder, it is no wonder that companies are willing to pay sums such as $200 million for access to a bank of patients' tissue for research on particular disorders.[58] Yet gene patenting poses potential harms to the tissue source, the health care system, and the research enterprise. These problems are sufficiently troubling that the American Society of Human Genetics and the College of American Pathologists oppose gene patents as threatening medical advances and patient care.[59] Still, tissue sources are generally not informed in advance of any research about whether genes discovered in their tissues (or related products created based on this genetic information) will be patented, how the patent will be licensed, and what the impact of the patent is likely to be on health care and research.

The tenets of the informed consent doctrine require disclosure of all "material" information, yet the commercial implications of patenting are not disclosed.[60] Therefore, patients cannot make a reasoned decision about whether to participate in research. When a gene is discovered in a tissue sample and patented, the gene patent holder can charge whatever it wants for a diagnostic test for mutations in that gene (or any other use of the gene). The patent holder can prohibit anyone else from performing a diagnostic test for the gene, and instead require all doctors to send their patients' blood for testing to the patent holder's own lab, which may be in another state or even another country. In fact, the tissue source whose gene is patented could find that she cannot afford the test or treatment created with her own gene or that she cannot get access to a genetic diagnostic test for a family member because the patent holder is restricting who may perform the test.

In the future, people might want to get a scan of their whole genome, all twenty thousand genes. The technology to do so, already technically available, cannot be implemented due to the financial and practical limitations put in place by gene patent holders. Myriad Genetics, which holds the patent on the BRCA1 and BRCA2 genes, charges nearly three thousand dollars for the test of those genes. Multiply the per gene cost by the twenty thousand genes in a person's body and it is clear that a whole genome scan would be unaffordable if every gene was patented and access to it was priced in the Myriad way. Already, one in four laboratories has stopped performing certain genetic tests because of patent restrictions or excessive royalty costs. Half have not developed a test for fear of running afoul of patent law.[61]

Patients—along with nonprofit foundations funding research—have gone to court when tissue is commercialized without consent, such as in the Canavan case in which the gene mutation causing the Canavan gene was patented. In that case, the doctor and hospital argued that the patients and foundations couldn't be trusted to exert rights over commercial use of their tissue and genetic information. The hospital brief said that, if patients had the right to dictate whether their genes were patented, the patients might decide to charge a lot of money for the test. The hospital brief also asked: "What if one contributor decided that he did not want the Canavan test made available to gay or elderly people—could the contributor dictate that the test be made available only to people whose lifestyle he approved?"[62]

These are ludicrous scenarios. It is gene patent monopolies given to the research institutions that let the institutions decide to discriminate about who gets the test and how much to charge. If the gene had not been patented, anyone could have offered the test. Also, the suggestion that patients will behave in an avaricious way contradicted the facts in this case: the families were suing to allow free and low-cost testing, while the researcher and his institution were battling to *limit* access and charge high fees.

There is no evidence that patients would use their legal rights in a way that would be against the public interest, for example, auctioning off their tissues to the highest bidder or setting unaffordable costs for gene tests. In litigation, they have instead fought to use their power in pro-public ways. Institutions, companies, and researchers have sought to profit from genetics research, or have refused to share samples and information. Giving property rights to investigators or institutions instead of to research participants creates a very high likelihood that the power will be used in anti-public ways, since institutions are highly motivated by money.

There are other examples of patients' willingness and desire to allow their tissue samples to be used in research for the public good. When film producer Jonathan Shestack discovered that researchers were unwilling to voluntarily share samples from autistic children and their families because each wanted to be the first to find an autism gene and patent it, he founded the organization Cure Autism Now and began a national bank of tissue samples from children who have autism and their families. His DNA bank allows access to any researcher whose planned study has Institutional Review Board approval. Sharon Terry and her husband undertook an alternative approach, founding PXE International to help uncover the gene responsible for their children's rare congenital disease. The Terrys campaigned to raise funds for research, and Sharon Terry provided technical assistance with DNA analysis on the samples. When the PXE gene was discovered, the gene was patented, and Sharon Terry was named as a coinventor.[63] Terry is in favor of patients acquiring property rights in genes because it gives the patients the ability to "ensure that licenses for any resulting genetic tests will be inexpensive and widely available."[64] Essentially, the patients get to be the ones "driving the boat."[65]

A policy that lists patients as coinventors—although better than their having no rights in a patent—still is not optimal. The transaction costs of obtaining patents divert money from research efforts. Generally patent attorneys are hired to undertake the patent application process, which can be lengthy and expensive, and the U.S. Patent and Trademark Office charges filing and other fees. Researchers who want to use the patented information have to seek permission from the patent holder. This is why the Canavan patients did not want to fight for patients' rights to be listed on the patents but instead wanted a policy prohibiting gene patents entirely.

Proponents of gene patents argue that the patents enhance medical care. They also encourage people with genetic diseases to support gene patents because, they claim, it will make the development of diagnostics and cures more likely. On the contrary, gene patents interfere with medical care. Gene patents have impeded the development of diagnostics and cures and increase the cost of the diagnosis and treatment of genetic diseases. For twenty years, a gene patent holder controls *any* use of "its" gene. Researchers who want to study a gene must obtain a license or infringe the patent and risk treble damages. The patent holder can charge whatever it wants for any test analyzing the patented gene—even if that test uses technology that was not invented by the patent holder—as evidenced by the high cost of the test for the genes owned by Myriad. Plus, when a single entity controls all testing of a gene sequence, it might not provide the highest quality test or it might decide, for commercial reasons, not to offer testing for all the known mutations in the gene sequence.

The federal district court for the Southern District of Florida held that the patients in the Canavan case and their families had no property right to their tissue. The Florida district court did not give the Canavan patients even the protection that the California Supreme Court had provided John Moore. The court in the Canavan case held that the researchers did not have a duty to disclose to patients in advance that they would be commercializing the tissue. However, the court ruled they could maintain a cause of action for unjust enrichment because "the facts paint a picture of a continuing research collaboration that involved [patients] also investing time and significant resources in the race to isolate the Canavan gene."[66]

Our analysis of the court cases dealing with research on tissue shows that the sources of the tissue—the patients—have been sorely disadvantaged. If the cases had dealt with any other item, the existing law would have led to a finding for the patients. A straightforward application of property law, informed consent law, human research law, or even criminal law would have led to findings in favor of the patients. For example, if Missouri gift law had been correctly applied in the *Catalona* case, the patients would have won—since there is no precedent that suggests that someone has made a gift (in this case, to the university) when they retain the right to destroy the gift. However, because these cases dealt with an unfamiliar item—human tissue—the courts deprived the people from whom the tissue was removed of basic legal protections that would have applied in all other instances.

The Policy Implications of Recognizing Patients' Rights to Control What Is Done with Their Tissue

A policy that recognizes people's right to control research on their tissue makes not only good moral sense but also good practical sense. More people are willing to participate in research when they can choose the type of research in which their tissue is used and can stop participating if they wish to. In one survey, 82 percent of people queried indicated they would be willing to let their tissue be used in cancer research, whereas barely one quarter would allow their tissue to be used for cloning research.[67] In another study, which asked people about their willingness to participate in biomedical research, of those surveyed who had a close family member or friend with an illness, 58 percent were willing to participate in medical research studies. Only 39 percent of those who did not have a family member or friend with a serious illness were willing to participate in medical research studies. Even among people who said they would not participate in research, a significant number said they would change their mind if they had the disease being studied.[68] Since many types of research require tissue from people with the particular disease being studied, it makes sense to encourage people to provide their tissue for research that affects them and their families. We would not have had a breakthrough in AIDS treatment if AIDS patients had not been able to choose the type of research that was done on them and their tissue. We would not have learned about the devastating disorder sickle-cell anemia if African Americans had not been allowed to choose to provide their blood for research on that particular disease.

Our proposed legal scheme for human research echoes those the legal system has in place for other types of altruistic behavior. Courts assure that when a decedent has designated in a will which people and which causes will receive his property, those designations are honored. When a person donates money to a charity for a particular purpose, that money cannot be used by another charity or for another purpose. It does not matter that it would do more good for society if a decedent's estate or a gift to a charity were used for another purpose. We do not eliminate people's right to choose merely because people might make choices that conflict with other public policy goals.

Potential research subjects will be less willing to participate if they cannot control what their tissue is used for or if they do not trust the researcher or institution. Already, one university has had to return a major NIH grant because, based on how Arizona State University treated the Havasupai, the Tohono-O'odham Tribe withdrew from an NIH-funded study. Decades after the Tuskegee syphilis study ended, the effects of the researchers' malfeasance is still having a negative impact on African Americans' decisions about whether to participate in research.[69] In one study about their views of research protocols, some African American participants said that their distrust of researchers was linked to the Tuskegee syphilis study, and that patients should "expect dishonesty and nondisclosure of research risk from investigators."[70] A study conducted by the Institute of Medicine found that of people who have been asked to have their personal medical information used in research and decided *not* to participate, 22 percent declined because they did not trust the people or organization conducting the research.[71]

Through legal briefs using scare tactics to convince judges that the research enterprise might be impeded if people were given the right to control what was done with their tissue, research institutions are winning the legal battle. But they may ultimately lose the war—for without the participation of humans, there will be no human research.

Specific Policy Proposals

Despite the high stakes involved (the future of medical research, access to health care, and questions of self-determination), few patients or patient groups bring these issues to court. Some patients never learn that their tissue has been used or their genes patented without their consent. Other patients cannot find lawyers to help them assert their rights or cannot afford to pay for a legal battle. In many instances, patient organizations have conflicts of interest because they don't want to alienate researchers or upset the pharmaceutical and biotech groups that fund some patient groups. It is a rare patient group, such as the People's Medical Society, that does not accept funding from industry.

To address the failure of courts to protect research participants, certain policy changes should be made. Courts should enforce the federal research regulations and the state property laws. Courts should recognize an individual cause of action under the regulations to allow participants to sue researchers directly, rather than rely on NIH to enforce the regulations by withdrawing funding. In addition, the regulations should be clarified to assure that researchers and institutions are not the owners of tissue that people provide for use in research and that participants cannot be asked to give up their property rights in their tissue.

The federal regulations should also be amended to apply to all research, not just federally funded research. As is currently true, the federal regulations would still provide minimum standards for protections for research participants, and states could enact provisions that would further protect people within their borders.

Patient groups should ensure that they truly advocate for patients instead of becoming bedfellows with the research enterprise or putting other interests above individual patient rights. Research is not about weighing interests to determine whether people must participate or not. If it were, we would not need informed consent; researchers could just take whatever they want without permission. But in research, people have the right to make individual decisions; we do not assume it is better for the public for everyone to participate in research and thus make them participate without their consent. This is intuitive in certain research situations: if someone decides to drop out of a pharmaceutical trial, we do not force them to continue to ingest the drug, even if arguably it would be better for the results of the trial to keep the number of participants consistent throughout the trial. But when it comes to research on people's tissue, this right to participate or not participate has been ignored by researchers, institutions, the government, and now the courts. This must change.

Patient groups should provide advice to potential subjects about what questions to ask before participating in research, including: What is the scope of the research? What types of research collaborations have the investigator and institution entered into and with whom? Will the subjects be notified if the researcher or institution enters into a research collaboration with industry subsequent to their decision to participate? If the research is genetics research, will the institution be patenting the genes discovered or other biological information? Will the samples and information be shared with other researchers, institutions, or biotech companies or used in secondary research? What happens to subjects' tissue if subjects change their mind? Who owns the tissue subjects provide?

Patient groups should further tell patients that they have the right to decline to participate in research and, if they so desire, can inform the researcher of the reason they are not participating (for example, "I do not want genetic information patented and will not participate in a study that will have this result" or "I do not agree to the sharing of my tissue or other information, even if my name has been removed from the sample"). Patients should be told that if they do agree to participate in research, they have the option of revising informed consent forms before they sign them, for example, crossing off sections they do not agree with or explicitly stating that their tissue may not be shared with other researchers.

Researchers and institutions should be required to disclose conflicts of interest, even conflicts that arise after the research begins, and should provide information about what they intend to do with research results. If they are hunting for a gene and intend to patent it, they should tell patients that the researcher and institution stand to profit from the discovery; that the patent will raise the price of genetic testing for the disease and will limit the availability of the test; and that intellectual property and other commercial interests have been documented to interfere with research into new therapeutics and diagnostics, and with the sharing of data and results.

In the past, physicians paternalistically made decisions for patients. Now this has changed. The same change is needed with respect to the relationship between researchers and research subjects.

The joint efforts of researchers and research participants led, in the AIDS and breast cancer contexts, to greater funding for research and laws protecting people from discrimination. When it becomes clear that not only money but also trust is key to successful biomedical research, perhaps researchers and participants will be able to join together again to create appropriate guidelines.

Notes

1. Gina Kolata, "Sharing of Profits Is Debated as the Value of Tissue Rises," *New York Times*, May 15, 2000.
2. Lars Noah, "Pigeonholing Illness: Medical Diagnosis as a Legal Construct," *Hastings Law Journal* 50 (1999): 291; Michael D. Greenberg, "AIDS, Experimental Drug Approval, and the FDA New Drug Screening Process," *New York University Journal of Legislation and Public Policy* 3 (2000): 296–297; Ziyad Hopkins, "'HIV' Testing Statutes: A Clash between Common Law and Public Health," *Northeastern University Forum* 2, (1997): 102–103; Sheila Taub, "Doctors, AIDS, and Confidentiality in the 1990s," *John Marshall Law Review* 27 (1994): 331.
3. On increased research funding, see Denise S. Wolf, "Who Should Pay for 'Experimental' Treatments? Breast Cancer Patients v. Their Insurers," *American University Law Review* 44 (1995): 2031–2032; on state laws, see, e.g., the efforts of the Breast Cancer Coalition and also Kathy L. Hudson, Karen H. Rothenberg, Lori B. Andrews, Mary Jo Ellis Kahn, and Francis S. Collins, "Genetic Discrimination and Health Insurance: An Urgent Need for Reform," 270 *Science* 270 (October 20, 1995): 391.
4. Lori Andrews, *Future Perfect: Confronting Decisions about Genetics* (New York: Columbia University Press, 2001).
5. H. K. Beecher, "Ethics and Clinical Research," 274 *New England Journal of Medicine* 274 (1966): 1354–1360.
6. *Trials of War Criminals before the Nuremberg Military Tribunals under Control Council Law No. 10* (Washington, D.C.: U.S. Government Printing Office, 1949), 2: 181–182.
7. "Basic HHS Policy for Protection of Human Subjects," 45 C.F.R. §§ 46.101(b)(4), 46.116.
8. Ibid., 45 C.F.R. § 46.116(a)(8).
9. Ibid., 45 C.F.R. § 46.101–46.409.
10. C. MacKay and G. S. Schatz, "The Unfinished Research Agenda," presentation to the National Institutes of Health Inter-Institute Bioethics Internet Group, June 7, 2004. This presentation led the secretary of health and human services to release a new guidance: Tommy G. Thompson, "Financial Relationships and Interests in Research Involving Human Subjects: Guidance for Human Subject Protection," Department of Health and Human Services, May 5, 2004, http://www.hhs.gov/ohrp/humansubjects/finreltn/fguid.pdf.
11. Until the 1980s, if a university or federal researcher discovered or invented something using federal funds, that advance belonged to the public. The researchers could not personally profit. But with the passage of the Bayh-Dole Act and the Stevenson-Wydler Act in 1980, and the Federal Technology Transfer Act in 1986, the rules changed completely.

    These legal measures were enacted to encourage the commercial development of government-funded research. The Bayh-Dole Act allows universities and nonprofit institutions to apply for patents on federally funded inventions and discoveries and provides significant tax incentives to companies that invest in academic research.

35 U.S.C. § 200–211 (2004). The Technology Transfer Act allows researchers in government facilities, including scientists at the National Institute of Health, to patent their inventions and keep up to $150,000 of the yearly royalties on top of their government salaries. 15 U.S.C. § 3710c (a) (3) (2004). The law also allows government researchers to enter into commercial arrangements (known as CRADAs—cooperation research and development agreements) with for-profit companies. 15 U.S.C. § 3701–3714 (2004).

Overnight, behavior that would have sent federally funded university researchers to the penitentiary in the 1960s and 1970s—personally profiting from research done at taxpayers' expense—was not just legal but encouraged. Leonard Hayflick, "Novel Techniques for Transforming the Theft of Mortal Human Cells into Praiseworthy Federal Policy," *Experimental Gerontology* 33 (1998): 204. Largely as a result of these legal changes, NIH patent applications increased nearly 300 percent. Sheldon Krimsky, "The Profit of Scientific Discovery and Its Normative Implications," *Chicago-Kent Law Review* 75 (1999): 22. But not all political leaders were convinced the law was a wise move. Then-congressman Al Gore argued that the arrangement was akin to "selling the tree of knowledge to Wall Street." Seth Shulman, *Owning the Future* (New York: Houghton Mifflin Company, 1999), 114.

12. Lori Andrews and Dorothy Nelkin, *Body Bazaar: The Market for Human Tissue in the Biotechnology Age* (New York: Crown Publishers, 2001), 34 (statement of Dr. Robert Murray).

13. Lori Andrews, "Body Science," *American Bar Association Journal* 13 (1997): 47.

14. Lori Andrews, *Future Perfect: Confronting Decisions about Genetics* (New York: Columbia University Press, 2001), 132.

15. Karen Honey, "GINA: Making it Safe to Know What Is in Your Genes," *Journal of Clinical Investigation* 118 (July 2008): 2369; Genetic Information Nondiscrimination Act of 2008, Public Law 110–233 (May 21, 2008).

16. Genetic Information Nondiscrimination, 42 U.S.C. §§ 2000ff—2000ff-1.

17. Ibid., 42 U.S.C. §§ 2000ff-1.

18. U.S. Dept. of Health and Human Services, Office for Human Research Protections, *Protecting Human Research Subjects: Institutional Review Board Guidebook*, chap. 5, "Biomedical and Behavioral Research: An Overview," sec. H, "Human Genetic Research," http://www.hhs.gov/ohrp/irb/irb_chapter5.htm.

19. Australian Associated Press, "'Warrior Gene' Blamed for Maori Violence," August 8, 2006, http://news.ninemsn.com.au/article.aspx?id=120718.

20. Jewish tradition maintains that as human beings were created in the image of God, in death the body should retain the unity of that image. Maurice Lamm, *The Jewish Way in Death and Mourning* (New York: Jonathan David, 1969), 10. If parts are removed, they must be returned and buried with the body. *Kohn v. United States*, 591 F. Supp. 568 (E.D.N.Y. 1984), citing Fred Rosner, "Autopsy in Jewish Law and the Israeli Autopsy Controversy," in *Jewish Bioethics*, ed. Fred Rosner and J. David Bleich (New York: Hebrew Publications, 1979), 332. Court cases have recognized that a patient's religious beliefs should be taken into consideration in determining proper handling of their bodies. See, e.g., *Lott v. State of New York*, 225 N.Y.S.2d 434 (Ct. Cl. 1962).

21. Henry Fitzgerald Jr., "Woman Awarded $1.25 Million in Suit; Funeral Home Must Compensate for Losing Mother's Amputated Legs," *Fort Lauderdale Sun-Sentinel*, May 16, 1997; this article also reported that when Menorah Gardens and Funeral Chapels lost the amputated leg of an Orthodox Jewish woman, it settled a lawsuit

by her daughter for $1.25 million. "Orthodox Jews believe that at the end of time, not only will a person's soul be resurrected, but the body as well. . . . It's important that the whole body, including blood, be buried" (ibid.). See also S. LaFee, "Einstein's Mind: His Brain Sits on a Shelf, Largely Unsought by the World," *San Diego Union-Tribune*, May 17, 1995.

22. Southern Baptist Convention, "Resolution on the Patenting of Animal and Human Genes," June 1995, http://www.sbc.net/resolutions/amResolution.asp?ID=570.

23. If a drug or device will be marketed, the FDA regulation will apply at some point. If the result of research is a genetic test, however, no FDA approval is necessary.

24. Hamilton Moses, E. Ray Dorsey, David H. M. Matheson, and Samuel O. Thier, "Financial Anatomy of Biomedical Research," *JAMA* 294 (2005): 1333–1342.

25. Harriet A. Washington, "Henrietta Lacks—An Unsung Hero," *Emerge* 24 (October 1994): 29. See also Harriet A. Washington, *Medical Apartheid* (New York: Doubleday, 2007); Rebecca Skloot, *The Immortal Life of Henrietta Lacks* (New York: Crown, 2010).

26. Golde also patented nine products made from the cell line. *Moore v. Regents of the University of California*, 249 Cal. Rptr. 494, 501 (1988).

27. Lori Andrews and Dorothy Nelkin, *Body Bazaar: The Market for Human Tissue in the Biotechnology Age* (New York: Crown, 2001), 28.

28. *Moore*, 249 Cal. Rptr. 494, 505, 508–509 (Cal. App. 2d Dist. 1988).

29. *Moore v. Regents of the University of California*, 793 P.2d 479, 493 (Cal. 1990).

30. *Moore*, 793 P.2d 479, 51 Cal. 3d 120, 160 (Cal. 1990) (Broussard, J. concurring in part, dissenting in part).

31. *Moore*, 793 P.2d 479 (Cal. 1990) (Mosk, J. dissenting).

32. Ibid., 490.

33. Ibid.

34. Ibid., 493.

35. *Hecht v. Superior Court of Los Angeles County*, 16 Cal. App. 4th 836, 846 n.4 (Cal. Ct. App. 1993).

36. *York v. Jones*, 717 F. Supp. 421, 426 (E.D. Va. 1989) (finding that a couple can have a property interest in their pre-zygote that limits a clinic's rights as bailee); *Hecht*, 850 (holding that sperm is property to be distributed by decedent's estate); *Whaley v. County of Tuscola*, 58 F. 3d 1111 (6th Cir. 1991) (next of kin have a "constitutionally protected property interest in the dead boy of a relative").

37. 1998 U.S. Dist. LEXIS 10307, at *16. In contrast, the state law precedent in Florida that was applied in the Greenberg case was *State v. Powell*, 497 So. 2d 1188 (Fla. 1986), in which "the Florida Supreme Court refused to recognize a property right in the body of another after death." *Greenberg v. Miami Children's Hospital Research Institute, Inc.*, 264 F. Supp. 2d 1064, 1075 (S.D. Fla. 2003).

38. Fla. Stat. Ann. § 760.40.

39. American Society of Human Genetics, "Statement on Informed Consent for Genetic Research," *American Journal of Human Genetics* 59 (1996): 471–474.

40. American Medical Association, "Code of Medical Ethics, Opinion 2.08, Commercial Use of Human Tissue," http://www.ama-assn.org/ama1/pub/upload/mm/Code_of _Med_Eth/opinion/opinion208.html.

41. Committee on Human Genome Diversity, Commission on Life Sciences, National Research Council, *Evaluating Human Genetic Diversity* (National Academy Press, 1997), 65.

42. Complaint at para. 14 and para. 53.

43. Testimony of Mr. James Ellis, *Washington Univ. v. Catalona*, Tr. 1:168–69 (April 11, 2005).
44. Testimony of Dr. Ellen Wright Clayton, Transcript vol. 1 at 122.
45. Andrews and Nelkin, *Body Bazaar* (some universities and hospitals sell access to patient's tissue to biotech companies).
46. Brief of Amicus Curiae AAMC Regarding the Legal Status and Use of Donated Biological Materials, *Washington University v. Catalona*, No. 03 CV 1065 (E.D. Mo. Apr. 6, 2005) at 6.
47. *Washington University v. Catalona*, 437 F. Supp. 2d 985, 1002 (E.D. Mo. 2006).
48. Ibid., 998.
49. Amici Curiae AAMC et al. in Support of Plaintiff-Appellee, *Washington University v. Catalona*, Nos. 06–2286 & 06–2301 (8th Cir. Aug. 31, 2006) at 7.
50. Brief for Amicus Curiae the American Cancer Society in Support of Plaintiff-Appellee and Affirmance, *Washington University v. Catalona*, Nos. 06–2286 & 06–2301 (8th Cir. Sept. 5, 2006) at 3.
51. Rayna Rapp, "Refusing Prenatal Diagnosis: The Uneven Meaning of Bioscience in a Multicultural World," *Science, Technology, and Human Values* 23 (1998): 45.
52. *Washington University v. Catalona*, 490 F.3d 667, 674–675 (8th Cir. 2007).
53. Ibid., 675.
54. National Congress of American Indians Resolution, "Supporting the Havasupai Indian Tribe in Their Claim against the Arizona Board of Regents Regarding the Unauthorized Use of Blood Samples and Research," National Congress of American Indians, October 1–6, 2006, http://www.ncai.org/ncai/resolutions/doc/SAC-06–019.pdf; Beverly Becenti-Pigman, Chairman Health and Human Resources Review Board: The Navajo Tribe, to Milton D. Glick, Executive Vice President and Provost at Arizona State University, March 21, 2006, author files; National Congress of American Indians Resolution, "Supporting the Havasupai Indian Tribe."
55. *Tilousi v. Arizona State University Board of Regents*, No. 04-CV-1290-PCT-FJM (Dist. Ariz. Mar. 3, 2005) (order denying in part and granting in part motion to dismiss).
56. Memorandum Opinion at 9–10, *Tilousi v. Arizona State University Board of Regents*, 3:04-CV-1290 (March 2, 2005). The court stated: "Despite plaintiffs' voluntary donation of the blood samples, which suggests plaintiffs had no right to immediate possession of the blood, plaintiffs claim defendants committed conversion by intentionally 'obtaining possession of a chattel from another by fraud or duress.'" However, the court held that since the plaintiffs failed to plead fraud with specificity, the count was dismissed.
57. The National Cancer Institute has emphasized the custodial nature of the institution's relationship to tissue samples, as opposed to a relationship characterized by ownership. National Cancer Institute, "Best Practices for Biospecimen Resources," June 2007, at C.1, http://www.allirelandnci.com/pdf/NCI_Best_Practices_060507 .pdf. The definition provided for "custodianship," is "the caretaking responsibility for a biospecimen collection, including management and documentation, as well as right to determine the conditions under which biospecimens are accessed and used." National Cancer Institute, "Best Practices," 33.

   Major research institutions such as Stanford University follow the federal research regulations and the OHRP's guidance, prohibiting informed consent document language that waives research participants' property rights in their tissue. Stanford University, "IRB Guidance: Basic Research Consent Requirements," http://humansubjects.stanford.edu/research/documents/ConsentGuidance.doc;

University of Nevada, Las Vegas, Office for the Protection of Research Subjects, http://www.unlv.edu/Research/OPRS/consent-exculpatory-language.htm; Illinois State University, http://www.rsp.ilstu.edu/research/exculpatory.shtml. That the entities that undertake the most cancer research in the country recognize that they cannot own patients' tissue brings into question researchers' admonition that recognizing patients' ownership rights in tissue will sound the death knell for research.

58. On the value of a gene patent, see S. M. Thomas et al., "Ownership of the Human Genome," *Nature* 380 (1996): 387–388; on the worth of access to a tissue bank, see R. Kunzig, "Blood of the Vikings," *Discover* 19 (1998): 90–99.

59. See College of American Pathologists, "Statement to the U.S. House of Representatives Subcommittee on the Internet and Intellectual Property, Hearing on 'Stifling or Stimulating—The Role of Gene Patents in Research and Genetic Testing,'" October 30, 2007, http://www.cap.org/apps/docs/advocacy/testimony/testimony_house _gene_patents.pdf.

60. *Grimes v. Kennedy Krieger Inst., Inc.*, 782 A.2d 807, 844 (Md. 2001).

61. Mildred K. Cho, Samantha Illangasekare, Meredith A. Weaver, Debra G. B. Leonard, and Jon F. Merz, "Effects of Patents and Licenses on the Provision of Clinical Genetic Testing Services," *Journal of Molecular Diagnostics* 5 (2003): 3.

62. Defendants Children's Hospital's Motion to Dismiss the Complaint, *Greenberg v. Miami Children's Hospital Research Institute, Inc.*, No. 00 C 6779 (E.D. Ill., Feb. 8, 2001).

63. Eliot Marshall, "Patient Advocate Named Co-Inventor on Patent for the PXE Disease Gene," *Science*, August 27, 2004, 1226.

64. Paul Smaglik, "Tissue Donors Use Their Influence in Deal over Gene Patent Terms," *Nature*, October 19, 2000, 821.

65. Marshall, "Patient Advocate Named Co-Inventor."

66. *Greenberg v. Miami Children's Hospital Research Institute, Inc.*, 264 F. Supp. 2d 1064, 1073–74 (S.D. Fla. 2003).

67. M. L. Goodson and B. G. Vernon, "A Study of Public Opinion on the Use of Tissue Samples from Living Subjects for Clinical Research," 57 *Journal of Clinical Pathology* 57 (2004): 136.

68. Jeanette M. Trauth, Donald Musa, Laura Siminoff, Ilene Katz Jewell, and Edmund Ricci, "Public Attitudes Regarding Willingness to Participate in Medical Research Studies," *Journal of Health & Social Policy* 12 (2000): 31–32.

69. Vicki S. Freimuth, "African Americans' Views on Research and the Tuskegee Syphilis Study," *Social Science and Medicine* 52 (2001): 797; Giselle Corbie-Smith, Stephen B. Thomas, Mark V. Williams, and Sandra Moody-Ayers, "Attitudes and Beliefs of African Americans toward Participation in Medical Research," *Journal of General Internal Medicine* 14 (1999): 541.

70. Corbie-Smith et al., "Attitudes and Beliefs of African Americans."

71. Har is Interactive Polls, "IOM Privacy and Research Studies for Dr. Alan F. Westin," September 11–18, 2007, 2, www.hca.wa.gov/hit/documents/westiniomsrvyreport 1107.doc.

Part II

From Individual to Collective

In the 1960s and 1970s, patient perspectives began to emerge as a more formative influence on U.S. health policy. The rise of social movements and demands for self-determination by formerly powerless groups created fertile ground for activism by patients and health care consumers. Greater attention to patient perspectives was also in part a consequence of emerging public policies explicitly intended to enhance the voice of individual patients, such as state-mandated grievance mechanisms for health insurance and the emergence of patient advocates as legitimate professionals within U.S. medicine. Also, new public policies and programs such as Medicare and Medicaid, though not intended to influence or amplify patient voice per se, nonetheless galvanized collective mobilization among patients and those intimately involved in their care.

The chapters in part 2 consider the ways in which patients have begun to have greater influence on policy by acting and speaking more directly and deliberately in the public sphere. The authors raise questions about how individual and collective identities can shape patients' roles as policy actors and suggest the many ways that aggregating patient voices can constitute a collective action. The first pair of chapters explores the impact of historical policy and social contexts on the collective mobilization of patient interests. The second pair addresses the challenges of translating individual patient grievances into effective system change in health insurance coverage and the possibilities for bringing together disparate measures of patient-consumer satisfaction to improve health care for all.

Collective Identity, Mobilization, and Representation

Over the past quarter century, collective action by patients and their allies has successfully altered health policy in a number of countries. These efforts often fall short of the groups' own aspirations. Nonetheless, they can effectively galvanize patient participation even within groups that are economically disadvantaged or heavily stigmatized by their medical diagnoses.

Public programs often provide a springboard over such hurdles. When a program targets the health needs of a distinct group, it facilitates mobilization in two ways. First it provides members of the target group with a shared identity as program recipients, along with certain legal rights to express their collective concerns to program administrators.[1] Second, by creating new funding streams, these programs raise the stakes for organizations providing health services, which can then advocate for their patients' collective interests (or at least for their interpretations of those interests).[2] Even the most favorable programmatic contexts, however, do not guarantee sustained, effective mobilization of patient interests. In some cases, patient needs, preferences, and experiences may be so diverse that a shared program proves insufficient grounds for collective identification. In other cases, effective representation may be displaced by a form of patient tokenism—the appointment of patients to advisory positions that lack any real influence over policy choices, or individual patients being asked to represent the interests of a larger group though they lack the resources, wherewithal, or information-gathering skills necessary to fulfill these expectations.

The two chapters that open this section explore the process of initial engagement by patients and their advocates with the infrastructure of health care and health policy making. Mental health patients were among the first to publicly question their treatment and demand a role in their own care. Their achievement—adding patient voices to the mental health system—is the focus of historian Nancy Tomes's essay, in which she argues that this movement's success is closely connected to its timing and historical policy context. Beatrix Hoffman's chapter considers, also from a historian's perspective, how the National Welfare Rights Organization in the 1970s worked to add the voices of poor women of color to health care policy making. When they acted collectively for a brief time, the poorest Americans had some success making themselves heard. Yet without powerful allies, greater resources, or a long-term organizational strategy, their voice and influence could not be sustained.

The Systemic Impact of Individual Initiative

For reasons explored in the first section of this volume, even when patients have become empowered consumers, that orientation often does not extend to collective identification and mobilization. Yet this reality does not necessarily obviate patients' role as policy actors. Even patients who do not intend to embark on collective action may influence the health care system and the policies that guide it.

Indeed, over the past fifteen years in the United States and abroad, public officials have begun to mine data on the behavior and attitudes of individual medical consumers to extract policy-relevant patterns. One early example used disenrollment rates from health plans as a way of identifying poorly performing plans.[3] Though this strategy proved disappointing in its impact—it was difficult for consumers perusing disenrollment data to discern why people were switching away from certain health plans—its widespread adoption clearly illustrates how patients' actions can be harnessed to create systemic interventions even when consumers act without intent beyond their personal needs and interests.

A broader array of U.S. policy innovations dating back as far as the 1970s sought to use patients' voicing of grievances regarding their own health care as a guide to identifying health system shortcomings. The earliest of these initiatives was the long-term care ombudsman program. Beginning in 1972, states were required to establish an ombudsman office charged with identifying consistent patterns of problems with long-term care facilities that affected multiple people and required systemic remediation.[4] Although some subsequent initiatives targeted similarly specified patient populations, it was not until the 1990s that policy makers in the United States and abroad strove to harness the voiced experiences of the average patient, primarily through attempts to accumulate information on grievances against clinicians and insurers.[5]

There has been, to date, only limited assessment of these efforts to interpret patterns of patient voice for policy purposes.[6] Most crucially, there has been no attention paid to the consequences of *using* patients' perspectives in the absence of a more concerted effort to encourage their own awareness of the collective implications of their voice. Connections between individual and collective action merit investigation, and the final two chapters in this section do just that.

Mark Schlesinger, a political economist, explores the policy relevance of patient voice in his discussion of individual consumer complaints and how they are aggregated. Using new data about consumers' health care experiences and their willingness and ability to complain about or praise that care, this chapter identifies the limitations in existing policy efforts to harvest meaning from individual patient voice, and contemplates what policies and mechanisms could best contribute to the creation of a "robust, representative public voice" for consumers.

Legal scholar Marc Rodwin focuses on a more specific set of public policies regarding grievances against managed care plans, considering whether and how consumers can exert a more sustained influence on private health insurance companies' practices. He argues that the backlash against HMOs in the 1990s represented a lost opportunity to enhance patients' power. Collective demands for redress when patients were denied treatments by their insurance companies were absorbed into an individualistic grievance system, which allowed outside review of individual cases but provided no mechanism for systemic change. This story is an example of potentially collective disputes being translated into individual ones, thus muting or even eliminating a potentially consequential policy-induced change.

Notes

1. Andrea Campbell, "Participatory Reactions to Policy Threats: Senior Citizens and the Defense of Social Security and Medicare," *Political Behavior* 25, 1 (2003): 29–50.
2. Colleen Grogan and Michael Gusmano, *Healthy Voices, Unhealthy Silence: Advocacy and Health Policy for the Poor* (Washington, D.C.: Georgetown University Press, 2007).
3. M. Schlesinger, B. Druss, and T. Thomas, "No Exit? The Effect of Health Status on Dissatisfaction and Disenrollment from Health Plans," *Health Services Research* 34, 2 (1999): 547–776.
4. C. Estes, D. Zulman, S. Goldberg, and D. Ogawa, "State Long Term Care Ombudsman Programs: Factors Associated with Perceived Effectiveness" *Gerontologist* 44, 1 (2004): 104–115.
5. R. Cauchi, "Making the Best of Managed Care: State Ombudsman, Report Card, and Profile Programs Aim to Aid Those Frustrated by HMOs," *State Legislatures* 27, 6 (2001): 22–24.
6. J. Gulland, "Second-Tier Review of Complaints in Health and Social Care," *Health and Social Care in the Community* 14, 3 (2006): 206–214; Estes et al., "State Long Term Care Ombudsman Programs."

From Outsiders to Insiders

The Consumer-Survivor Movement and Its Impact on U.S. Mental Health Policy

This chapter represents an attempt to think more systematically and critically about the "patient factor" in policy making by focusing on a particularly important example of change: the impact of the patient empowerment movement on the mental health field. Since the 1970s, so-called consumer-survivors have gained new visibility as expert patients whose voices matter in policy decision making. Although breast cancer and AIDS activism are better known examples of powerful advocacy, the consumer-survivor movement has arguably had as great a policy influence.

At first glance, this influence seems hard to explain. People with severe mental disorders hardly conform to the definition of a powerful interest group: they suffer from a highly stigmatized disability, often have critical views of health care professionals who might otherwise be their allies, and depend on a fragile network of social services in order to maintain their independence. Yet despite these disadvantages, consumer-survivors have played a key role in spearheading the therapeutic emphasis on recovery and rehabilitation now dominant in the mental health field. Today, for example, consumer-survivors sit on state mental health councils, work for mental health agencies, and serve on treatment policy committees.[1]

By taking an explicitly historical approach to the subject, this chapter shows how consumer-survivor groups benefited from important trends that originated outside the mental health field, including the consumer health revolution and the disability rights movement. I also relate their growing influence to the travails of institutional psychiatry and public mental health policy over the past half century. Consumer-survivor advocates emerged in the

aftermath of deinstitutionalization, an example of disastrous policy implementation that placed a premium on low-cost fixes to a system in crisis. In the
midst of this brutal downsizing, patient voices gained a hearing that in more
prosperous, settled times had been denied them.

The history of the consumer-survivor movement suggests a more general
model for explaining the ebb and flow of the "patient factor" in health care
policy as an interaction between therapeutic and economic imperatives. To be
sure, such generalizing has to be done carefully. The extent of downsizing in
institutional psychiatry has few counterparts in the history of U.S. health care.
But this case study provides some insight into the seeming paradox that serious efforts at cost containment often require greater attention to patient concerns
and priorities.

In what follows, I use the term "consumer-survivor" to describe my subjects,
fully aware that it carries a heavy load of historical baggage. Changing views
of health care rights have prompted many attempts to replace the word
"patient" with a better term to describe that role. In the mental health field,
this quest has been a particularly long and painful one. Trying to alleviate the
stigma associated with madness, nineteenth-century reformers replaced the
term "lunatic" with "insanity"; a generation later, for the same reasons, "insanity" was replaced by "mental illness." More recently, the term "biologically
based mental illness" has emerged as part of an effort to break down what
advocates see as an invalid and harmful distinction between mental and physical disease. Starting with the upheavals of the 1960s, activists rejected the
term "patient," which they felt was irredeemably tainted with medical paternalism, and tried out terms such as "survivor," "consumer," and "client."
Ideological battles over terminology continue to this day, for reasons I explore
in this chapter. Meanwhile, most people served by the mental health specialty
sector still refer to themselves as "patients" rather than as "consumers" or
"survivors." Nonetheless, the term "consumer-survivor" has gained wide usage
in the mental health field, so I have chosen to use it here.[2]

The Origins of the Modern Consumer-Survivor Movement

The consumer-survivor movement in mental health emerged as part of a larger
questioning of medical authority in the 1960s. Its genesis reflects the convergence of two traditions until then largely separate: the legal tradition of protecting patients' constitutional rights, and the economic tradition of protecting
their consumer, or market-based, rights. During the turbulent 1960s, these two
traditions fused into a new kind of patient empowerment, characterized by an
overt rejection of medical paternalism, an assertion of self-determination, and

a critique of limiting stereotypes. The consumer-survivor movement, along with women's health and disability rights activism, represented the extreme edge of what became a broader, more moderate kind of health consumerism in the 1970s.

That the mental health field would produce one of the earliest and most radical of the angry patient movements should come as no surprise. As Howard Brody noted in a 1985 account of the new mental health consumerism, psychiatry is the medical specialty charged with "identifying and classifying people whose behavior leads others to suspect their mental competence and capacity for autonomous action," and on the basis of that classification, "recommending their removal from free civil life to confinement in special institutions." From its inception in the mid-1800s, the modern mental hospital has generated criticism for precisely those reasons. Among its first critics were Elizabeth Packard, an Illinois housewife who in the 1870s pressed for asylum reform after what she felt was her wrongful confinement, and Clifford Beers, a Connecticut businessman who in the early 1900s protested against the abuses he encountered while a patient in several hospitals. Both Packard and Beers are frequently referred to as forerunners of the modern consumer-survivor movement.[3]

The mental hospital's record as an extremely expensive and often ineffective form of treatment led to a "cyclical pattern of reform and retrenchment, of hope and despair," as Joseph P. Morrissey, Howard H. Goldman, and Lorraine V. Klerman have termed it, which reached a new pitch of intensity in the post–World War II period. Revelations about patient abuse in state mental hospitals, dramatized in Hollywood films such as *The Snake Pit*, coupled with new currents in therapeutic reform, set the stage for a radical restructuring of the U.S. mental health system, starting with the 1955 Mental Health Study Act. As new antipsychotic drugs became available, alternatives to prolonged hospitalization seemed more feasible. The premise that patients would be better cared for in the community, under less restrictive conditions, gained popularity both as a therapeutic and an economic resolution of the seemingly intractable problems of institutional psychiatry. Widening legal conceptions of patients' rights and the intellectual critiques associated with the antipsychiatry movement also contributed to the growing enthusiasm in the 1950s and 1960s for the policy that came to be called "deinstitutionalization."[4]

The rise of the community health center, the legal rethinking of institutional commitment, and the critique of psychiatric authority all contributed to the rise of the consumer-survivor movement. But although those developments profoundly affected the status of people with serious mental disorders, they were largely expert-driven shifts, spearheaded by psychiatrists, lawyers, and academics, rather than by ex-patients. For example, while founded by the ex-patient Clifford Beers, the National Mental Health Association, the main advocacy organization in the field, had long been dominated by its professional constituencies. Likewise, people with severe mental illnesses played no direct role in the passage of the landmark Community Mental Health Centers Act of 1964 or in the early debates over commitment law. In sum, until the 1960s, mental patients figured primarily as objects rather than agents of policy making.[5]

The Mental Patients' Liberation Movement

In 1970, the claim to have special expert knowledge of mental disease by having experienced it was a novel one. It was on precisely these grounds that ex-patients, as individuals and in groups, began to assert a new entitlement to speak on their own behalf. What its founders christened the "mental patients' liberation movement" was strikingly different from earlier efforts to speak on behalf of mental patients, in that it was militantly antimedical in orientation, fiercely committed to operating outside the mental health establishment, and critical of accommodationist attitudes among fellow patient activists.[6]

Movement historians usually cite the Oregon Insane Liberation Front, founded in late 1969 or early 1970, as the first rights group run by consumer-survivors. Other groups soon followed in New York, Boston, and San Francisco. With the founding in 1972 of the newsletter *Madness Network News*, the sense of a broader movement with common goals began to develop. This early survivor movement bore the imprint of 1960s radicalism. As an early participant recalled, its leaders "dressed like hippies and talked like militants."[7]

The movement drew heavily on the intellectual traditions of antipsychiatry, particularly the works of R. D. Laing and Thomas Szasz. In their speeches and writings, ex-patient activists portrayed madness not as an illness but as an alternate state of being that challenged the sane community, much as feminism frightened male chauvinists and gay rights offended homophobes. Inspired by other liberation movements of the era, they celebrated "mad pride." The route to wholeness, movement leaders suggested, lay in accepting the mad person's unique perspective and changing society so that their differences could be accepted rather than used as grounds for involuntary confinement and repressive treatment regimes. While indebted to antipsychiatry theorists such as Laing and Szasz, activists had no hesitation in asserting the superiority of their own opinions, on the grounds that they had the ultimate insiders' understanding of what it meant to be mad.[8]

The 1970s survivor movement aimed not at influencing the mental health system, but at developing a viable alternative to it. That spirit is well illustrated in Judi Chamberlin's landmark 1978 book, *On Our Own: Patient-Controlled Alternatives to the Mental Health System*, often referred to as the bible of the new empowerment philosophy. The core principle of the "mental patients' liberation movement," as Chamberlin termed it, was the issue of power in the therapeutic relationship: the right of patients and ex-patients to get the help they needed without giving up their basic human rights to self-determination. "Many ex-patients are angry," she wrote, because of the "neglect, indifference, dehumanization, and outright brutality we have seen and experienced at the hands of the mental health system." This "distrust of professionals" she continued, "is not irrational hostility, but is the direct result of their treatment of us in the past."[9]

The key to improving the mental health system, Chamberlin argued in her book, was giving patients control over their therapeutic fates. Unlike the orthodox mental health system, which fostered patient compliance through their taking medication and conforming to hospital regimen, consumer-survivor-run groups stressed measures designed to lead to recovery, that is, being able to live fully and independently. Participation was voluntary; the clients chose the providers of service, and those providers often included other ex-patients. Most importantly, clients shared in deciding all aspects of the organization's operation.

Chamberlin's book helped galvanize the creation of consumer-survivor groups, both in the United States and elsewhere. Their number increased dramatically during the 1980s: in the late 1980s, sociologist Robert E. Emerick found over a hundred self-help groups for consumer-survivors in existence. Most of those groups shared Chamberlin's core assumptions: that consumers needed to take charge of their own care, that consumer-run self-help programs were essential to their well-being, and that the goal of treatment was a broadly conceived state of recovery rather than a more medically defined cure.[10] At the same time, consumer-survivor groups differed greatly in their conception of advocacy. Emerick found that about 60 percent of the groups he surveyed took what he termed an outer-focused "social movement" approach, compared to 40 percent with a more conservative, inner-focused, or "individual therapy" approach. (Examples of the latter include Recovery, Inc. and Emotions Anonymous.) Advocacy groups (the main focus in this chapter) also differed in their stance toward separatism, that is, the necessity to exclude mental health professionals and other non-consumer-survivors from their groups. Along the same lines, they disagreed over the degree to which they rejected the medical model of mental disease and the value of its therapeutic modalities. Finally, groups differed over whether consumers should be paid for their work with

the early 1970s. Consumer-survivor perspectives were closely associated with the antipsychiatry critiques of Thomas Szasz, described by one contemporary as "a barbed thorn in [the psychiatric profession's] flesh."[15]

Yet larger changes were at work that gradually created more receptivity to consumer-survivor perspectives. On the one hand, research into the biochemical basis of mental illness suggested the promise of more effective drug treatments, a view reinforced by the introduction of the antidepressant selective serotonin reuptake inhibitors (SSRIs) in the late 1980s. On the other hand, few people believed that pharmaceutical breakthroughs would eliminate the need for other supportive programs. Meanwhile, the continued trend toward deinstitutionalization created pressing needs for new forms of community support for the chronically ill. The accelerating closures of state mental hospitals created enormous pressure for rethinking the direction of mental health policy. In this context, policy makers gradually became more willing to listen to consumer-survivor suggestions for change.[16]

The first signs of this receptivity came in the Commission on Mental Health established by President Jimmy Carter soon after he took office in 1977. Initially, activists complained about the consumer-survivor's limited representation on the commission, which included only one ex-patient, Priscilla Allen, who did not have a history of involvement in the new patient movement. But Allen proved to be an effective representative for consumer-survivor interests, while the commission's open hearings gave activists the opportunity to participate in its deliberations.[17]

But it was not so much activism as economics that created the opportunity for consumer-survivor groups to make a more substantive contribution to policy debates. In the 1970s, the policy agenda was increasingly dominated by the general problem of health care costs. As Medicare and Medicaid programs expanded, federal and state governments had compelling reasons to try to limit health care costs. Likewise, in a largely employment-based system of private health insurance, employers wanted to slow the growth of health expenditures. These economic developments also fostered a new attention to the user's views of health care. Battles over what procedures did or did not get covered highlighted the general problems that consumers faced in making health care choices.[18]

In the mental health field, these problems were complicated by the special economic burdens of caring for people with severe and persistent mental illnesses. Often impoverished by virtue of their illness, many lacked adequate housing and food, much less medical treatment. The 1970s expansion of social security disability payments for the mentally ill helped some survive outside the hospital, but that safety net was a fragile one, always vulnerable to cost-cutting efforts. By the late 1970s, many policy makers had become aware that the transition from hospital to community-based care was not being done well, and that people discharged from institutional care were left too much to fend for themselves. This recognition was reflected in passage of the 1980 Mental Health Systems Act, which called for a more integrated system of community care, but the election of Ronald Reagan as president prevented its implementation. In 1981, the new administration reduced federal funding to mental health services by 25 percent and instituted a new block system of funding that forced states to decide what cuts to make.[19]

Faced with an urgent need to find more effective as well as economically viable programs of community support, policy makers began to display a growing receptivity to consumer-survivor perspectives. A key locus of this change was the Community Support Program (CSP) of the National Institute of Mental Health, set up in 1977 with the charge to respond to the problems surrounding deinstitutionalization. Starting in 1978, the CSP began to invite consumer-survivor advocates to take part in its annual Learning Conferences. Impressed by the ideas shared at these meetings, the CSP had by 1984 adopted "self-determination" and "consumer empowerment" as part of its mission. In addition to funding consumer-run programs, the CSP began to sponsor an annual Alternatives Conference to bring consumer-survivors together to share experiences and develop policy ideas.[20]

This greater receptivity to consumer-survivor perspectives was likely influenced by the growing power of consumer health groups more generally. In the 1970s, the women's health and disability rights movements gained new visibility with philosophies that questioned medical authority, promoted self-determination, and resisted demeaning stereotypes. In the 1980s, AIDS activists took grassroots mobilization to a new level of sophistication, both in public protests and political networking. Thus by the mid to late 1980s, the consumer-survivor movement had peer groups making arguments about autonomy and experience very similar to their own. Victories won by one group were increasingly cited by the others as their due as well. Moreover, the growing attention to cancer and AIDS survivors created new pressures for parity in the treatment of physical and mental disorders.[21]

The 1990s to the Present: Finding Places at the Policy-Making Table

Over the next two decades, consumer-survivor engagement in decision making increased at all levels, including individual therapeutic choices, institutional planning, and consultation and research initiatives. Perhaps the most notable success of the movement was the growing acceptance of the recovery concept, which moved into the mainstream of mental health discourse in the 1990s.

The recovery model, as it matured in the 1990s, offered a view of severe mental illness as a chronic disability and lifelong challenge. In part, as Nora Jacobson has noted, the success of the recovery model came from the multiple meanings that came to be ascribed to it. For some consumer-survivors, the term "recovery" embodied the objective of "learning to live well despite the continuing symptoms of mental illness." For others, it signified the need to empower consumers to resist forms of medical and state authority that robbed them of autonomy. For family members, it promised something else, namely, more patient compliance with treatment (a point explored further in a moment).[22]

Whatever its definition, there was widespread agreement that promoting recovery required a better-coordinated system of medical and social services. Without that integration, people with severe mental illness found it difficult to survive outside a mental hospital. Thus many states began in the 1990s to try to improve the coordination of services to the mentally ill. For example, Wisconsin undertook a sweeping review of the state's social and mental health services aimed at creating a more recovery-oriented culture of care. An integral part of its reform was the creation of working groups in which consumer-survivors participated as full and valued partners.[23]

As state-level experiments gained momentum, the recovery model gained important national endorsements, first in the 1999 surgeon general's report on mental health and then in the 2003 report of the New Freedom Commission. Created by President George W. Bush to review the nation's mental health care system, the New Freedom Commission's use of the recovery model marked a new high point in its visibility. Its Subcommittee on Consumer Issues, headed by Daniel Fisher, himself an ex-patient, came out strongly in favor of a "recovery oriented mental health system." The subcommittee's final report stated that "the culture of mental health care must shift to a culture that is based on self-determination, empowering relationships, and full participation of mental health consumers in the work and community life of society." Building such a system, the report emphasized, required "meaningful involvement" of people with mental illnesses at every level of policy making and implementation.[24]

In important ways, such meaningful involvement did develop in the 1990s. One tangible sign of consumer-survivors' growing influence was their inclusion on the planning councils increasingly required by federal and state mental health laws. A major accomplishment of patient activists was convincing policy makers that such planning bodies needed to have equal numbers of patient-consumers as well as family members. Thus the 1986 State Comprehensive Mental Health Plan Act and the 1992 restructuring of federal government that created the Substance Abuse and Mental Health Services Administration (SAMHSA) made consumer representation a requirement for federal funding. Over the next two decades, consumer-survivors became involved in state planning boards, mental health task forces, state offices of consumer affairs, and other mental health agencies. In a survey done in the late 1990s, fifty-one U.S. states and territories reported that their mental health authorities met regularly with "empowerment groups," including affiliates of NAMI.[25]

Faced with the imperative of cost cutting while simultaneously improving services, mental health institutions and agencies saw the value of not only consulting but also hiring consumers. By 1998, twenty-seven states had paid positions for consumers on their staffs in positions ranging from program evaluator to community support worker. Some public agencies began to hire consumers to be service providers themselves, as case managers, peer counselors, and crisis workers. This practice both provided a form of supported employment for a person in recovery and saved money, in that consumers usually worked for lower salaries than professional staff.[26]

Consumer-survivors also became involved in research initiatives, particularly those designed to evaluate treatment outcomes. Here again, the general pressure to rethink investments in specific treatment modalities resulted in unexpected opportunities for their input. In the 1990s, the growing interest in health systems research and quality assurance focused new attention on outcome measurement in health care. Within the medical profession, similar concerns prompted the rise of interest in evidence-based medicine. Given limited economic resources and multiple treatment options, policy makers had an obvious interest in getting objective information on what treatments and practices worked best.

Initially, these initiatives were expert driven: the original implementation of quality assurance and evidence-based medicine did not account for the possibility that patients might define outcomes differently than health care professionals did. But consumer-survivors quickly made exactly this point and successfully pushed for a role in developing and reviewing the processes used to compare treatments, in order to ensure that goals particularly valued by consumers, such as the ability to live independently or to hold a job, were included as outcome measures. By helping to move outcomes research from a narrow focus on symptom cessation to a broader focus on recovery, consumer involvement played a critical role in redefining the definition of effective treatment.[27]

Other studies examined the value of self-help programs, including those run by consumers. In 1998, SAMHSA began funding a multisite study known as the Consumer Operated Services Program (COSP) that compared peer-run organizations with more traditional service providers. The study's findings offered empirical evidence that peer-run groups were both cost effective and therapeutically valuable. Members of the program's Consumer Advisory Committee collaborated to write a book showcasing the eight peer programs included in the COSP study, whose title *On Our Own Together* paid tribute to Chamberlin's seminal 1978 book.[28]

Growing empirical as well as anecdotal evidence that consumer participation improved policy making at many levels reinforced the willingness of local and state agencies to adopt more collaborative practices. As evident in the working papers posted on Web sites of state mental health agencies and patient advocacy groups, there is now widespread acceptance of the basic principles of recovery: that self-determination is a core principle of treatment; that treatment plans have to be individualized to reflect patients' different states of "readiness" in its pursuit; that integrated programs of community support, including housing, employment, and supportive peer groups, as well as medication, are essential to long-term recovery; and that adequate public funding of medical and social services is essential to the successful implementation of deinstitutionalization.[29]

Focusing consumer efforts on educating providers has emerged as one of the most promising avenues for development. As noted in a 2005 study, a serious barrier to the use of available support services lies in mental health professionals' "negative attitudes toward rehabilitation and mutual support" and tendency to "underestimate consumers' interest in collaborative treatment." In a study conducted in five large community health centers, researchers found that a consumer-led program, featuring educational outreach, technical assistance, and clinician-client dialogues, significantly improved the likelihood that patients received a wide range of supportive services.[30]

As consumer-survivor advocates have gained greater visibility in certain policy arenas, they have provoked resistance as well. Nowadays it is possible to find self-identified consumer-survivors on every side of current debates in the mental health field. Perhaps inevitably, the growing prominence of consumers in positions of influence has increased the amount of consumer-versus-consumer conflict. Asserting a position based on personal experience alone has become less and less compelling, as illustrated in a 2002 exchange in *Psychiatric Services* in which both parties to an argument cited their experience in recovering from schizophrenia.[31]

This diversity is complicated by consumer advocates' relationships to other stakeholders in the field. A case in point is the funding of patient advocacy groups by pharmaceutical companies. In recent years, the extent of pharmaceutical influence on both providers and consumers has generated ethical and political concern throughout the health care field. The role of so-called astroturf groups—patient advocacy groups supported by pharmaceutical companies—has been especially unsettling in the mental health field, given its long and difficult history of debates about the dangers of antipsychotic medications. As states have tried to cut back on health care expenditures by requiring the use of less expensive drugs, pharmaceutical companies have helped fund protests by consumer-survivor groups against such cost-saving measures, often with great success. As one state official put it: "Antipsychotics are the third rail of Medicaid politics." He continued: "If you try to confront this issue, you get hit with these strange bedfellows of the Trotskyite lawyers for patient advocacy groups being allied with the plutocratic lawyers for drug companies." Thus arguments about the authenticity of consumer perspectives are now further complicated by accusations and counteraccusations about undue corporate influence.[32]

Even closer to home, literally as well as figuratively, are the persistent differences of opinion between consumer-survivor and family advocacy groups. As mentioned earlier, consumer-survivor groups tend to be more critical of biomedical approaches and more concerned about mental patients' civil rights. In contrast, the family-oriented National Alliance for the Mentally Ill strongly favors the biological model of mental disease and favors more restrictive commitment and involuntary treatment laws.[33]

Involuntary treatment represents perhaps the sharpest point of controversy between consumer-survivors and family members. Since the 1960s, legal advocates for people with severe mental illnesses have pressed the courts to limit the circumstances under which they can be forced to have treatment without their consent. Some critics of these trends argue that the consumer-survivor movement has created such hostility both to medication and to involuntary treatment that many people who might benefit from new drug regimens are left to suffer with devastating mental disorders. Others respond by suggesting that an overemphasis on compulsory medication programs diverts funding away from more integrated approaches to recovery that require investment in housing, employment, and other social services.[34]

Similar fault lines show up in conceptions of recovery. Although both consumer-/survivor and family advocates find the recovery ideal appealing, they often differ in their interpretation of its goals. As Nora Jacobson has observed, for NAMI and similar groups, "recovery is a phenomenon of clinical improvement and functional normalization made possible by ensuring access to new medications and cutting-edge service delivery models—the 'best practices' of elite professionals." But for many consumer-survivor activists, recovery is "a political experience . . . with the potential to transform the world through its practice of linking consciousness-raising and social action."[35]

Although fundamental tensions between the two wings of the mental health consumer movement remain, the two have shown a growing ability and willingness to work together in recent years. One example is the growing push for parity in insurance coverage of mental health care. As the managed care movement gained ground in the 1980s, many health plans began to limit their options for mental health treatment. As of the mid-1990s, over 60 percent of all health maintenance organizations (HMOs) and preferred provider organizations (PPOs) specifically excluded treatment for those with severe mental disorders; only 37 percent of all health insurance policies provided inpatient coverage for mental diseases as generously as for other illnesses; and only 6 percent did the same for outpatient treatments.[36]

Led by NAMI, a broad coalition of advocacy groups played a key role in convincing legislators to pass laws forbidding such discriminatory policies. They had success first at the state level; by the mid-1990s, thirty-seven states had passed so-called parity laws. In 1996, the U.S. Congress passed the Mental Health Parity Act requiring comparable coverage for mental and physical illnesses. The support of lawmakers with family members suffering from severe mental illness was crucial to its passage. To be sure, it was a limited victory, in that the 1996 law applied only to insurance plans that already offered behavioral care benefits. But its passage heralded a slow expansion of insurance coverage, most recently with the 2008 Mental Health Parity and Addiction Equity Act, which forbids group health plans and insurance issuers to make coverage of mental health and substance use disorders more restrictive than that of medical and surgical conditions.[37]

Unfortunately, like many other forms of consumer empowerment, the benefits of insurance parity have accrued primarily to affluent Americans with private insurance plans. Meanwhile, the economic difficulties of the past decade have fallen disproportionately hard on people with severe mental illnesses who are also poor, elderly, or nonwhite. Even before the fiscal crisis of 2008, federal and state budget cuts had greatly diminished the medical and social services available to them. These cuts reduced communities' ability to provide residential facilities, outpatient support staff, and other services required to support people in recovery. Among the outcomes were a growing number of mentally ill people among the homeless and the growing use of correctional facilities as the "de facto institution for the mentally ill." Since 2008, the downturn now referred to as the Great Recession has exacerbated an already dire situation.[38]

Conclusion

Consumer/survivor involvement in policy making has increased significantly over the past two decades, with many positive results. Perhaps inevitably, these developments have generated criticism and resistance. Although barely begun, the idea of according consumer-survivors a privileged role in policy making has prompted expressions of concern. There are worries that the "wrong" consumer perspectives are being accorded too much policy weight, that their views are insufficiently evidence based, and that they inject too much "political correctness" into medicine.

In a more general sense, the consumer-survivor movement has been linked to what Steven Sharfstein, current president of the American Psychiatric Association, has described as the "crisis of credibility" facing psychiatry. In his 2005 acceptance speech to the APA membership, he observed that a "blizzard of policy proposals . . . sits unadopted, because nobody has the moral authority to pull together a winning political coalition." He noted that psychiatry now competes with the consumer movement, the pharmaceutical industry, and the insurance industry in its bid to exercise leadership in the mental health field.[39] Sharfstein's lament suggests some of the ways that the inclusion of consumer-survivor perspectives is regarded not only as a force for positive change but also as a source of the fragmentation that continues to hamper real progress in the mental health field.

But as this overview suggests, the networks of influence used by consumer-survivor advocates hardly have the policy weight commanded by the pharmaceutical industry, the insurance industry, government health care agencies, or the medical profession. What Judi Chamberlin observed in 1990 is still true twenty years later: the term "consumer," she wrote then, "implies an equality of power which simply does not exist."[40] Hence to hold consumer-survivors responsible for policy outcomes, good or bad, seems untenable. Nor does it seem accurate to suggest that growing receptivity to consumer-survivor perspectives has created fragmentation and policy gridlock where none existed before. The difficult array of economic and treatment issues facing the mental health field today would have come about had no such movement ever developed. Indeed, the biggest threat to the gains won over the last thirty years comes not from consumer-survivors' fractiousness but instead from the massive funding cutbacks that now imperil the health and safety of many Americans.

The growing attentiveness to consumer perspectives has largely been a consequence, not a cause, of radical restructuring of the mental health field. Consumer perspectives entered policy discourse in the wake of policy failures and have flourished in a climate of perpetual crisis and tight budgets. Because it has been such a contested arena for so long, the field of mental health has produced some refreshingly honest, insightful discussions of the problems inherent in patient empowerment and the need to consider cost effectiveness along with therapeutic value. Thus as Colleen Barry and her colleagues argued recently in the *American Journal of Psychiatry*, its battles are worth studying for the insights they may hold for how health care reform will unfold now that the Patient Protection and Affordable Care Act of 2010 has been signed into law.[41]

As this history suggests, the empowerment initiative in mental health has had to contend with the jagged edges of change: a long tradition of mistrust between physicians and patients, a plethora of advocacy groups with very different philosophies and priorities, intense disagreements over treatment modalities, fiscal limitations on available resources, and the entrenched stigma and discrimination that surround mental disease. Yet the more hopeful aspects of these debates need also to be acknowledged. Precisely because the field is still deeply divided, it has been forced to grapple with basic conflicts rather than deny that they exist.

Out of these struggles have emerged some thoughtful and creative experiments in patient-centered medicine and consumer-driven health care very different from concepts such as the medical savings account. This process might best be described as policy innovation on the edge of desperation, by imperfect actors facing intensely frustrating circumstances. But despite being underfunded, divided among themselves, and subject to intense hostility and suspicion from other stakeholders, consumer-survivors have nonetheless succeeded in turning the field of mental health in more patient-centered directions.

Notes

1. U.S. Department of Health and Human Services [hereafter HHS], *Mental Health: A Report of the Surgeon General* (Washington, D.C.: U.S. Government Printing Office, 1999), 92. Several useful overviews of the mental patient empowerment movement have appeared in the last few years. For a synthesis oriented toward practical applications of the empowerment concept, see Donald M. Linhorst, *Empowering People with Severe Mental Illness: a Practical Guide* (New York: Oxford University Press, 2006). For a sympathetic account of the consumer-survivor movement based on oral

histories and participant observation, see Linda J. Morrison, *Talking Back to Psychiatry: The Psychiatric Consumer-Survivor/Ex-Patient Movement* (New York: Routledge, 2005.) For an excellent study of the recovery model and its impact on mental health policy in Wisconsin, see Nora Jacobson, *In Recovery: The Making of Mental Health Policy* (Nashville: Vanderbilt University Press, 2004)

2. A study done in Canada found that the majority of recipients of service (55 percent) preferred the term "patient," 29 percent "client," and only 10 percent either "survivor" or "consumer." See Verinder Sharma, Diane Whitney, Shahe S. Kazarian, and Rahul Manchanda, "Preferred Terms for Users of Mental Health Services among Providers and Recipients," *Psychiatric Services* 51, 2 (February 2000): 203–209. On activists' thoughts about terminology, see Morrison, *Talking Back*, esp. 126–129.

3. Eugene B. Brody, "Patients' Rights: A Cultural Challenge to Western Psychiatry" *American Journal of Psychiatry* 142, 1 (January 1985): 59. For a longer discussion of Packard and Beers, see Nancy Tomes, "From Patients' Rights to Consumers' Rights: Some Thoughts on the Evolution of a Concept," in *Making History: Shaping the Future*, Proceedings of the 1998 Conference, Mental Health Services of Australia and New Zealand (Balmain, Australia: Mental Health Services, 1999), 39–48.

4. Joseph P. Morrissey, Howard H. Goldman, and Lorraine V. Klerman, "The Enduring Asylum," in *The Enduring Asylum: Cycles of Institutional Reform at Worcester State Hospital,* ed. Joseph P. Morrissey, Howard H. Goldman, and Lorraine V. Klerman (New York: Grune and Stratton, 1980), 281. For historical background on these developments, see Gerald N. Grob, *From Asylum to Community* (Princeton, N.J.: Princeton University Press, 1991); and Norman Dain, "Psychiatry and Anti-Psychiatry in the United States," in *Discovering the History of Psychiatry*, ed. Mark Micale and Roy Porter (New York: Oxford University Press, 1994), 415–444.

5. On Beers and the NMHA, see Norman Dain, *Clifford W. Beers: Advocate for the Insane* (Pittsburgh: University of Pittsburgh Press, 1980). My focus here is on independent ex-patient organizations, so I do not discuss the NMHA and its affiliates, although they eventually became important allies for the consumer movement. See Athena McLean, "From Ex-Patient Alternatives to Consumer Options," *International Journal of Health Services* 30, 4:831–832. For a good overview of the intellectual and political context of change in the 1950s and 1960s, in particular the legal challenge to commitment laws, see Phil Brown, "The Mental Patients' Rights Movement and Mental Health Institutional Change," in *International Journal of Health Services* 11, 4 (1981): 532–540.

6. Morrison, in *Talking Back to Psychiatry*, provides the first book-length history of the consumer-survivor movement in the United States. Other useful short accounts include Brown, "The Mental Patients' Rights Movement"; Judi Chamberlin, "The Ex-Patients' Movement: Where We've Been and Where We're Going," *Journal of Mind and Behavior* 11 (1990): 323–336; Harriet P. Lefley, "Impact of Consumer and Family Advocacy Movements on Mental Health Services," in *Mental Health Services: A Public Health Perspective*, ed. Bruce L. Levin and John Petrila (New York: Oxford University Press, 1996), 81–96; McLean, "From Ex-Patient Alternatives," 821–847; David P. Moxley and Carol T. Mowbray, "Consumers as Providers," in *Consumers as Providers in Psychiatric Rehabilitation*, ed. David P. Moxley, Carol T. Mowbray, C. A. Jasper, and L. L. Howell (Columbia, Md.: International Association of Psychosocial Rehabilitation, 1997), 2–34; and "Overview of Consumer and Family Movements," in HHS, *Mental Health*, 92–97. For parallel developments in

Canada, see Barbara Everett, *A Fragile Revolution* (Waterloo, Ont.: Wilfrid Laurier University Press, 2000).

7. Sally Clay, "A Personal History of the Consumer Movement," http://www.sallyclay .net/Z.text/history.html, accessed October 25, 2010. See also Chamberlin, "The Ex-Patients' Movement," esp. 326–328; Gerald N. Grob, "Public Policy and Mental Illnesses: Jimmy Carter's Presidential Commission on Mental Health," *Milbank Quarterly* 83, 3 (2005): 425–456, 428.

8. The early movement's counterculture ideology is well illustrated in Sherry Hirsch, ed., *The Madness Network News Reader* (San Francisco: Glide Publications, 1974).

9. Judi Chamberlin, *On Our Own: Patient-Controlled Alternatives to the Mental Health System* (New York: Hawthorn Books, 1978), xi, xiv.

10. Robert Emerick, "Self-Help Groups for Former Patients," *Hospital and Community Psychiatry* 41, 4 (1990): 401–407.

11. Mary O'Hagan, *Stopovers on My Way Home from Mars* (London: Survivors Speak Out, 1993), 31, 76.

12. HHS, *Mental Health*, 94.

13. For an overview of the NAMI's history, see HHS, *Mental Health*, 96. On NAMI's conflicts with consumer-survivor activists, see Morrison, *Talking Back*, esp. 148–155. On NAMI and its state affiliates, see McLean, "From Ex-Patient Alternatives," 831–832.

14. The contrast with the developmentally disadvantaged is instructive on this point. In a 1992 study, David Braddock documented that in the 1980s, spending on community services for the mentally retarded increased four times as rapidly as community spending for the mentally ill, a disparity he attributed to the stronger, more unified voice of the parents of the retarded. Their Association for the Retarded Citizens of the United States is both older and better organized than NAMI, and does not face competition from groups run solely by the developmentally disabled themselves. See David Braddock, "Community Mental Health and Mental Retardation Services in the United States," *American Journal of Psychiatry* 149, 2 (February 1992): 175–183.

15. Morrison, *Talking Back*, 69; for a good description of the 1970s, see 66–80.

16. Grob, *From Asylum to Community*; Gerald N. Grob and Howard H. Goldman, *The Dilemma of Federal Mental Health Policy: Radical Reform or Incremental Change?* (New Brunswick, N.J.: Rutgers University Press, 2006).

17. Chamberlin, "The Ex-Patients' Movement," 329, notes that activists "packed" the public hearings held by the commission panels. On the 1978 commission more generally, see Grob, "Public Policy and Mental Illnesses."

18. David Mechanic and D. McAlpine, "Mission Unfulfilled: Potholes on the Road to Mental Health Parity," *Health Affairs* 18, 5 (1997): 1533–1537; David Mechanic, *Mental Health and Social Policy: Beyond Managed Care*, 5th ed. (Boston: Allyn and Bacon, 2007); Richard G. Frank and Sherry A. Glied, *Better but Not Well: Mental Health Policy in the United States since 1950* (Baltimore: Johns Hopkins University Press, 2006).

19. Grob, "Public Policy and Mental Illnesses."

20. McLean, "From Ex-Patient Alternatives," 826–827, 832–834.

21. Carol S. Weisman, *Women's Health Care: Activist Traditions and Institutional Change* (Baltimore: Johns Hopkins University Press, 1998): Sandra Morgen, *Into Our Own Hands: The Women's Health Movement in the United States, 1969–1990* (New Brunswick, N.J.: Rutgers University Press, 2002); Steven Epstein, *Impure*

Science: AIDS, Activism, and the Politics of Knowledge (Berkeley: University of California Press, 1996), and Joseph P. Shapiro, *No Pity: People with Disabilities Forging a New Civil Rights Movement* (New York: Times Books, 1993).

22. Jacobson, *In Recovery*, x; see also esp. chap. 4.

23. Jacobson, *In Recovery*.

24. See "President's New Freedom Commission on Mental Health," http://www .mentalhealthcommission.gov/, accessed October 25, 2010. For the "Report of the Subcommittee on Consumer Issues: Shifting to a Recovery-Based Continuum of Community Care, March 5, 2003," click the link for subcommittees and open the file labeled "Consumer Issues." That takes you to a PDF of the subcommittee's report, accessed October 25, 2010.

25. McLean, "From Ex-Patient Alternatives," 835; Linhorst, *Empowering People*, 167–202; Jeffrey Geller, Julie-Marie Brown, William H. Fisher, Albert J. Grudzinskas, Jr., and Thomas D. Manning, Jr., "A National Survey of 'Consumer Empowerment' at the State Level," *Psychiatric Services* 49, 4 (1998): 498–503. Like other Great Society legislation, the 1963 Community Mental Health Centers Act had a provision for citizen participation, which some family members used to participate in their deliberations. McLean, "From Ex-Patient Alternatives," 826. The enthusiasm for citizen-consumer participation in general health care planning diminished by the late 1970s, when it failed to have the transformative effect its proponents had hoped for. See Barry Checkoway, *Citizens and Health Care Planning* (New York: Pergamon Press, 1981). The importance of consumer participation in planning activities appears to have lasted much longer in the mental health field than elsewhere, and to have been more easily revived in the 1990s as a result.

26. Geller et al., "A National Survey." On the rationale for consumer employment, see Laura Van Tosh, *Working for a Change* (Rockville, Md.: Center for Mental Health Services, 1993). For overviews of consumer-provided services, see P. Solomon and J. Draine, "The State of Knowledge of the Effectiveness of Consumer Provided Services," *Psychiatric Rehabilitation Journal* 25, 1 (2001): 20–27; and Sally Clay, ed., *On Our Own, Together: Peer Programs for People with Mental Illness* (Nashville: Vanderbilt University Press, 2005). See also Linhorst, *Empowering People*, 203–242 and 269–298.

27. On consumers' role in research initiatives see HHS, *Mental Health*, 95; Jean Campbell, "How Consumer/Survivors Are Evaluating the Quality of Psychiatric Care," *Evaluation Review* 21 (1997): 357–363; and Linhorst, *Empowering People*, 243–268. On consumers and evidence-based medicine in New York State, see "Infusing Recovery-Based Principles into Mental Health Services," September 2004, www .omh.state.ny.us/omhweb/statewideplan/2005/appendix4.htm, accessed October 25, 2010. Note that consumer input has been suggested in the next revision of the *Diagnostic and Statistical Manual of Mental Disorders*. See J. Z. Sadler and B. Fulford, "Should Patients and Their Families Contribute to the DSM-V Process?" *Psychiatric Services* 55, 2 (2004): 133–138. For a critical response, see R. L. Spitzer, "Good Idea or Politically Correct Nonsense?" *Psychiatric Services* 55, 2 (2004): 113.

28. Clay, *On Our Own, Together*. See also J. Campbell, C. Lichtenstein, G. Teague, M. Johnsen, B. Yates, and L. J. Sonnefeld, *The Consumer Operated Service Programs (COSP) Multi-Site Research Initiative: Final Report* (St. Louis: Coordinating Center at the Missouri Institute of Mental Health, 2006).

29. For two examples of such documents and working papers, see Michigan Department of Community Health, "Dialogue on Self Determination," March 5, 2003,

http://www.michigan.gov/documents/PathwaysDialogue_70246_7.pdf, accessed October 25, 2010. "Infusing Recovery-Based Principles into Mental Health Services."

30. Alexander S. Young, Matthew Chinman, Sandra L. Forquer, Edward L. Knight, Howard Vogel, Anita Miller, Melissa Rowe, and Jim Mintz, "Use of a Consumer-Led Intervention to Improve Provider Competencies, " *Psychiatric Services* 56, 8 (2005): 967–975.

31. "Evidence Based Practices and Recovery," *Psychiatric Services* 53, 5 (2002): 632–634. The hiring of consumers as advocates and providers has also brought complaints about their behavior from other consumers. See, for example, Mary Gibson-Leek, "Client versus Client," *Psychiatric Services* 54, 8 (2003): 1101–1102.

32. Gardiner Harris, "States Try to Limit Drugs in Medicaid, but Makers Resist," *New York Times*, December 18, 2003. See also Andrew Herxheimer, "Relationships between the Pharmaceutical Industry and Patients' Organizations," *BMJ* 326, 7400 (2003): 1208–1210, doi:10.1136/bmj.326.7400.1208, accessed October 25, 2010. A consumer lobbyist testified before Congress: "I don't think there is a patient-advocacy group in America that does not receive some level of funding from a pharmaceutical company." See Jim Drinkard, "Drugmakers Go Furthest to Sway Congress," *USA Today*, April 4, 2005, http://www.usatoday.com/money/industries/health/drugs/2005–04–25-drug-lobby-cover_x.htm, accessed October 25, 2010. Note that some survivor advocacy groups remain resolutely opposed to compulsory medication and have long accused psychiatrists of being overly influenced by the pharmaceutical industry. See, for example, the Web site maintained by MindFreedom International, which regularly features articles critical of psychiatric medication practices, http:/www.MindFreedom.Org, accessed October 25, 2010.

33. Robert Sommer, "Family Advocacy and the Mental Health System," *Psychiatric Quarterly* 61, 3 (Fall 1990): 208; see also Morrison, *Talking Back*, 149–150.

34. These arguments are evident in the pages of *Psychiatric Services*. See, e.g., "Evidence Based Practices and Recovery"; E. F. Torrey, "Psychiatric Survivors or Non-Survivors," *Psychiatric Services* 48, 2 (1997): 143; and the letters in response to it, in *Psychiatric Services* 48, 5 (1997): 601–605.

35. Jacobson, *In Recovery*, 164.

36. David Mechanic, *Mental Health and Social Policy: the Emergence of Managed Care*, 4th ed. (Boston: Allyn and Bacon, 1999), 30.

37. Colleen L. Barry, "The Political Evolution of Mental Health Parity," *Harvard Review of Psychiatry* 14, 4 (July–August 2006): 185–94; "Fact Sheet: The Mental Health Parity and Addiction Equity Act of 2008," http://www.dhcs.ca.gov/provgovpart/Documents/Waiver%20Renewal/01292010_MHPAEA_factsheet_FINAL%5B1%5D.pdf, accessed October 25, 2010.0.

38. Peter Cunningham, Kelly McKenzie, and Erin Fries Taylor, "The Struggle to Provide Community-Based Care to Low-Income People with Serious Mental Illness," *Health Affairs* 25, 3 (May–June 2006): 697.

39. Steven Sharfstein, "Advocacy for Our Patients and Our Profession," *American Journal of Psychiatry* 162, 11 (2005): 2045, 2046. For more full-bodied criticisms of the consumer movement, see Sally Satel, *PC, M.D.* (New York: Basic Books, 2000), esp. chap. 2.

40. Chamberlin, "The Ex-Patients' Movement," 334.

41. Colleen Barry, Howard H. Goldman, Richard G. Frank, and Haiden A. Huskamp, "Lessons for Healthcare Reform from the Hard-Won Success of Behavioral Health Insurance Parity," *American Journal of Psychiatry* 166, 9 (September 2009): 969–971.

"Don't Scream Alone"

The Health Care Activism of
Poor Americans in the 1970s

The poor are among the most silent and disempowered of actors in U.S. society, the poor and sick even more so. Yet there have been attempts by poor and sick Americans to change health care policy from below. This chapter looks at one important example: the health care activism of poverty groups in the early 1970s.

Unlike many of the activist groups discussed in this book, which tend to focus on a single disease, condition, or policy, the National Welfare Rights Organization (NWRO) tried to transform the fundamental nature of the U.S. health care system. It did this by targeting specific health care institutions, including Medicaid and hospitals, but always with a broader goal in mind—the elimination of the two-tier health care system in the United States, which offers access to care for those who can pay and inferior or no care for those who cannot. Although the group did not reach this ambitious goal, the creative and multifaceted tactics of welfare rights activists left permanent marks on the health system, most importantly hospitals' adoption of patients' bills of rights.

This chapter looks at how the National Welfare Rights Organization came to develop its critique of the American health care system and the tactics it deployed to change it. The NWRO, which grew from a convergence of the civil rights movement with local antipoverty efforts, was active from 1966 through 1973. Although its lifespan was brief, it was momentous. At its peak in 1969, the organization had only about twenty-two thousand dues-paying members, but thousands more participated in its actions throughout the country.[1]

Inspired by academic social scientists Frances Fox Piven and Richard Cloward, the NWRO aimed to organize welfare recipients to demand the full benefits to which they were entitled, and in so doing to disrupt the system enough to bring about lasting social change, including greater political power for the poor.[2] The group's founder, charismatic civil rights leader George Wiley, was a middle-class academic, but several influential leaders, including Johnnie Tillmon and Beulah Sanders, and the vast majority of the membership were women of color who were or had been on welfare. Because most people receiving welfare payments were women, the NWRO was also a feminist organization, both contributing to and critiquing the growing women's movement.[3]

The health care activism of African American women has an honorable history. Early in the twentieth century, middle-class black women's organizations created National Negro Health Week and vigorously campaigned for public health improvements.[4] Despite this tradition, the NWRO was slow to adopt health care as an issue. For the first few years of its existence, the movement concentrated on adding the maximum number of eligible poor people to the rolls and wresting the maximum benefits from local welfare authorities. Cash and in-kind benefits were the priorities, possibly because these were items that poor mothers needed every day, while the need for medical care was more sporadic.

No study of the NWRO discusses the organization's approach to the health care system.[5] However, the antipoverty movement did engage in some significant health care campaigns during the early 1970s. Women on welfare were crucial actors in forcing hospitals to begin fulfilling their obligations to provide some free care to impoverished patients. The NWRO also pressured hospital organizations to include representatives of the poor on their governing boards. Its most successful campaign, as noted, was to demand that the major hospital organizations, the Joint Commission on the Accreditation of Hospitals and the American Hospital Association, adopt a patients' bills of rights.

Compared to the predominantly middle-class health activism around issues like breast cancer and AIDS, the poor people's health care movement of the 1970s was far less successful. Patients' bills of rights did become ubiquitous, but they were watered-down versions of the NWRO's demands, with no mechanisms for enforcement. The free-care campaign was at best partly successful, creating only a very limited obligation for hospitals to advertise free care, and demands for a more accessible and expanded Medicaid program met with defeat. Social movements of and on behalf of the poor face tremendous obstacles in the U.S. political system, particularly due to lack of resources and lack of connections to powerful institutions and lawmakers.[6] Yet, as the story told in this chapter shows, activism by the poor carried a particular kind of power. When women on welfare stood up to challenge entrenched health care institutions, not all their demands were met, but their voices could not be ignored.

Poor People's Medicine

Medical care for the poor in the United States has its roots in a long tradition of charity medicine dating back to the 1601 Elizabethan Poor Law of England. The ideology and structure of charity and welfare programs have deliberately excluded the poor from becoming policy actors; indeed, they have been designed to stigmatize and disempower the poor rather than to empower them. County and municipal medical programs, with their strict eligibility and residency requirements, imposed restrictions on poor people's freedom of movement, privacy, and individual choice. While public welfare programs at least conferred some rights to benefits, the private medical system required the poor to rely entirely on the impulses and traditions of charity and voluntarism in their quest for medical care. Free or reduced-cost care was given at the discretion of physicians and hospitals, with no place for patient voice or agency. After World War II, states and the federal government modestly expanded their roles in health care provision for the poorest of the poor, but this resulted not from agitation by poor people themselves, but from medical providers' demands for more stable reimbursement.[7]

The creation in 1965 of Medicaid, the national insurance program for the poor, did not move the United States very far from the tradition of charity medicine, despite creating a greater role for the federal government in indigent care. Medicaid was categorical (including only those eligible for other welfare programs), imposed strict income and other requirements, and allowed states to determine the level of benefits. While Medicare for the elderly was deliberately constructed as an honorable entitlement, Medicaid continued to be a stigmatized welfare program. Although its benefits would eventually become more generous than Medicare's in most states, provider reimbursements were so low that there was (and continues to be) a chronic shortage of doctors willing to accept Medicaid patients.[8]

Histories of Medicaid do not include discussions of poor people's reaction to the new program. Yet Medicaid was created at a time when the voices of the poor were beginning to be heard due to civil rights and welfare activism. When the Department of Health, Education, and Welfare held hearings across the country in 1968 and 1969 to gauge the public response to Medicaid, poor women came forward to describe their experiences and also to offer powerful criticism of the program. They were clearly a minority at the hearings—most of the testimony came from physicians and health officials, and some hearings included no statements from poor women at all. Still, at most of the events at least one woman identified as a Medicaid recipient or a member of a welfare rights organization testified, about a dozen in total. Most were members of the

NWRO or a local affiliate, but some came on their own, and a few were brought to the hearings by their doctor or preacher. The participation of these women at the Medicaid hearings received virtually no notice in the press and no specific response from government, but their testimony (found in transcripts held at the Lyndon B. Johnson Presidential Library in Austin, Texas) marks the beginning of the welfare rights movement's critique of the health care system and its ideas about how it needed to change.

Poor women's words at the hearings show a surprisingly uniform response to Medicaid. Almost without exception, the women expressed gratitude for the existence of the program. Bessie Goodwin of Bedford-Stuyvesant in Brooklyn, who identified herself as a "Medicaid cardholder," was typical but especially articulate. "My statement today is based upon what Medicaid has personally meant to me and members of my community," Goodwin stated. "With all of its problems and costs, for the first time in my life I am able to get medical care like other Americans for myself and the members of my family. Since Medicaid, I do not have to wait until someone falls seriously ill before we rush to see the doctor, which was usually in the emergency room of the nearest hospital."[9]

But welfare recipients at these hearings also began to testify that Medicaid exacerbated the indignity of being poor and continued to put up barriers to obtaining medical care. In Atlanta, several women and their minister described conditions at Grady Hospital, the city hospital, which was the only place in the city that would accept Medicaid cards. As a result, overcrowding was horrendous. Emergency-room waits ranged from eight to ten hours. Many Medicaid recipients lived far from the hospital and did not have transportation to get there. They were denied certain drugs, as well as glasses and other items they needed. After the women had told their stories, the Reverend Austin Ford asked the hearing: "Why should not these people be as free to go to any hospital as to go to Grady?"[10] He raised an issue central to the critique of welfare medicine: in a system and culture that worshipped free choice of physician or hospital, the poor were denied that choice.

Even hospitals and clinics that did accept Medicaid treated welfare patients separately from and differently than others. Lucy Priggs of Washington, D.C., who was diabetic, described waiting for two hours at D.C. General Hospital to get syringe needles while dozens of private pay patients got to go ahead of her and received their needles.[11] Most of the women also spoke of the stigma of the separate line that Medicaid clients had to stand in, among them Odell Young of Columbus, Ohio: "When I went in the [University Hospital] clinic you are sick to start with and here stands a line of paid customers here (indicating); here is the welfare customers here. . . . What I would like to talk about," she continued, "is the poor people having a little more human dignity. We poor people that are on welfare everywhere we go we stand in line. We are marked by people [for] holding a card. 'You are welfare. You go to the clinics. That is what you do.'"[12]

One of the biggest problems facing poor women seeking health care was a shortage of doctors willing to accept Medicaid. Young told of a doctor she knew who "has got a big sign up on his door, 'Welfare Clients Monday and Wednesday Only.' Tuesday, Thursday, and Friday you can die simply because he doesn't get his money."[13] A welfare rights activist in Washington, D.C., testified that she had called dozens of doctors on a list of those accepting Medicaid, and only a few agreed to make an appointment with a Medicaid client. Several other women at the Washington hearing also testified that doctors who claimed to take Medicaid either limited the number of their Medicaid patients or refused them altogether.[14]

Especially moving testimony came from a Mexican migrant worker at the San Francisco hearing. She spoke of the importance of Medicaid to herself and her family after she was badly burned in a fire: "I don't know what I'd do without Medi-Cal . . . I had no money, no insurance, when I received the Medi-card, I was losing the arm, it cost $1,200. So you see, I didn't lose my arm, so I'm proud of the Medi-card. . . . So I say, everybody needs it." But she went on to tell the audience that about three months earlier, her ten-year-old boy, who was born with severe defects, suddenly "got trouble with [his] bladder, and he [could] not make water. And we were so afraid, and we took him [in] the morning, about 9:30, we took him to five doctors in Morgan Hill, and nobody wanted to take him. He was all night and all those hours not making water, and he was all swollen. He would just holler and holler. And we went to these five doctors, and they don't want to see him. I say, 'I've [got] the Medi-card'; they say 'No.'"[15]

Apart from the doctor shortage that plagued Medicaid recipients, an aspect of the program that received notice at the hearings was the strict eligibility requirements that excluded a great proportion of the nation's poor and virtually all the working poor. A Mrs. Flanagan of Baltimore, with ten children, spoke of her oldest girl, who had her left lung taken out at age two. Local welfare programs helped pay her medical bills of several hundred dollars a year until Flanagan went back to work. "So, since I went to work they cut me off from medical assistance . . . when I was on my medical assistance, the other children, they were able to eat the things that other children had, able to wear the type of clothes. . . . I have a boy, he is five. He had a fractured skull in May. So I still owe for his hospital bill and I have taken him back for these stitches to be removed and they said, 'Mrs. Flanagan, how much money do you have?

To remove the stitches will be $10." So I said I only had $6. So they refused to take the stitches out. So I brought my child back and removed the stitches myself from his ear." This at-home medical practice occurred because Flanagan made too much money to qualify for Medicaid, even though she could not afford ten dollars for her son's stitches to be removed. Her complaint typified some of the most frequent comments of people testifying at the hearings: concern that medical bills hit hardest the working poor and lower middle class, who were not eligible for any aid whatsoever. Panelists recognized the problem, and one at the Washington hearing actually asked Flanagan whether she had considered leaving her job and her husband to qualify for Aid to Dependent Children and Medicaid. She replied proudly: "No. My family has never been broken up."[16]

As Medicaid recipients and poor women told stories of the impact of poverty medicine on their lives, several of them offered a deeper, more systematic critique of Medicaid and U.S. health care itself. One powerful theme identified state rather than federal control of poverty medicine as the source of many of its inequities. A San Francisco welfare activist declared that "the Federal Government should take more responsibility for the Medicaid program and not leave it up to the States to set up their own eligibility requirements. Many States exploit and abuse low-income people. Governors and State Legislators and administrators often try to deprive poor people of basic necessities. This happened in California when Governor Reagan tried to cut back on the Medi-Cal program. The Federal Government should provide for equal standards of medical care in all States."[17]

The problem with Medicaid, insisted Etta Horn, a D.C. activist, was that it was a welfare program rather than a health care program. In the United States, any program that served only the poor would be stigmatized and inferior. "Hospitals and doctors know that all Medicaid patients are poor and many of us are black, and will therefore often discriminate against us by refusing us service," Horn said. "Experience has taught us that we will only get good service when there are also middle-class people participating in the same program. We therefore advocate that the Federal government begin now to move toward a National Health Insurance that will guarantee that all Americans will be able to pay for hospitalization and chronic illness."[18]

Welfare rights representatives at the Medicaid hearings turned their experiences as poor women seeking health care for themselves and their families into a critique of welfare medicine itself. They took to task the two pillars of the U.S. welfare state—federalism and categorical eligibility, or nonuniversalism—that kept programs scattered and fragmented and set the interests of the poor and the middle class against each other. Their critique, coming only three years after the creation of Medicaid, struck at the foundations of the U.S. welfare and health systems. As the NWRO began to officially campaign for health care rights for the poor, its focus would shift to specific health care institutions, especially hospitals, but welfare activists never lost sight of the primary goal of equality of access.

The National Welfare Rights Organization Takes on Health Care

Women's testimony at the Medicaid hearings was organized locally, not by the national WRO. The NWRO throughout the late 1960s emphasized signing up new welfare clients and demanding better treatment and benefits for people on welfare but did not officially address health care until 1970, when it created a National Health Rights Committee.

By then, leaders thought the time was right for the organization to make health care a major issue. "NWRO has the potential to lead in this struggle," Cincinnati organizer Ronald Arundell wrote to George Wiley, noting that welfare recipients "spend a great deal of their time in health institutions" and that some welfare rights groups had already been involved in local health care campaigns. Another reason for the timing was that welfare rights was tapering off as a major rallying point; organizers felt the NWRO had gone as far as it could in demanding more benefits and better treatment from the welfare system. Health care could be an especially valuable issue for organizing "in those areas where local WROs have gotten as much from the Welfare Dept as they possibly can," Arundell suggested.[19]

The Health Rights Committee was a bold step forward in the NWRO's theory and practice. As the name announced, the committee insisted that health care be treated as a right: "Just as all people have *welfare rights*, we believe they also have *health rights*. . . . NWRO maintains that quality health care, both in prevention and treatment, is a basic right and should be provided for all people on the basis of need rather than the basis of income."[20] Although other organizations had called for health rights since the 1940s, the NWRO was the first to explicitly conceptualize access to care as a central right of the poor.[21]

The Health Committee's first step was to launch an attack on the undemo-cratic nature of the U.S. hospital system, specifically one aspect of it: hospital accreditation, which was managed by a single nonprofit organization, the Joint Commission on the Accreditation of Hospitals (JCAH). Without JCAH accredi-tation, hospitals could not function; they would lose their eligibility for Medicare and Medicaid funds. Despite its central role in the health care system, the accreditation process was opaque and, NWRO argued, not accountable to the public. According to Laurens Silver, an attorney who worked with NWRO, JCAH seemed a "natural target" due to its "quasi-governmental function."[22] The newly formed Health Rights Committee decided to "press an attack on JCAH to force the inclusion of the voice of low income and welfare recipient persons."[23]

In April 1970, Johnnie Tillmon of NWRO wrote to John Porterfield, director of JCAH. The Joint Commission was nearly finished revising the standards for hospital accreditation and planned to submit the new standards to its board of delegates meeting in Chicago. "It has been brought to our attention that, although experts from many medical organizations were involved" in revising the standards, wrote Tillmon, "there has been no general 'consumer' participation or consultation incorporated. . . . As representatives of an estimated 75,000 families on welfare who are organized to fight for their rights to a decent standard of living and adequate health care, we are concerned that the needs of large numbers of health consumers—specifically, those dependent on the Medicaid system—have not been taken into account by the JCAH." Tillmon insisted that JCAH defer adopting its new standards until it held hearings for consumers and appointed consumer representatives to its board of delegates. The board at the time consisted of representatives from medical and hospital associations but no consumers or patient advocates—indeed, no one outside the provider organizations.[24]

The commission at first responded with "its traditional position that the public could not attend executive meetings of the JCAH." However, it then relented, inviting NWRO members to make a presentation to the board of delegates before the vote in Chicago on the final accreditation standards. There had never been a JCAH meeting quite like the one of April 25, 1970. The board moved the meeting from its traditional location at Chicago's exclusive Lake Shore Club to the nearby Drake Hotel. Bertha Johnson of Detroit, a welfare recipient, spoke for the NWRO. She apologized for being a "nervous wreck," and then went on to ask for seven seats on the JCAH Board for welfare rights and other consumer representatives. The JCAH commissioners sat "grim-faced" and "somewhat disconcerted by the presence of these welfare mothers" (in the words of one observer) as other NWRO members told them "that their new standards were completely inadequate from the patients' perspective [and] that there were no standards that would assure that patients would be treated with dignity or given an adequate level of care."[25]

Following the meeting, the JCAH commissioners continued to reject direct consumer representation or participation in the accreditation process. But the welfare rights speakers did convince the commission that it had to incorporate some type of consumer voice in its operations. In June 1970, the JCAH Board of Delegates held a meeting for consumer organizations that resulted in Beulah Sanders of NWRO being named "Acting Chairman of a Consumers Advisory Council to the JCAH." JCAH leaders assured activists that "the Board would listen to the recommendations of the Council."[26] However, within a year, the council left to form an independent organization, the National Consumer Coalition on Health Care, denouncing JCAH as "elite" and "secretive," and arguing that an organization run by the very hospitals it reviewed suffered from a central conflict of interest.[27]

The greatest change brought about by National Welfare Rights Organization's targeting the Joint Commission on the Accreditation of Hospitals came not in consumer representation but in a new and sudden acknowledgment of the rights of hospital patients. Immediately following the Chicago meeting, JCAH adopted a "Preamble" to the new standards that included the first "patients' bill of rights." The preamble declared that patients were entitled to "equitable and humane treatment at all times and under all circumstances." It made reference to the patients' individuality and dignity and adopted the NWRO demand that hospital patients had the right to know the identities of the physicians responsible for their care, as well as additional rights to information about treatment and prognosis. Most groundbreaking, the JCAH included language opposing discrimination by hospitals, including discrimination on the basis of "nature of the source of payment for care"—clearly a response to NWRO demands for equal treatment of Medicaid patients.[28] The inclusion of the preamble in the new JCAH standards implied, although it did not state specifically, that attention to these patient rights would be required for hospital accreditation. Like the other JCAH standards, the patients' bill of rights was advisory and voluntary, and no mention was made of mechanisms for enforcement. Still, the preamble represented a major change in thinking about hospitals' duties to the public. With one meeting, the NWRO had brought the language of patients' rights into the health care system.

In July 1970, fresh from their JCAH victories, NWRO members met in Pittsburgh to prepare a broader strategy for health care activism. Delegates made a list of the problems that they "were most concerned about." Their complaints ranged from everyday difficulties with access to highly political critiques of the medical establishment. Problem number one was "doctors not taking welfare recipients as patients." NWRO members brought up rejections by clinics; poor care in nursing homes; poor or no mental health care, dental care, or drug treatment; racial discrimination; problems with Medicare and Medicaid; lack of ambulance and abortion services; and experimentation on prisoners. Delegates also spoke of a "lack of dignity" for poor patients and "the AMA and its lack of interest in welfare recipients' care," and contended that the "health care system [is] killing welfare mothers and children."[29]

During the conference, NWRO members came up with demands that would make the medical system more responsive to poor people's needs. They fell into two general categories: better access to basic care, and more respect toward patients from medical professionals. For better access, delegates wanted walk-in clinics, waiting times of no more than half an hour, after-hours telephone consultations, and transportation to doctors' offices. For an improved doctor-patient relationship, they asked that primary physicians stay with patients for at least a year, that all hospital medical staff wear name tags, that patients have the right to see medical bills, and that limits be set on the use of poor patients as teaching material.

These goals do not seem overly ambitious—there is no call for universal health insurance, for instance—yet the medical system and medical professionals had long resisted such demands. The delegates' suggestions for how to achieve their goals were equally modest. They emphasized, first, that poor people should be able to participate in existing decision-making bodies, and second, that institutions with substantial government funding should increase their accountability to poor patients. The organization should promote health advocates to help poor people navigate the medical system; "get NWRO members on controlling boards" of hospitals; "watch Federal grants and be sure the people have a say in who is going to get this money and how it is to be spent"; and "mak[e] all doctors accept Medicaid patients or find . . . doctors who won't do their duty." There were also more radical suggestions: "attack AMA and ask for control of some of the money it spends" and gain "community control of health service facilities." Overall, though, the NWRO's political strategy centered on pressuring existing organizations, as it had with JCAH, and tapping existing sources of funding, rather than on schemes for a major redistribution of money and power in the health system or for a rethinking of health care itself.

Yet the delegates at the Pittsburgh convention did hit an on idea that could have far-reaching implications for the medical system. This was the idea that collective action by the poor might change the way health care was delivered. The convention called on NWRO members to "fight the notion patients have that 'If I scream too loud, the doctor won't take care of me.' The answer is: 'Don't scream alone!'" Physicians or hospital committees might disregard one poor patient, but they would not dare ignore a group of them. "Don't be fooled by being invited to meetings to talk things over where you are the only WRO person," the delegates advised. "Take the group along even if you are only ten people."

The NWRO took this advice to heart at the September 1970 convention of the American Hospital Association (AHA), the largest hospital organization in the country. NWRO members traveled to Houston to picket the convention and confront AHA delegates. To avoid further disruption of the proceedings, AHA leaders agreed to give Mrs. Geraldine Smith, financial secretary of NWRO, a time to speak.

In her speech to the assembled delegates, Geraldine Smith launched an attack on the AHA from the perspective of poor mothers on welfare. "The American Hospital Association is hypocritical, selfish, parochial, and patronizing," she declared. It "hides behind a screen of concern for the disadvantaged," while perpetuating "a dual system of health care" and "preaching freedom of choice." Smith then presented the AHA with a list of demands from the NWRO. The demands included more outpatient clinics; 51 percent community membership on boards; formal patient grievance mechanisms; open medical staff privileges; making admissions and collections policies available to the public; opening JCAH survey reports to the community; including unaffiliated physicians on utilization review and evaluation and audit committees; transferring patients only on medical indications; translation services; and keeping patients informed. Several demands addressed the right of access for the poor, including the stipulations that ward patients receive equal treatment and that hospitals "not refuse Medicaid, Medicare or medically indigent" patients.[30]

Geraldine Smith's blistering speech was met with silence from the AHA delegates—"courteous attention," according to one report, but afterward "the house proceeded to conduct its business without further reference to the NWRO complaints."[31] Although the welfare mothers' presence did not change the meeting's agenda, the AHA journal reported on the protest and speech, with photographs. Shortly afterward, the AHA began to draft its own version of a patients' bill of rights.

Pressure from welfare rights activists forced the AHA into action, but the bill of rights approved by the association's members in 1973 would bear little resemblance to Geraldine Smith's demands. Its twelve provisions included rights like informed consent and medical privacy, which were important to middle-class and wealthy patients as well as to the poor. But the bill listed no rights that might cost hospitals money or that would involve shifting control from hospitals and physicians to patients. Rights to consumer participation in governance and especially enforceable rights to access were not included. Point 7 of the AHA Patients' Bill of Rights did stipulate that "the patient has the right to expect that within its capacity a hospital must make reasonable response to the request of a patient for services."[32] The vagueness of this statement was both self-evident and deliberate.

Hospitals did not exactly rush to implement the AHA's bill of rights, either. Many were slow to adopt it, some refused altogether, and the American Medical Association registered its displeasure with the concept.[33] But, as hospital attorney John F. Horty argued, as consumers became more demanding and rights talk permeated political debates, it was probably in hospitals' best interest to adopt the AHA bill or aspects of it, as it guaranteed maximum flexibility and was entirely voluntary and unenforceable. Horty, writing in the AHA journal *Modern Hospital*, warned members to adopt the bills "or the courts will tell them what it means." Hospitals could pick and choose among the rights they would advertise to patients, Horty noted: "If the hospital feels that a Patient's Bill of Rights serves its purpose, it should carefully review the language and delete any portions of points or entire points which are not applicable to the institution." He especially cautioned against point 7, which threatened to guarantee care, and also a provision requiring continuity of care.[34] Despite the built-in flexibility of the AHA's bill of rights, eighteen months after it was announced only about one-third of the nation's seven thousand hospitals had adopted it in one form or another.[35]

There was no national grassroots organization pressuring hospitals to accept the bill of rights because by the end of 1973, the NWRO had disbanded due to weakened leadership and internal disagreements (as well as the general political backlash against the War on Poverty).[36] The language of rights promulgated by the poor people's movement would, perhaps ironically, become a central theme of the more middle-class consumer movements of the 1970s, particularly individual rights like informed consent and privacy. Rights to access and to equal treatment, however, fell off the radar without a strong poor people's movement to advocate for them.

The missing voice of the poor is evident in the fate of hospital patients' bills of rights in the twenty-first century.[37] Bills of rights have been incorporated into the market-based approach to health care, emphasizing the relationship between hospital and individual consumer. In 2003 the American Hospital Association actually discontinued its Patients' Bill of Rights, replacing it with a list entitled "The Patient Care Partnership: Understanding Expectations, Rights, and Responsibilities." The only "rights" specified in this document are a patient's right to know the identity of practitioners; the right to

consent to or refuse treatment; and the right to decide to participate in a
research study. The original point 7, about the right to care, has completely
vanished, replaced by requirements that the patient provide information about
insurance coverage. The only promise made by the hospital is that it will assist
in filing billing claims.[38] In today's hospital-patient "partnership," welfare
rights activists would recognize only the faintest echoes of their original
demands for dignity, participation, and rights to access.

The welfare rights movement's health care campaigns won some short-term
victories but did not transform the system. Poor women were able to speak out
at Medicaid hearings, and to pressure the AHA and the hospital accreditation
organization to include consumers on some committees and to adopt patients'
bills of rights. They also, via a series of lawsuits, were able to force hospitals
into greater compliance with longstanding federal regulations on uncompensated care.[39] However, poor women's critiques did not lead to Medicaid reforms;
consumer participation in hospital decision making was limited; patients'
bills of rights were watered down and eventually eliminated; and free care to
the poor is still provided mostly at hospitals' discretion rather than as a right.

Yet poor people's activism did create some permanent changes. The
welfare rights movement left behind what Steven Epstein in his chapter in this
volume calls "cultural effects"—most significantly, broad acceptance of the
language of patient rights. Patients' bills of rights may not have alleviated the
two-tier nature of the health system, but they meant that powerful stakeholders, including hospitals and government, had for the first time to acknowledge,
discuss, and define the rights of patients.

Although they had no official national organization after 1973, poor
people and their local organizations have continued to pursue legal remedies
to discrimination in health care, and the National Health Law Program, a group
of public interest lawyers working on behalf of the poor in the health care system, still exists.[40] It may be that poor people have been able to have a lasting
impact only when they have collaborated with middle-class professionals and
organizations.[41] When welfare activists declared, "Don't scream alone," they
intended poor women to get together and use their numbers and their expertise as health care consumers to bring change to the system. In the U.S. health
system and political culture, however, the poor are alone, even when they are
many. Thus their screaming may become transformative only when they can
scream in concert with more politically powerful actors who have more
money, influence, and resources.

Since the U.S. health care system so clearly divides patients and consumers
by race and economic status—separating, for example, Medicaid recipients

from the privately insured—it makes it especially difficult for the poor and middle class to see common interests and to work together. Once again, Etta Horn, Medicaid recipient and NWRO member, spoke to the heart of the matter: "Experience has taught us that we will only get good service when there are also middle-class people participating in the same program."[42] Until middle-class and low-income patient-consumers identify the ways both groups could benefit from health care transformation and begin to act on them together, the poor will continue to scream alone.

Notes

1. Felicia Kornbluh, *The Battle for Welfare Rights: Politics and Poverty in Modern America* (Philadelphia: University of Pennsylvania Press, 2007), 2; Mark Toney, "Revisiting the National Welfare Rights Organization," *Color Lines: The National Magazine on Race and Politics*, November 2000, http://www.colorlines.com/archives/2000/11/revisiting_the_national_welfare_rights_organization.html, accessed June 11, 2010. NWRO occasionally claimed up to seventy-five thousand members, but this included participants who were not paying dues.
2. Guida West, *The National Welfare Rights Movement: The Social Protest of Poor Women* (New York: Praeger, 1981), 23; Frances Fox Piven and Richard A. Cloward, *Poor People's Movements: Why They Succeed, How They Fail* (New York: Pantheon, 1977).
3. Kornbluh, *The Battle for Welfare Rights*, 2–3.
4. Susan L. Smith, *Sick and Tired of Being Sick and Tired: Black Women's Health Activism in America, 1890–1950* (Philadelphia: University of Pennsylvania Press, 1995).
5. Kornbluh, *The Battle for Welfare Rights*; West, *The National Welfare Rights Movement*; and Martha F. Davis, *Brutal Need: Lawyers and the Welfare Rights Movement, 1960–1973* (New Haven: Yale University Press, 1995), do not discuss health care. One work that briefly mentions health care in the context of welfare rights is Premill Nadasen, *Welfare Warriors: The Welfare Rights Movement in the United States* (New York: Routledge, 2004), 200.
6. Constance A. Nathanson, "The Limitations of Social Movements as Catalysts for Change," in *Social Movements and the Transformation of American Health Care*, ed. Jane Banaszak-Holl, Sandra Levitsky, and Mayer N. Zald (New York: Oxford University Press, 2010).
7. Robert Stevens and Rosemary Stevens, *Welfare Medicine in America: A Case Study of Medicaid*, rev. ed. (Piscataway, N.J.: Transaction, 2003).
8. Colleen Grogan and Eric M. Patashnik, "Between Welfare Medicine and Mainstream Entitlement: Medicaid at the Political Crossroads," *Journal of Health Politics, Policy, and Law* 28, 5 (October 2003): 821–858; Jonathan Engel, *Poor People's Medicine: Medicaid and American Charity Care Since 1965* (Durham, N.C.: Duke University Press, 2006); Stevens and Stevens, *Welfare Medicine in America*.
9. Testimony of Mrs. Bessie Goodwin, "US Dept of Health, Education and Welfare, Public Medicaid Hearings, New York City, December 27, 1968," 484–485, Box 1, Papers of Wilbur J. Cohen, Lyndon Baines Johnson Presidential Library, Austin, Texas (hereafter Cohen Papers).

10. Testimony of Ethel Mae Matthews, Pin Ria Stinton, and Rev. Austin Ford, all of Atlanta, "Public Hearing on Medicaid, Atlanta, Georgia, December 20, 1968," 16–28, Box 1, Cohen Papers.

11. Testimony of Mrs. Lucy Priggs, "Hearings on Medicaid, Washington D.C., December 30, 1968," 181, Box 2, Cohen Papers.

12. Testimony of Mrs. Odell Young, "HEW Hearings on Medicaid, Columbus, Ohio, December 30, 1968," 167–168, 171, Box 3, Cohen Papers.

13. Ibid.

14. "Hearings on Medicaid, Washington D.C., December 30, 1968," 181–188, Box 2, Cohen Papers.

15. "Hearings on Medicaid, San Francisco, December 27, 1968," 108–110, Box 3, Cohen Papers.

16. Testimony of Mrs. Flanagan, "Hearings on Medicaid, Washington D.C., December 30, 1968," Box 2, Cohen Papers.

17. Mrs. Espanola Jackson, "Hearings on Medicaid, San Francisco, December 27, 1968," Box 3, Cohen Papers.

18. "Hearings on Medicaid, Washington, D.C.," 189–190.

19. Ronald M. Arundell to George Wiley, August 12, 1970, Records of the National Welfare Rights Organization, unprocessed collection, Moorland Spingarn Research Center, Howard University (hereafter NWRO Papers).

20. "Conference Committee on Health Rights, Recommendations to NWRO National Executive Board, ca. 1970," NWRO Papers.

21. On other organizations, see Alan Derickson, *Health Security for All: Dreams of Universal Health Care in America* (Baltimore: Johns Hopkins University Press, 2005).

22. Laurens H. Silver, telephone interview with author, June 9, 2010.

23. "Conference Committee on Health Rights."

24. Johnnie Tillmon to John Porterfield, April 9, 1970, NWRO Papers.

25. Carl M. Brauer, *Champions of Quality in Health Care: A History of the Joint Commission on Accreditation of Healthcare Organizations* (Lyme, Conn.: Greenwich Publishing Group, 2001), 58; Laurens H. Silver, "MCHR and Consumer Groups Attack JCAH," n.d., NWRO Papers.

26. "Report on Health Actions to Health Committee and Executive Committee from Phyllis Robinson, June 29, 1970," NWRO Papers.

27. Brauer, *Champions of Quality*, 63.

28. Ibid., 59.

29. "Report on NWRO Conference Committee Meetings on Health Rights, Pittsburgh PA July 23, 24, 1970," NWRO Records. This report is the source for the information about and quotes from this meeting in the succeeding text.

30. *Modern Hospital*, October 1970, 30–32.

31. Ibid.

32. For the full text of the 1973 Patients' Bill of Rights, see George J. Annas, *The Rights of Hospital Patients* (New York: Avon Books, 1975), 25–27.

33. "Acceptance Held Lagging on Patients' Bill of Rights," *Hospital Practice* 9 (February 1974): 56.

34. John F. Horty, "Hospitals Must Adopt Patient Bill of Rights," *Modern Hospital*, June 1973, 33–34.

35. Lee Dembart, "Follow-Up on the News," *New York Times*, June 16, 1974, 29.

36. The organization also never recovered from George Wiley's departure and untimely death in 1973. Kornbluh, *The Battle for Welfare Rights*, chap. 7; Silver interview.

37. I do not discuss here the so-called patients' bill of rights proposed in the 1990s specifically to protect managed care consumers; see Marc Rodwin's chapter in this volume for an analysis of this.

38. American Hospital Association, "The Patient Care Partnership," http://www.aha.org/aha/issues/Communicating-With-Patients/pt-care-partnership.html, accessed June 12, 2010.

39. Legal services lawyers and local welfare rights organizations in the early 1970s brought a series of class action lawsuits on behalf of welfare recipients who had been denied care at hospitals that accepted federal Hill-Burton construction dollars. The Hill-Burton regulations included a requirement that hospitals provide some uncompensated care to the poor. James F. Blumstein, "Court Action, Agency Reaction: The Hill-Burton Act as a Case Study," *Iowa Law Review* 69 (1981): 1227–1261; Michael A. Dowell, "Hill-Burton: The Unfulfilled Promise," *Journal of Health Politics, Policy, and Law* 12, 1 (Spring 1987): 153–175.

40. See the National Health Law Program Web site, www.healthlaw.org.

41. Nathanson, "The Limitations of Social Movements."

42. "Hearings on Medicaid, Washington, D.C.," 189–190.

The Canary in Gemeinschaft

Using the Public Voice of Patients to Enhance Health System Performance

Until March 2006, Larry Welby thought himself healthy. Forty-five years old and hardly ever inside a doctor's office—even if he did smoke some . . . and indulge a bit at mealtimes. But then things changed. First there was a cough that just wouldn't go away, even after Larry found his way to a doctor for some help. After a few weeks, it started getting hard to breathe at all, especially at night. During the next three months Larry went to all sorts of medical specialists, only afterward discovering that his health plan wouldn't pay for some of them. Even though these physicians seemed really smart and attentive to his symptoms, his health seemed worse after each new visit. Pretty soon Larry had a hard time even getting out of bed a couple of days each week.

Larry and his wife, Lois, began wondering if they might be better off switching doctors, finding a new health plan, or both. Then one night, Larry sounded so bad that Lois drove him to the ER—and that led to three days in the hospital. Larry's health seemed to improve after that, though his medical treatment really hadn't changed much. Over the next six months, the breathing problems eased. By spring of 2007 Larry was back at work on a regular basis.

Larry's yearlong adventure into medical wonderland left behind a few calling cards: some symptoms never really went away, and a stack of unpaid medical bills piled up on the kitchen table. So did some nagging questions, which Larry wished he could get answered just for his own peace of mind. Had his doctors mismanaged his care, or was his condition just tricky to treat? Having read newspaper accounts of medical errors, Larry couldn't help wondering if someone had actually made *mistakes* in his treatment. And there were all those bills. Was his insurer playing hardball with those specialist charges or was this the way all health insurance worked? What could he have done to avoid all this? Quit smoking? Found a better doctor or more generous insurer from the get-go? Had any of them really listened carefully enough to his concerns? Might he have expressed them more clearly—or sought out someone who knew medical-speak and could better advocate on his behalf?

Most perplexing of all: to whom could Larry turn for some honest answers? He'd liked his doctors—but maybe they were part of the problem, so could he trust their answers? He'd talked to Lois and a couple of close friends—but what did they really know about medical care? Not enough to answer these questions. Or even to know if these were reasonable questions to be asking in the first place. Or whether getting them answered was worth the time and effort.

The Public Voice of Patients

This Larry Welby doesn't exist—not literally. But there are millions of Americans like him. Each year, roughly half of all adult Americans experience some problem with their medical care or financing.[1] Roughly a third report that they or their family have at some point experienced "errors" in their medical care;[2] they see their doctors as at least partly culpable for 70 percent of these adverse events.[3] Of those who experience shortcomings with health care, fewer than half have them resolved to their satisfaction.[4]

This sorry track record persists in part because many problematic experiences, even those inducing a serious subsequent decline in health or imposing substantial out-of-pocket expense, are never reported through any formal grievance mechanism.[5] People do talk frequently to family and friends about such matters, fairly often to their own doctor.[6] But rarely do these conversations yield formal complaints that get recorded in any way. Most Americans aren't even aware that grievance mechanisms exist, let alone how to make use of them.[7] As a result, most complaints go unheard by public officials, making it hard for authorities to discern how many problematic experiences occur, how they might use this information to better diagnose systemic shortfalls in health system performance, or how to design effective remedies.

Unresolved and unvoiced problems thus remain persisting aspects of the typical American's medical encounters. It might therefore seem odd that this chapter opened with a hypothetical vignette, rather than a real case history. This was no arbitrary choice. Even though examples of frustrated patients and problematic medical care do make it into the popular media, these individual anecdotes rarely represent the ways in which most Americans experience their medical care or respond to distressing experiences.[8] My goal in this chapter is to explore how patients' voices might be aggregated in a more true-to-life manner. Like the hypothetical case of Larry Welby, the analyses presented herein abstract from the particulars of individual real-world cases, constructing a composite portrait that more accurately represents the experiences of U.S. patients.

By so doing, I explore here what one can learn from pooling complaints that patients and their advocates file with government authorities. I refer to this as patients' public voice, since these grievances are expressed in a public forum rather than in private conversations. What insights emerge from the aggregation and analysis of these sorts of complaints that would not be evident from individual patient narratives? Several hold promise.

First, a more representative assemblage of patient grievances can provide a more accurate assessment of the shortcomings in health care and insurance, dispelling the oft-voiced myth that Americans get the best health care in the world.[9] Second, understanding how patients respond to problematic episodes can belie the impression that Americans are litigious whiners. In fact, Americans rarely seek legal recourse even for grievous health care failings and complain rather less frequently than do patients with comparable experiences in other countries.[10] Third, statistical analysis of patterns in complaints can help explain why many Americans' voices are so muted, by identifying the characteristics of groups who less regularly articulate their concerns or less frequently get their problems resolved.

Despite this promise, aggregate representations of patient experiences have had far less influence on U.S. health policy than have the exceptional, media-worthy cases.[11] That's in large part because aggregations of complaints are typically presented as counts, rather than accounts—tabulations of numbers, rather than explanations for why the grievances emerged. Counts of complaints always feel cold and lifeless compared to compelling individual narratives, unless there are parties tasked with bringing them to life, translating the numbers into meaningful terms that can motivate public officials and the public at large.

Furthermore, cumulated patient grievances have not had more of an impact because there simply have been too few of them—too few relative to the prevalence of serious problems and too few to grab the attention of policy makers. And too few from some groups of patients who are having the most frequent or most severe problems. I illustrate this bias by drawing upon two national surveys that are representative of patient experiences, using them as a benchmark against which to compare the grievances that get reported to government authorities. To gain a better sense of both promises and shortcomings, we need first to consider more carefully what policy makers might aspire to learn from patients' health care experiences.

There are some striking parallels (along with meaningful distinctions) between what we might now expect from patients' public voice and why miners long ago carried canaries to test the air in mineshafts. As with expiring canaries, aggrieved consumers might warn the rest of us about impending threats—an accumulation of complaints signaling a bad doctor, health plan, or hospital. Like the canaries (who died, so that miners could live), consumers who complain to public officials are expected to do so not so much to gain recourse for themselves, which would be better served by talking directly to their clinicians or insurance representatives, but to protect others from similar problems.[12]

But in other ways the analogy between canaries and consumers breaks down. First, canaries didn't have much choice about being air quality monitors. By contrast, contemporary patients clearly have more options—and that may shape their propensity to voice complaints. Patients experiencing problems might see switching providers or insurers as their best bet. Choosing to fly away might obviate any perceived need for voicing concerns yet could also encourage it, since complaining patients who have left are less vulnerable to retaliation.

Second, miners didn't expect their caged birds to analyze the components of the lethal vapors, identify their origins, or determine the parties culpable for their emission. Simply dropping to the bottom of the cage was adequate. But in the exercise of public voice, we ask far more of patients.[13] When deciding whether to complain to authorities, patients must first conclude that there has been a blameworthy event and make sense of the causes of the problem in question.[14] These assessments call for knowledge, judgment, *and* awareness.

Finally, poisoned by noxious gases, canaries didn't decide whether to keel over—it just came naturally. Exposed to problematic medical care, however, consumers must decide whether it's worth the effort to voice their dissatisfaction. Since the primary beneficiaries of public voice are all the patients who might in the future get care or insurance in that same setting, patients' motivation will depend in part on their sense of connectedness and obligation to future patients. Ferdinand Tönnies, the nineteenth-century German sociologist, referred to social orders in which such obligations were dominant as "gemeinschaft." Tönnies expected that shared commitments would be most pervasive in simple, homogeneous societies. He saw the process of modernization and commodification as shifting social norms toward greater individual self-interest, producing a need for more laws and regulations to foster good behavior, a social order he termed "gesellschaft."

Contemporary medical care exhibits many features of gesellschaft. Patients are encouraged to make the best-informed choices for themselves, while providers and insurers face extensive regulation of quality and cost.[15] Yet in many countries, a shared system for financing medical expenses creates a countervailing reinforcement of social solidarity, a contemporary form of gemeinschaft involving reciprocal commitments regarding health care and medical spending.[16] By contrast, both the delivery and financing of medical care in the United States are fragmented into thousands of separate subsystems. The question is whether this fragmentation discourages public voice, because Americans think less in terms of collective benefit or know few people who would directly benefit from their public grievance.

Past Policy Initiatives to Enhance Patients' Public Voice

The earliest voice-enhancing policies in the United States date back about forty years, though most emerged several decades later and in most other advanced market economies about ten to fifteen years ago.[17] These initiatives reflected a cross-national embrace of consumer empowerment in health care, as policy makers grew frustrated with the shortcomings of other forms of intervention. Empowerment seemed most attractive for promoting caring and humane treatment, since these were more difficult to assess through standardized measures.

Policy makers were also recognizing the inevitability of failures and errors in medical care.[18] No matter how much was spent on care, how broadly patients were insured, or how generously their treatment was reimbursed, citizens in every country continued to report prevalent problems of quality, access, and financial insecurity.[19] Patient grievances were seen both as a way to document these failings and to identify clusters of problems that demanded remediation.

Empowerment policies were designed to enhance patients' capacity to assess their medical experiences and either exit (switching providers or insurers) or voice (expressing their dissatisfaction) in response to problems. Over the past ten years, policies to promote patient voice have been incorporated into health systems in New Zealand, Australia, the United Kingdom, Denmark, and Finland.[20] These go by various names in different polities, including grievance mechanisms, complaint systems, and ombuds programs and tend to elide the protection of individual patients with efforts to improve health system performance.

This merging (and muddling) of aspirations for voice also characterized U.S. policies, beginning with ombudsman demonstration programs for nursing homes in the early 1970s.[21] Voice-enhancing policies gradually spread as ombudsmen were incorporated into the Older Americans Act in 1978, extended to mental health services during the 1980s, adopted as state-administered insurance reforms during the 1990s, and made a part of Medicare in 2003.[22] Federal support for state-administered ombuds programs was incorporated into the recently enacted Patient Protection and Affordable Care Act. These voice-enhancing initiatives have received surprisingly little evaluation.[23] The handful of existing studies do, however, document the limits of patients' willingness and ability to voice their concerns to public authorities.

What Do We Know about Public Voice Stemming from Health Care Problems?

In both the Commonwealth countries and the United States, fewer than one in ten episodes of problematic care are ever reported to public authorities. How much this limited response affects the usefulness of these complaints depends crucially on our aspirations for how policy makers should use this information.

Infrequent Public Voice in the Commonwealth Countries

Even in countries with established national systems to collect patient complaints, such grievances are rarely reported. One study of adverse events in New Zealand hospitals found that only 0.4 percent yielded a formal complaint to government.[24] When patients identified adverse events that seemed preventable—"medical errors"—complaints were more frequent but still uncommon. Only 4 percent of the preventable adverse events led to a formal complaint. Public complaints in the United Kingdom were also scarce—a survey of patients who experienced problems found that only 5.2 percent complained to government: "neither elected officials nor advice agencies were contacted frequently, despite them often being presented as an essential part of the armoury of dissatisfied citizens."[25]

The number of formal grievances may, of course, understate the number of patients who wanted to complain if aggrieved individuals were daunted by the logistics of the grievance process.[26] But the primary constraints on grievances in other countries appear to be more attitudinal than logistical. English patients given hypothetical problem scenarios were not disposed to file a formal complaint: only 2.3 percent of those contemplating problems in primary care and 10.7 percent of those considering problems related to hospital care thought it sensible to report these to government officials.[27]

Extrapolating from these findings, one would expect that some 6–8 percent of all patients might consider it worthwhile to complain to public authorities.

This is a bit higher than the measured rates for complaint reporting, so perhaps public voice could be increased a bit by making the logistics easier. But that leaves nine in ten problems unreported, most patients seeing too little gain from complaining.[28]

Limited Public Voice in the U.S. Health Care System

The United States has a multilayered mesh of ombuds programs and grievance systems, laid down over the past several decades and differing in particular by program and particular health service.[29] Their use in response to problematic patient experiences can be assessed using two national surveys fielded after most such policies were enacted.

The first of the surveys was formulated by the Kaiser Family Foundation in 1999, the second by researchers from Yale University and the New York Academy of Medicine (NYAM) in 2002. The first survey collected data from 2,500 people, the second from 5,000. The Yale-NYAM survey was explicitly designed to build upon the Kaiser survey, using the same core of questions regarding patient experiences and problems, but incorporated a larger set of questions about the context and patients' understanding of health care problems. Both surveys collected information only from Americans who had health insurance, since the surveys were intended to explore how patients attributed blame and responsibility among various actors, including insurers.

Both the Kaiser and Yale-NYAM surveys indicate that problems occur in medical care and payment arrangements on a regular basis. Just under half (49.5 percent) of the respondents on the Kaiser survey indicated that they had experienced at least one problem in the past year, 48.2 percent on the later Yale-NYAM survey. Yet very few of these problems were reported to state agencies, though slightly more were in the second survey. In 1999, only 2.6 percent of the problems experienced by patients were reported to state authorities. By 2002, this had more than doubled to 5.8 percent, though this remains a tiny portion of all problems, even as the public grew more away of voice-enhancing state regulations enacted during the 1990s.

The increase in patient complaints to state agencies between 1999 and 2002 was accompanied by comparable increases in other forms of written grievance, including filing a formal grievance with that plan and contacting a lawyer (figure 7.1). Formal complaints to health plans more than doubled and contacts to lawyers more than tripled in these three years. By contrast, there was very little change in informal health plan contacts; in this same time period 55 percent of respondents who experienced problems in 1999 informally contacted their health plan, 59 percent in 2002.

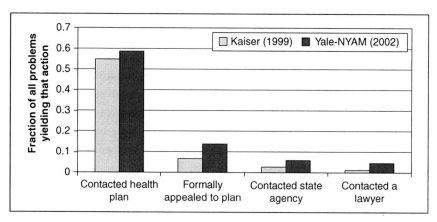

Figure 7.1 Forms of Patient Voice in 1999 and 2002
Source: Author's calculations from Kaiser and Yale-NYAM survey data.

Given Americans' image as demanding consumers of health care and their evident willingness to complain about faulty nonmedical products, it might seem surprising that U.S. patients are complaining to government no more frequently than are their counterparts in the United Kingdom or New Zealand.[30] Certainly it is *not* because Americans are happier with their medical care—they report more frequent and more serious problems than do their counterparts in these other two countries.[31] But limited voice is only half the story. As infrequently as Americans report contacting state agencies, those agencies register even fewer cases in their official records.

Consider Connecticut as a case in point.[32] The state established its Office of the Healthcare Advocate in 1999; the program became fully operational in 2001. In that year the health advocate recorded 800 complaints from health plan enrollees. That number grew to just over 1,500 by 2004 and peaked at 2,019 in 2006. With more than 2.5 million adult (twenty-one and older) residents in the state, one would expect (extrapolating from the rate of health care–related problems reported on our two surveys) Connecticut residents, in any given year, to experience more than one million problems. If they reported these to the state at the rate indicated by respondents on the Kaiser survey, one ought to have seen roughly 25,000 complaints. At the rate reported on the Yale-NYAM survey, there ought to have been more than 50,000 complaints.

Then why did so few complaints become actions for the state's health care advocate? The answer involves the nature of medical problems, the aspirations of such state officials, and the often challenging circumstances under which patients must make sense of their medical experiences.

What Sort of Problems Merit Reporting to Public Authorities?

Of course, an endless proliferation of minor complaints is not ideal. If every Connecticut resident reported every little miscommunication, misunderstanding, and misstep in medical settings, public officials would be swamped by millions of plaints each year. But that leaves open the question of what problems *should* be conveyed to public officials. One could imagine several possible criteria—some relatively uncontroversial, others seemingly sensible at first but open to contestation on closer examination. Trivial mishaps and temporary misunderstandings might arguably be best left unreported, unless repeated with such frequency that their sheer number becomes a deterrent to patients seeking medical care in a timely fashion. For different reasons, it may serve little purpose to report problems that had consequential effects but were outside the control of clinicians or plan administrators—for example, acts of God or quirks of fate for which no one is really to blame. Finally, problems that can be fully resolved by dealing with more proximate parties such as doctors or plan administrators might also be deemed less relevant to report, since they can be more effectively and efficiently remedied through other channels.

To assess the adequacy of patients' public voice, one could therefore start by identifying all the bad experiences that ought not be reported. But each of these three exclusionary criteria raises some challenging questions about the appropriate scope of state authority in resolving health care problems; we will return to these later in the chapter.

Moreover, even if these exclusionary criteria are perfectly sensible, they can serve as reasonable benchmarks for public voice only if patients can reliably determine whether their own experiences represent problems that are trivial, transitory, or better remedied by other parties. Discerning the immediate impact of the problem (larger out-of-pocket costs, feeling too sick to go to work) isn't hard, so problems with trivial consequences ought to be reliably left out of public voice. But longer-term harms (e.g., not really recovering as expected from an illness) are impossible to ascertain quickly—and thus harder to link back to medical experiences. It gets even harder for the other criteria. Which bad outcomes are blameworthy? Who is really to blame?[33] Which problems were really resolved—which might it crop up again in the future?

Problem Severity and Public Reporting

These challenges are least daunting for assessing problem severity. Not surprisingly, problem severity is consistently and positively associated with complaints to authorities. In New Zealand, for example, adverse medical events that resulted in permanent disability were five to ten times as likely (depending on

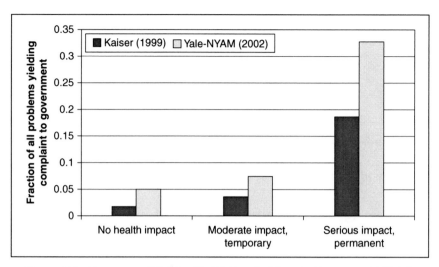

Figure 7.2   Frequency of Voicing Health Care Problems to Government Officials by Severity of Health Harm

Source: Author's calculations from Kaiser and Yale-NYAM survey data.

the degree of disability) to induce a grievance to government than were events that had only temporary health consequences.[34] The same pattern holds true in the United States.

This pattern is evident in both surveys. The Kaiser survey measured three consequences: additional out-of-pocket spending on medical care, subsequent declines in health, and time lost from work (or other social responsibilities) due to persisting ill health. The Yale-NYAM survey assessed only the first two of these consequences. The findings convey both good news and bad.

On the positive side: the more severe the consequences of the problem, the more likely that it will be reported to public authorities (figure 7.2). And it appears that patients are becoming more discriminating in their reporting over time, since there appears to be a sharper relationship between problem severity and reporting to state authorities in the later of the two surveys.

But there are two downsides also evident. Even for the most severe harms (permanent serious declines in health; medical expenses or lost earnings totaling thousands of dollars), no more than one in three get reported to public authorities. For some serious outcomes, even fewer get reported. For example, health care problems that resulted in a loss of two or more weeks of work (5 percent of annual income if there's no paid sick leave) get reported to state authorities less than 15 percent of the time (figure 7.3).

Moreover, even though each severe problem is more often reported than each trivial problem, there are a lot more trivial problems than severe ones.

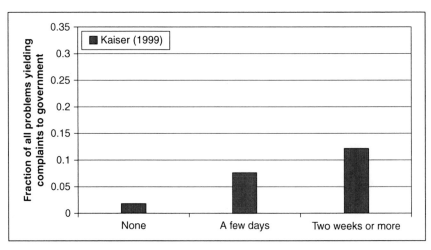

Figure 7.3   Frequency of Voicing Health Care Problems to Government Officials
by Time Lost

Source: Author's calculations from Kaiser survey data.

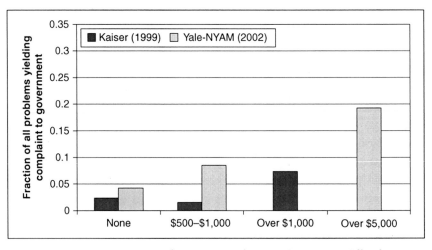

Figure 7.4   Frequency of Voicing Complaints to Government Officials
by Financial Harm

Source: Author's calculations from Kaiser and Yale-NYAM survey data.

Consequently, about half the grievances filed with state authorities involve relatively trivial concerns. Under these circumstances, it's easy to see how patterns of serious problems might get lost in the background noise of complaints about less consequential matters. State agencies might exhaust their limited resources dealing with trivial complaints, leaving some serious problems unaddressed.

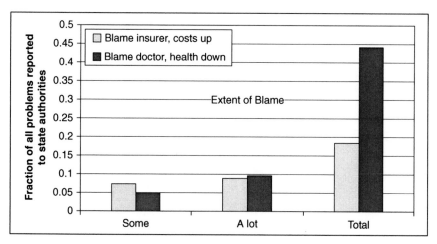

Figure 7.5 Relationship of Blame and Problematic Outcomes for Public Voice
Source: Author's calculations from Yale-NYAM survey data.

State authorities' burdens would be lessened if patients complained only about problems for which providers and plans were culpable. But this requires that patients be able to assess blame accurately. Many patients think they can: roughly two-thirds (63.5 percent) of those who experienced a problem indicated on the Yale-NYAM survey being confident that they could identify the blameworthy party or parties. When patients believed that one party was primarily to blame for a problem (doctors for worsening health, health insurers for unpaid medical bills), patients were far more likely to report these problems to state officials—all else equal.[35] Compared to problems that were equally severe but with no clear culpability, the frequency of patients' public voice was three times as high for blameworthy problems related to health plans' coverage choices, nine times as high for blameworthy problems involving physicians' impact of patient health (figure 7.5).

This again seems like good news about patients' public voicing, since it makes sense to notify authorities about problems that could have been avoided or mitigated by more responsive plans and providers. But how good it really is depends on how confident we are that patients are able to attribute blame in a consistent and unbiased manner—a question to which we'll return shortly.

Finally, when consumers believe that a problem—whatever its nature or initial severity—has been satisfactorily resolved, they are much less likely to bring the problem to the attention of state officials. The impact of problem resolution is substantial and appears to be growing over time. In 1999, problems that were resolved were somewhat less likely to be reported to government officials, but this relationship was inconsistent across types of problems. By 2002, the relationship had become stronger and more consistent. For problems that increased patients' out-of-pocket spending by five thousand dollars or more, 15 percent were reported to state officials if the problem remained unresolved, but only 3.6 percent if the patient felt that it had been rectified. For problems associated with serious declines in health, a quarter were reported to state officials if the problem remained unresolved, but this dropped to 2.8 percent if the patient felt it had a satisfactory resolution.

If patients *are not expected* to complain to state authorities about problems that are less severe, of unclear blame, or already resolved, this might explain, in part, why so few cases make it to the offices of state health advocates. Let's return to our Connecticut example. Although more than a million residents each year experience a problem with their medical care or insurance, extrapolating from our survey data one would expect that fewer than 15 percent of these would have caused severe harm. Taken together, this yields roughly 138,000 cases with serious harms.

The survey data further suggest that about half of these be judged to involve blameworthy behavior by physicians or health plans. Since relatively few of these severe and blameworthy problems are resolved to the patient's satisfaction (10–15 percent, depending on the nature of the problem), one would expect to have about 58,000 cases, all told, that arguably should have come to the attention of the state's health care advocate.

This is a big reduction from one million problems each year. Yet even in the most productive year for Connecticut's health advocate office, that agency identified and dealt with only about two thousand cases. In other words, 97 percent of the episodes that arguably deserved public voice never made it to the state agency charged with their resolution. What are some additional factors that inhibit public voice?

Why Is Public Voice So Limited in Health Care?
Barriers, Biases, and Points of Leverage

Our distinctions between canaries and consumers offer a helpful typology for the factors that inhibit public voice. Consider them in the order that they would be experienced by aggrieved patients: first, discerning whether disappointing health outcomes reflect problems that merit a response; second, choosing whether to exit or voice; third, assessing whether the benefits of public voice merit the effort of filing a complaint; and fourth, for patients who endeavor to complain, how to negotiate the grievance process.

The Discerning Consumer: Complexities of Attribution

Two forms of attribution appear most consequential in health care settings. The first involves deciding whether a given problem involved coverage issues (the responsibility of health insurers) or was caused by quality shortcomings (the domain of clinicians' responsibility). How patients categorize the problem influences how they voice a response.[36] Put simply, most patients never think to complain to their health plan about quality of care, because they don't consider treatment quality to be within the purview of health plan administrators.

The impact of these attributions is amplified by states' voice-enhancing policies. When most states established their ombuds programs and external arbitration systems for grievances, they required that enrollees exhaust the internal grievance processes at their health plan before contacting a state agency. This seemed a sensible enough requirement, given concerns that state agencies would otherwise be deluged by trivial complaints best rectified by the plan itself. However, if patients think that health plans are not responsible for the quality of medical care, they would never even consider filing a grievance with their health plan about such matters.[37] This is exactly what we observe in the survey data. Two-thirds of the respondents on the Yale-NYAM survey who had not contacted their health plan about a treatment-related problem said that they didn't see how the plan could help. By contrast, only 21 percent of those with problems that involved coverage or benefit issues offered this explanation for not contacting their plan. The result is that problems related to medical care are far less likely to induce grievances to state agencies (2.2 percent of all such problems) than are problems related to access barriers (7.2 percent of all such problems) or inadequate insurance coverage (6.9 percent of all such problems), even for problems of equal severity.

A second relevant attribution involves blame. If patients are *unsure* about whom to blame, they are much less likely to contact a state agency, even for problems with severe consequences. Consider respondents who reported substantial harms, either paying a thousand dollars or more in additional out-of-pocket expenses, or suffering a serious and permanent decline in their health (figure 7.6).

There's a strong relationship between being sure about the attribution of blame for these severe outcomes and reporting them to state authorities. (That's not an error in the graph—respondents who were very unsure about blame filed *no* grievances at all.) Since roughly a third of all respondents indicated that they were unsure about blame, this attribution is a frequent deterrent to public voice. This seems decidedly counterproductive, since the very confusion evidenced by unclear attribution of blame arguably represents the patients most in need of external assistance.

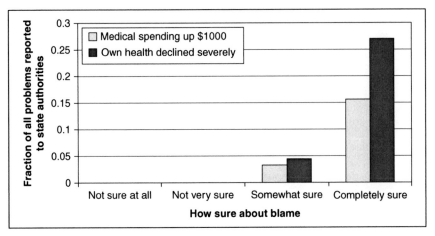

Figure 7.6 Certainty of Blame Attribution and Propensity to Voice

Source: Author's calculations from Yale-NYAM survey data.

Patients' being able to make sense of their health care experiences—especially the problematic ones—is a vital aspect of good medical care. Roughly 75 percent of the respondents on the Yale-NYAM survey indicated that when they contacted their health plan after a problem, they did so in part to obtain an explanation. It seems ironic, therefore, that patients who are most confused by their circumstances are least likely to publicly voice their grievances. Put differently, a health care system that befuddles patients with its complexity also inhibits their expression regarding its shortcomings—hardly a prescription for enhancing health system performance through public voice.

Being There: The Choice to Exit or Stay, and Its Implications for Public Voice

Studies of consumer behavior regarding nonmedical goods and services suggest that exit and voice can interact in complex ways.[38] On the one hand, by reducing the threat that a problem might reoccur, exit may reduce complaint rates. On the other hand, if consumers hesitate to voice grievances because they fear retaliation from the parties that caused the problem, the opportunity to get away may reduce their inhibitions about complaining.

Switching health plans or physicians in response to a health care problem proves to be relatively rare: the propensity to change health plans in response to perceived problems was 4.8 percent in 1999, 5.7 percent in 2002. Physician switching due to problems doubled over these three years, from 6.4 percent to 13.1 percent. Though infrequently exercised, exit does appear to be associated

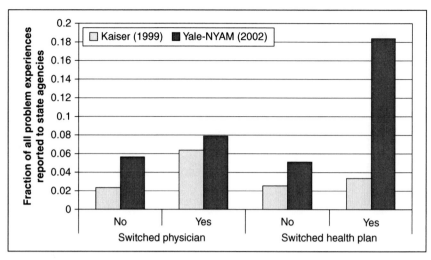

Figure 7.7 Association of Exit and Voice as Responses to Problematic Health Care Experiences

Source: Author's calculations from Kaiser and Yale-NYAM survey data.

with the propensity for public voice—in a positive way (figure 7.7). The magnitude of this relationship appears to vary a bit by year and the nature of the harm caused by the problem, but the overall pattern persists: those who switched health plans or clinicians are also more likely, all else equal, to complain to a state agency about the problem.[39]

Thus at least to some extent exit appears to enhance—not discourage—public voice. Which in turn suggests that when patients are not given a choice of health plans (as the majority with employer-sponsored insurance are not) or when they feel that they cannot leave their current doctor without disrupting vital continuity of care, these constraints on switching will significantly inhibit public voice.[40]

Volition and Voice: Perceptions of Collective Commitments in Medical Care

Few patients turn to government for immediate succor from problems. Half of all problems with medical care or financing induce patients to first contact their health plan. Patients also turn to their doctor for initial assistance and—for those with employer-based health insurance—to benefit managers at work. Seeking these sources of support is growing more common. In 1999, 13 percent of patients who experienced a problem contacted their employer about it, whereas 33 percent said something to their physician. Just three years later, 28 percent of all problems were discussed with employers, 48 percent with doctors.

Patients typically complain to government only after these initial efforts have faltered. They take this next step only if they see government as having a stake in their medical experiences. In countries with national health insurance or national health services, where the government pays for or administers medical care, this association comes naturally. In the United States, this is less often the case. Because much of the government financing for medical care in the United States is indirect and hidden, Americans are less likely to hold government responsible for health system performance and less likely to turn to government for succor in time of distress.[41]

We can get some sense of the impact of Americans' failure to associate government with health system performance by comparing the propensity for public voice of Americans covered by government insurance to those enrolled in private insurance. Two forms of government insurance are most common: Medicaid (the primary program for low-income households, covering about twelve million adults during this time period) and Medicare (the primary insurance for the aged and disabled, covering about thirty-three million). Medicaid is a closer analog to the role of government in a country with national health insurance, since state governments administer both Medicaid and the grievance process. This turns out to make quite a difference: people who are enrolled in Medicaid are five times as likely as those in other forms of insurance to complain to the state, for problems of similar severity.

Medicare beneficiaries are also more likely to complain to state authorities than are those with private insurance: 8.3 percent of Medicare beneficiaries with health care–related problems complained to state government, compared to 5.2 of the privately insured. Although a smaller impact than for Medicaid, this pattern is in some ways more intriguing. It suggests that seeing government as responsible for health system performance promotes public voice, though it involves two different levels of government (Medicare being a federal program).

Government could be held responsible for health system performance even if it wasn't footing the bill. But for this to translate into enhanced public voice, people must be aware of this government role. And this is no sure thing. In 2002 roughly 70 percent of Americans were residents of states that mandated external grievance arrangements to which plan enrollees could appeal. Yet only 37 percent of those enrolled were aware that their state had such a law. Now this might not be a problem, were it the 37 percent who actually needed to know—that is, those who had problems of sufficient severity that contacting the state might make sense. In fact, however, precisely the opposite is true: respondents with the most severe problems were less likely than other citizens (26 percent versus 35–40 percent) to be aware that their state offered external review of health plan denials.

Capabilities: The Burdens of the Voicing Process and the Availability of Social Support

No matter how friendly and inviting ombuds programs or grievance arrangements are designed to be, relatively few patients feel prepared to make use of them. Many who do so report being confused by the process and disappointed at the results.[42] In the last ten years, the grievance arrangements in both the United Kingdom and New Zealand were redesigned to make them more readily understood and easily used by the average patient.[43] Citizens in these countries favor further simplification, including greater use of telephone and the Internet to facilitate the complaint process.[44]

By contrast, complaint-reporting systems in the United States appear to have been designed to make public voice as complicated as can be imagined (or more so). In many countries with formal grievance arrangements, patients have an explicit legal right to contact the public advocate as soon as they experience problems and are encouraged to do so.[45] By contrast, virtually all U.S. states in the offer external arbitration for disputes only after consumers exhaust opportunities for appeal within the plan.[46] In many states, residents are discouraged from even contacting the agency with oversight responsibilities until they have pursued every other grievance option. For example, the Web site of the Office of the Healthcare Advocate for Connecticut describes the process that consumers should follow before filing a complaint with the state:

> You should expect a formal written response from the health plan acknowledging your complaint and a description of what the health plan will do to resolve it. You should be advised in writing of the health plan's decision. This response should tell you what was decided and why. You should also be told what to do if you wish to appeal a decision you feel is not fair. . . . If your appeal has been denied, you also need a copy of the second denial letter. This letter will outline the process for the next level of appeal. This second level of appeal will, typically, be reviewed by a different group of people at the managed care plan. The second denial letter may instruct you that if you wish to initiate a second level appeal you must submit another appeal packet with *new* information specifically addressing the current reason for denial.[47]

All this before the good citizens of Connecticut can even contact the state's health advocate. Might this seem just a bit daunting, particularly for patients debilitated by serious illness? If the state's assistance seems so far out of reach, why even start the appeals process to begin with?

To be sure, requirements of this sort may be useful in discouraging some complaints about trivial matters. This said, using a multistage grievance process to filter complaints in this manner has some real liabilities. Consumers who have difficulty negotiating the plan's internal grievance mechanisms are effectively disempowered from public voice. Roughly one in five respondents to the Yale-NYAM survey expressed some doubts about being able to use their health plan's grievance arrangements. And those who expressed such doubts were only half as likely to have voiced problems with their medical care to state agencies, for a given severity of problem.

Even those who understand how to file a grievance may be deterred by the prospect of an extended multistage complaint process. A long administrative process can feel taxing even to those in good health. When patients are severely debilitated by illness, injury, or medical insult, they may need to depend on friends or family to serve as their advocates in a grievance process. Roughly a third of all complaints filed with the National Health Service in the United Kingdom, for example, are submitted by family members.[48] Family and friends may also help with making sense of patients' medical experiences, researching the grievance process, or providing other support that makes public voice easier for the patients themselves.

The association of social support with public voice is evident in the behavior reported on our surveys. Respondents who talked about their health care problems with family and friends were about twice as likely as those who did not to eventually report those problems to state authorities. These differences were even more pronounced for patients whose health care problems caused the largest harms. Under those circumstances, patients who discussed matters with family, friends, or both were three to five times more likely to voice those complaints to the state. This suggests that more socially isolated patients may find public voice too daunting.

Persisting Differences in Propensity for Public Voice in Health Care

These factors inhibiting voice can reinforce one another. We illustrate this compounding process with two examples. The first involves education: patients who stayed longer in school are significantly more likely to voice problems with medical care to state agencies.[49] More-educated patients are more aware of state laws that promote public voice. They can also better deal with the administrative requirements of a multistage grievance process: in the Yale-NYAM survey, just over half of respondents with less than a high school education expressed confidence at using their health plan's internal grievance procedures, compared to 88 percent of those who had completed a graduate degree after college.

All this makes for substantial differences in voice across educational strata.[50] Strikingly, this is most pronounced among patients who had a graduate degree—all else equal, they were about twice as likely to complain to state officials as were patients with similar problem experiences but less education. Because patients with graduate training were significantly more likely to publicly voice complaints than those who had completed college, it seems unlikely that it is limited literacy, numeracy, or other basic skills that are inhibiting public voice. Perhaps it is more linked to social status and perceived self-efficacy, both of which have been shown to enhance voice in health care settings.[51]

A second crosscutting attribute involves the influence of chronic health conditions. Patients with chronic illness have more opportunities to learn how to make sense of their health care experiences, reducing the challenges of blame attribution. They have ample opportunity to learn how to effectively deal with doctors and insurers, to discover how best to negotiate grievance arrangements, and to become informed about relevant state laws.

Although patients with chronic illness are only slightly more likely to report being informed in each of these ways, the cumulative effect of all these modest differences leads to substantial disparities in public voice. Patients reporting chronic conditions on the Kaiser survey were three times as likely to grieve to a state agency as were patients with acute health conditions, twice as likely on the Yale-NYAM survey.

Enhancing and Rebalancing the Public's Voice in Medical Settings

Every year, tens of millions of real-life Larry Welbys have health care episodes that seemingly go awry, adding to their medical expenses, threatening their health, or both. Inadequate knowledge, blurred attributions, problems seen as outside government's purvey—these all help to explain why so few health care problems (even those that cause quite substantial harm) are brought to the attention of state authorities. Millions of Americans experience problems with serious consequences annually, yet these induce no public voice. The immensity of this silence is striking. Yet sheer numbers should not cause us to forget that each complainant is a person, each complaint an episode of pain, fear, confusion, anger.

The profound impact of these experiences on peoples' lives needs to be acknowledged, not lost in a body count of harmful events. Grievance mechanisms, rightly structured and sensibly interpreted, have the capacity to put a more human face on the shortcomings of U.S. health care. To do this, however, public officials must acknowledge complaints as stories, rather than simply as numbers. Consequently, state agencies charged with collecting and responding to grievances have the responsibility to do more than count. They can and must learn from these narratives.

Public officials who take on this role must learn also how to more powerfully recount the stories behind the complaints and translate statistical counts into more meaningful accounts of the true suffering, confusions, dilemmas, and fears that patients experience when something goes awry with their medical care or financing. In other words, agencies that collect and respond to patient grievances should take their inspiration as much from Studs Terkel as from Ralph Nader—and far more from both these advocates than from the social epidemiologists who aspire only to count the prevalence of problems of different sorts.

To be sure, personal anecdote has always played a crucial role in health policy, as in other policy domains. As commonly deployed, however, personal anecdotes can frequently distort policy making by reducing the complexities and heterogeneity of medical experiences to a few iconic cases.[52] And precisely because these anecdotes come disproportionately from patients with particular types of health problems and certain sociodemographic backgrounds, they can also bias our collective understanding of health care's strengths and limitations.

A well-designed system that collects patients' complaints can do better, because its inherent design is to assemble a *cumulative* (and therefore richer) portrait of the problems that emerge in the course of providing medical care. To overcome existing biases in the motivation to complain, states' complaint arrangements need to more actively solicit patients' experiences with medical care, rather than waiting passively for the patients to contact the state.

Of course, individual patients' voices are not the only way of representing patient experiences: numerous disease advocacy groups have arisen in recent years and have grown increasingly influential politically. The voice embodied by disease advocacy groups, though often fraught with its own problems of representation (see chapters by Steven Epstein, Rachel Grob, and Elizabeth Mitchell Armstrong and Eugene DeClercq in this volume), has the capacity to capture a collective experience that can never be adequately assessed or conveyed through individual grievances. But patients' personal experiences offer some unique insights into medical care. Before considering how this voice might best be elicited, it's useful to return the question with which this chapter began: what sorts of problems ought to be seen as within the purview of a well-functioning grievance system?

How Large a Chorus of Voices? Defining the
Appropriate Scope of State Responsibility

Even limiting the purview of state oversight to problems that generate serious harms leaves a daunting task: can state officials invest sufficient resources to accurately identify, interpret, and identify patterns in 2.5 million cases that annually meet these criteria? But states could have a different scope of authority. Perhaps identifying and tracking every serious complaint should fall to an advocacy system composed of private agencies that contract with the state to investigate complaints. The state authority could then aggregate these individual cases and look for patterns at the level of providers, insurers, or community. For these functions, it may be sufficient to collect information on a *sample* of complaints, as long as these are representative of patients' experiences.

There are other reasons for the state to delegate advocacy for individual cases. Americans have limited enthusiasm for government as an active player in their medical care.[53] Nonprofit agencies might be seen as more appropriate for taking on the individual patient advocacy role because Americans view nonprofits as a more trustworthy source of information regarding medical care.[54] Establishing one such nonprofit in each locale would provide just the sort of locally embedded guidance that has proven most useful in assisting patients to navigate medical care.

Were such a system in place, the requirements for patients' public voice involving state agencies would be substantially transformed. The newly established network of nonprofit patient advocacy agencies could be created with a mandate that each agency synthesize and analyze their individual cases to identify patterns in health system shortcomings, which they would then report on a regular basis to the state's health advocacy agency.[55]

With such a network of nonprofits in place to conduct case-level advocacy, state patient advocacy offices could turn their full attention to the vital task of interpreting patient voice to improve health care at the system level. These state agencies could be charged with overcoming reporting biases, so that patients who have less education, acute rather than chronic medical conditions, and limited social support are no longer underrepresented in the chorus of public voices. Some of the provisions of the Patient Protection and Affordable Care Act seem consistent with this sort of multitiered advocacy infrastructure, though the proof will be in the implementation of the so-called patient navigator provisions in the bill—which remains several years in the future.

Building a Better Mouthtrap: Ensuring that
Patients' Public Voice Is Representative

To overcome these biases, states' patient advocacy offices would need to take on three initiatives. The first would involve adopting arrangements to help patients make sense of their health care experiences. Help lines of this sort already exist in a handful of jurisdictions, but their scope (and public awareness of their presence) would need to be expanded. The British National Health Service has had a comparable help line (NHS-Direct) in operation for about a decade, with growing evidence that it is effective at reducing patients' confusion and at least somewhat enhancing their capacity for making sound choices.[56]

A second essential change involves eliminating the prerequisites that currently require consumers to exhaust the internal grievance procedures of their health plan before contacting the relevant state agency. An advocacy infrastructure should help patients address their confusion, not require them to do so before they can even make contact with public officials. It should most aggressively protect the frailest and most vulnerable patients, not discriminate against them. And it should encourage the voicing of problems that are related to quality of care, not inhibit them.

Third, any arrangement that aspires to accurately assess patient complaints cannot passively rely only on complaints that patients initiate, since they will do so unevenly as a reflection of their checkered motivation and diverse circumstances. The creation of robust, representative public voice can be accomplished only if state agencies actively *solicit* accounts from patients who have problematic experiences. One promising approach would be to survey a relatively large cross-section of citizens in each state every year. Some relatively simple questions regarding respondents' experiences could serve as useful screening items to identify patients who have problems worth learning more about. For example, the Kaiser survey asked patients to assign their health plan a letter grade, and the Yale-NYAM survey asked whether they would recommend their health plan to friends or family members. Either question could identify subgroups of aggrieved patients.

To illustrate: 6.9 percent of respondents assigned their health plan a grade of D or F on the Kaiser survey. As revealed in figure 7.8, these responses are about twice as effective as unsolicited complaints at identifying problems that led to substantial increases in out-of-pocket medical spending (but not much

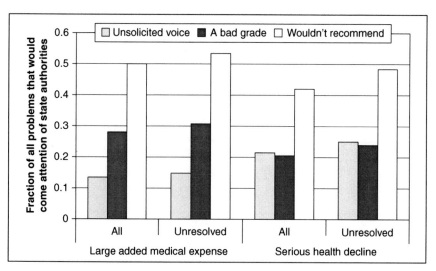

Figure 7.8   Eliciting Dissatisfaction to Identify Problematic Experiences
Source: Author's calculations from Kaiser and Yale-NYAM survey data.

more effective than unsolicited complaints at identifying problems that harmed patients' health).

To be clear, I am *not* suggesting substituting such survey questions for information regarding the specifics of patient complaints. What I'm proposing is that surveys be used to identify, in a low-cost manner, patients who've had some serious issues with their medical care. The state advocacy agency would then solicit from them the details regarding their specific grievances. Although one cannot predict how many of these patients would willingly respond to such solicitation, a similar approach has proven quite successful in hospital-based programs for patient advocacy. In one program, for example, interviews conducted by the hospital's patient advocate with 1,233 patients identified 695 previously unvoiced concerns with the care provided. During this same time period, these patients filed a rather smaller number of complaints with the hospital's formal grievance system—twelve, to be exact.[57] To do their job effectively, state offices of patient advocacy need to adopt a similarly active role in eliciting the experiences of patients in their state's health care system.

Concluding Thoughts: Aspirations for the Future of Public Voice

Policy makers have favored quantitative measures for assessing health system performance. As a result, the subtler dimensions of humane treatment have been given short shrift in collective efforts to make health care more accountable and responsive. Because patients' experiences must, by definition, *always* remain vital aspects of humane health care, the effective elicitation of and response to patients' public voice must become as vital to health policy as those caged canaries were to the miners who carried them to work.

In this case, however, policy makers ought to care about more than whether these human canaries have survived their journeys into the depths of the U.S. health care system. They must pay attention to motives, must take into account to whom and how these uncaged birds sing. Only by so doing can public officials really learn from, and appropriately interpret, the broader meanings of this multiplicity of patient experiences. By giving government a clearer, more supportive role in this process and a more constructive way to respond to expressed concerns, more patients will see the value in conveying their grievances to state authorities. Moreover, the very act of listening more carefully to patients' experiences will enhance patients' sense of solidarity— leading patients to see themselves as having collective interests that they can further by expressing their grievances. This ought to further encourage them to take seriously the responsibility to give public voice to their concerns. And by so doing, to recognize the deeper communal connections that are fundamental to all health care, the caring portion of which is inherently a social good, not simply an individually purchased service.

Notes

1. Shannon Mitchell and Mark Schlesinger, "Managed Care and Gender Disparities in Problematic Healthcare Experiences," *Health Services Research* 40, 5 (2005): 1489–1513; Mark Schlesinger, Shannon Mitchell, and Brian Elbel, "Voices Unheard: Barriers to the Expression of Dissatisfaction with Health Plans," *Milbank Quarterly* 80, 4 (2002): 709–755.
2. Kaiser Family Foundation/Agency for Healthcare Research and Quality, *2006 Update on Consumers' Views of Patient Safety and Quality Information* (Menlo Park, Calif.: Kaiser Family Foundation, September 2006); Kaiser Family Foundation/ Agency for Healthcare Research and Quality, *National Survey on Consumers' Experiences with Patient Safety and Quality Information* (Menlo Park, Calif.: Kaiser Family Foundation, November 2004).
3. Kaiser Family Foundation, *National Survey on Consumers' Experiences*, 19.
4. Kaiser Family Foundation, *Consumer Experiences with Health Plans Survey* (Menlo Park, Calif.: Kaiser Family Foundation, October 1999).
5. Schlesinger et al., "Voices Unheard."
6. Ibid.
7. Ibid.
8. John McDonough, "Using and Misusing Anecdote in Policy Making," *Health Affairs* 20, 1 (2001): 207–212.
9. For example, Americans are more likely to report having experienced errors with their medical care than are patients in most other countries in the Organization for Economic Cooperation and Development. Cathy Schoen, Robin Osborn, Michelle Doty, Meghan Bishop, Jordan Peugh, and Nandita Murukutla, "Toward

Higher-Performance Health Care Systems: Adults' Health Care Experiences in Seven Countries, 2007," *Health Affairs* 26, 6 (November–December 2007): w717–w734.

10. Fewer than 10 percent of the problems that patients identify as medical errors lead to malpractice actions. Kaiser Family Foundation, *National Survey on Consumers' Experiences*, 20; Marlynn L. May and Daniel B. Stengel, "Who Sues Their Doctors? How Patients Handle Medical Grievances," *Law and Society Review* 24, 1 (1990): 105–120.

11. Barron Lerner, *When Illness Goes Public: Celebrity Patients and How We Look at Medicine* (Baltimore: Johns Hopkins University Press, 2006).

12. Patients know that most complaints will not resolve their own problems. See Linda Mulcahy and Jonathan Q Tritter, "Pathways, Pyramids, and Icebergs? Mapping Links between Dissatisfaction and Complaints," *Sociology of Health and Illness* 20, 6 (1998): 825–847. On complaints as a means of preventing similar problems for others, see Ron Paterson, "The Patients' Complaints System in New Zealand," *Health Affairs* 21, 3 (2002): 70–79; Roland Friele and Emmy Sluijs, "Patient Expectations of Fair Complaint Handling in Hospitals: Empirical Data," *BMC Health Services Research* 6 (2006): 106.

13. It is sometimes sufficient for consumers simply to keel over: policy makers often use an excessive mortality rate as a marker of substandard quality. See Peter Rivard, Stephen Luther, Cindy Christiansen, Shibei Zhao, Susan Loveland, Anne Elixhauser, Patrick Romano, and Amy Rosen, "Using Patient Safety Indicators to Estimate the Impact of Potential Adverse Events on Outcomes," *Medical Care Research and Review* 65, 1 (2008): 67–87.

14. Marsha Rosenthal and Mark Schlesinger, "Not Afraid to Blame: The Neglected Role of Blame Attribution in Medical Consumerism and Some Implications for Health Policy," *Milbank Quarterly* 80, 1 (2002): 41–95.

15. Mark Schlesinger, "The Dangers of the Market Panacea," in *Healthy, Wealthy, and Fair*, ed. James Morone and Lawrence Jacobs (New York: Oxford University Press, 2005), 91–136; Aggie Paulus, "Market Competition: Everybody Is Talking, but What Do They Say? A Sociological Analysis of Market Competition in Policy Networks," *Health Policy* 64 (2003): 279–289.

16. Francesco Paolucci, Andre Den Exter, and Wynand Van de Ven, "Solidarity in Competitive Health Insurance Markets: Analysing the Relevant EC Legal Framework," *Health Economics, Policy, and Law* 1, 2 (2006): 107–126.

17. Schlesinger, "Dangers of the Market Panacea"; Paulus, "Market Competition," 279–289; Nancy Tomes, "Patients or Health-Care Consumers? Why the History of Contested Terms Matters," in *History and Health Policy in the United States*, ed. Rosemary Stevens, Charles Rosenberg, and Lawton Burns (New Brunswick, N.J.: Rutgers University Press, 2006), 83–110.

18. Lucian Leape and Donald Berwick, "Five Years After to Err Is Human: What Have We Learned?" *JAMA* 293, 19 (2005): 2384–2390.

19. Cathy Schoen, Robin Osborn, Phuong Tranh Huynhm, Michelle Doty, Kinga Zapert, Jordon Peugh, and Karen Davis, "Taking the Pulse of Health Care Systems: Experiences with Health Problems in Six Countries," *Health Affairs* 5 (Web exclusive, 2005): w510–w523; Robert Blendon, Cathy Schoen, Catherine DesRoches, Robin Osborn, and Kinga Zapert, "Common Concerns Amid Diverse Systems: Health Care Experiences in Five Countries," *Health Affairs* 22, 3 (2003): 106–121.

20. For New Zealand and Australia, Paterson, "Patients' Complaints in New Zealand"; for the United Kingdom, V. Entwistle, J. Andrew, M. Emslie, K. Walker, C. Dorrian,

V. Angus, and A. Conniff, "Public Opinion on Systems for Feeding Back Views to the National Health Service," *Quality and Safety in Health Care* 12 (2003): 435–442; and Mulcahy and Tritter, "Pathways, Pyramids, and Icebergs?"; for Denmark, Erling Segest, "The Ombudsman's Involvement in Ensuring Patients' Rights," *Medicine and Law* 16, 3 (1997): 473–486; for Finland, I. Pahlman, T. Hermanson, A. Hannuniemi, J. Koivisto, P. Hannikainen, and P. Ilveskivi, "Three Years in Force: Has the Finnish Act on the Status and Rights of Patients Materialized?" *Medicine and Law* 15, 4 (1996): 591–603.

21. Carroll Estes, Donna Zulman, Sheryl Goldberg, and Dawn Ogawa, "State Long-Term Care Ombudsman Programs: Factors Associated with Perceived Effectiveness," *Gerontologist* 44, 1 (2004): 104–115; Elma Holder and Barbara Frank, "Advocacy for Residents in Long-Term Care: Lessons and Challenges," in *Patient Advocacy for Health Care Quality*, ed. Jo Anne Earp, Elizabeth French, and Melissa Gilkey (Boston: Jones and Bartlett, 2008), 387–418.

22. Holder and Frank, "Advocacy for Residents"; Clarence J. Sundram, "Implementation and Activities of Protection and Advocacy Programs for Persons with Mental Illness," *Psychiatric Services* 46, 7 (1995 July): 702–706; Richard Cauchi, "Making the Best of Managed Care: State Ombudsman, Report Card, and Profile Programs Aim to Aid Those Frustrated by HMOs," *State Legislatures* 27, 6 (2001): 22–24.

23. For a few exceptions, see David Evans, Jane Powell, and Tanya Cross, "Patient Advice and Liaison Services: Results of an Audit Survey in England," *Health Expectations* 11 (2008): 304–316; Marie Bismark, Troyen Brennan, Ron Paterson, Peter Davis, and David Studdert, "Relationship between Complaints and Quality of Care in New Zealand," *Quality and Safety in Health Care* 15 (2006): 17–22; Alicia O'Cathain, Jackie Goode, Donna Luff, Tim Strangleman, Gerard Hanlon, and David Greatbatch, "Does NHS Direct Empower Patients?" *Social Science and Medicine* 61, 8 (2005): 1761–1771; Estes et al., "State Long-Term Care Ombudsman Programs," 104–115.

24. Bismark et al., "Complaints and Quality of Care."

25. Mulcahy and Tritter, "Pathways, Pyramids and Icebergs?"

26. Sarah Nettleton and Geoff Harding, "Protesting Patients: A Study of Complaints Submitted to a Family Health Authority," *Sociology of Health and Illness* 16 (1994): 38–61.

27. Entwistle et al., "Public Opinion on Systems."

28. Mulcahy and Tritter, "Pathways, Pyramids, and Icebergs?"

29. See Robert Blendon, Mollyann Brodie, John Benson, Drew Altman, Larry Levitt, Tina Hoff, and Larry Hugick, "Understanding the Managed Care Backlash," *Health Affairs* 17, 4 (1998): 80–94; Mark Peterson, ed., "The Managed Care Backlash," *Journal of Health Politics, Policy, and Law* 24, 5 (special issue, 1999): 873–1218.

30. Regarding Americans as demanding consumers of health care, see Ellie Lee, *Abortion, Motherhood, and Mental Health: Medicalizing Reproduction in the United States and Great Britain* (Hawthorne, N.Y.: Aldine de Gruyter, 2003); Paul Dutton, *Differential Diagnoses: A Comparative History of Health Care Problems and Solutions in the United States and France* (Ithaca, N.Y.: Cornell University Press, 2007). Regarding complaining about faulty nonmedical products, the Kaiser Family Foundation, *National Survey of Consumer Experiences with Health Plans*, Publication No. 3025 (Menlo Park, Calif.: Kaiser Family Foundation, 2000), asked respondents whether they, having "experienced a serious problem with [a company's] products or services," generally found it "worth the time and effort to complain to someone." Two-thirds of respondents indicated that it generally was.

31. Schoen et al., "Toward Higher-Performance Health Care Systems."

32. Kevin Lembo, *Office of the Healthcare Advocate: 2007 Annual Report* (Hartford, Conn., Office of the Healthcare Advocate, 2007).

33. Rosenthal and Schlesinger, "Not Afraid to Blame"; Kelly Shaver, *The Attribution of Blame: Causality, Responsibility, and Blameworthiness* (New York: Springer-Verlag, 1985).

34. Bismark et al., "Complaints and Quality of Care."

35. The findings reported in this chapter are generally kept to simple bivariate relationships, to make them more accessible to readers who are not trained in statistics. However, the relationships described in the text were also analyzed using more statistically sophisticated multivariate regression models; the results reported in the text are those that retained significant relationships with public voice in these more complex models (unless explicitly noted in the text or endnotes).

36. Rosenthal and Schlesinger, "Not Afraid to Blame"; Kelly Shaver, *The Attribution of Blame.*

37. Studies of enrollees' complaining to their health plan have found that problems related to quality of care are less likely to induce complaints than are concerns about administrative matters or coverage issues. See Rosenthal and Schlesinger, "Not Afraid to Blame"; Schlesinger et al., "Voices Unheard."

38. Dan Farrell, "Exit, Voice, Loyalty, and Neglect as Responses to Job Dissatisfaction: A Multidimensional Scaling Study," *Academy of Management Journal* 26 (1983): 596–607; Karen Boroff and David Lewin, "Loyalty, Voice, and Intent to Exit a Union Firm: A Conceptual and Empirical Analysis," *Industrial and Labor Relations Review* 51, 1 (1997): 50–62.

39. The patterns evident in figure 7.7 may also reflect unmeasured aspects of problem severity that lead to greater exit and voice, but our measures of severity and blame are sufficiently robust that these aspects are not likely to be the primary explanation for this positive relationship.

40. On the limited exit from health plans, Brian Elbel and Mark Schlesinger, "A Neglected Aspect of Medical Consumerism: Responsive Consumers in Markets for Health Plans," *Milbank Quarterly* 87, 3 (2009): 633–682; Mark Schlesinger, Benjamin Druss, and Tracey Thomas, "No Exit? The Effect of Health Status on Dissatisfaction and Disenrollment from Health Plans," *Health Services Research* 34, 2 (1999): 547–576.

41. Jacob Hacker, "Privatizing Risk without Privatizing the Welfare State: The Hidden Politics of Social Policy Retrenchment in the United States," *American Political Science Review* 98, 2 (2004): 243–260; Christopher Howard, "The Hidden Side of the American Welfare State," *Political Science Quarterly* 108, 3 (1993): 403–435.

42. Mulcahy and Tritter, "Pathways, Pyramids, and Icebergs?"

43. Paterson, "Patients' Complaints in New Zealand"; Mulcahy and Tritter, "Pathways, Pyramids, and Icebergs?"

44. Entwistle et al., "Public Opinion on Systems."

45. Paterson, "Patients' Complaints in New Zealand"; Pahlman et al., "Three Years in Force"; Mulcahy and Tritter, "Pathways, Pyramids, and Icebergs?"

46. Carole Gresenz, David Studdert, Nancy Campbell, and Deborah Hensler, "Patients in Conflict with Managed Care: A Profile of Appeals in Two HMOs," *Health Affairs* 21, 4 (2002): 189–206.

47. Office of the Healthcare Advocate, Connecticut, http://www.ct.gov/oha.

48. Mulcahy and Tritter, "Pathways, Pyramids, and Icebergs?"

49. It should be noted that this is explicitly an effect related to education, not income. A household's financial resources appear to be unrelated to a propensity toward public voice.

50. May and Stengel, "Who Sues Their Doctors?"; Jane Kolodinsky, "A System for Estimating Complaints, Complaint Resolution, and Subsequent Purchases of Professional and Personal Services," *Journal of Consumer Satisfaction, Dissatisfaction, and Complaining Behavior* 5 (1992): 36–44; Jagdip Singh, "Determinants of Consumers' Decisions to Seek Third-Party Redress," *Journal of Consumer Affairs,* 23, 2 (1989): 329–364.

51. Schlesinger et al., "Voices Unheard."

52. John McDonough, "Using and Misusing Anecdote in Policy Making," *Health Affairs* 20, 1 (2001): 207–212. See also Rachel Grob's chapter in this volume for an explication of this point, drawn from recent policy debates over the expansion of newborn-screening panels in the United States.

53. Mark Schlesinger, "Reprivatizing the Public Household? Medical Care in the Context of American Public Values," *Journal of Health Politics, Policy, and Law* 29, 4–5 (2004): 969–1004.

54. Kaiser Family Foundation, *National Survey on Consumers' Experiences.*

55. Nancy Davenport-Ennis, "Access to Healthcare: Using Data from a Nonprofit Advocacy Practice to Drive Policy Change," in *Patient Advocacy for Health Care Quality,* ed. Jo Anne Earp, Elizabeth French, and Melissa Gilkey (Boston: Jones and Bartlett, 2008), 419–444.

56. O'Cathain et al., "Does NHS Direct Empower Patients?"; Emma Knowles, James Munro, Alicia O'Cathain, and Jon Nicholl, "Equity of Access to Health Care: Evidence from NHS Direct in the UK," *Journal of Telemedicine and Telecare* 12 (2006): 262–265.

57. Jane Garbut, Diana Bose, Beth McCawley, Tom Burroughs, and Gerold Medoff, "Soliciting Patient Complaints to Improve Performance," *Joint Commission Journal on Quality and Safety* 29, 3 (2003): 103.

Patient Appeals as Policy Disputes

Individual and Collective Action in Managed Care

Patients and medical consumers often confront powerful, organized actors and institutions who have focused interests.[1] As individuals, patients usually lack comparative resources and clout. However, acting as a group, patients increase their power, expand their choices, and can often affect policy. This chapter recounts the situation that patients-consumers confronted in the 1980s and 1990s when the growth of managed care created problems for them, particularly the denial of services. They could not solve these problems individually; however, through collective action they secured legislation to address them. State legislation created a right for patients to appeal health plans' denial of services to an independent physician, who decided the dispute.

Ironically, resolving disputes individually through such appeals limited patients' collective influence. Nevertheless, information from these appeals has the potential to yield benefits for patients as a group. But that would require making certain information public that most states either do not collect or do not disclose. Federal policy should require the collection of information from individual patient complaints and appeals so that this aggregated data can reveal problems with health plans and create pressure for these plans to improve their performance and change their policies.

The Potential for Collective Action in Insurance Markets

Individuals have little choice when purchasing health insurance. Insurers sell standard policies that they can accept or reject. Lawyers call these *contracts of adhesion* because purchasers cannot modify the terms. Health plans are unconcerned that a few individuals may opt for a competitor as long as they retain a significant market share. Often, health plans control a sufficient market share to set the market price.[2]

The situation changes when patient-consumers act collectively. Aggregating purchasing decisions creates a countervailing power to that of health plans.[3] A group decision to switch to another insurer has significant effects on a health plan's income. When unions or cooperatives purchase insurance on behalf of members and when employers purchase policies for their employees collectively, patient-consumers can bargain over contract terms.

Grievance and Litigation

Many obstacles impede patients from seeking redress if their health plan does not reimburse medical bills or authorize medical treatment. Patients may be unaware that they have grounds for complaint and that remedies exist, or may think they are unlikely to prevail. They may lack resources to finance a grievance or lawsuit. The cost of taking action might be greater than the benefit it would yield to the individual. Some individuals may retain a lawyer under a contingency fee agreement, but such arrangements exclude many with claims that have merit, because lawyers only accept contingency payment when they can earn high fees in relation to the time they spend and when they have a strong chance of success. Even then, lawyers typically require clients to pay expenses (fees for court filing, expert witnesses, court reporters, etc.).

However, class-action lawsuits allow one lawyer to represent all similarly situated individuals as a group. Many claims that are not profitable for lawyers to pursue individually then become lucrative. Moreover, only a few individuals need to become involved as the named plaintiffs. Thus, efforts by a few individuals create remedies for all individuals with similar problems in the group.

Advocacy groups can facilitate litigation by pooling resources and developing strategy. They can fund litigation to change health plan practices without seeking compensation, lawsuits that lawyers paid by contingency fees will not take. They can also support individual litigation to produce collective benefits. In Anglo-American law, appellate court decisions create precedents that bind courts deciding the same issue in the future. Thus, individual lawsuits can establish a rule that makes policy.

Legislation

As individuals, patients may vote, contribute funds to political campaigns, and support legislation that can change the rules within which markets operate, can create patient rights, or can establish obligations for other parties. However, patients have more influence when they act through organized advocacy groups and in coalitions. Through groups, patients can marshal resources and develop expertise. Contemporary U.S. democratic politics relies on organized groups to represent competing interests. However, not all interests are organized or represented. A key challenge for certain groups—including patients—is that they are often unable to participate in policy making because barriers prevent their forming interest groups, as seen in part 1 of this book. Even then, their resources cannot match those available to major corporations.

The Managed Care Backlash: Aggregating
Individual Complaints into a Policy Dispute

In the 1980s, employers and policy makers began to rely on managed care to control medical spending. Managed care health plans mediated the relationship between individual patients and providers through rules, financial incentives, and contracts. They set practice guidelines, oversaw physicians, and refused payment for services that they deemed unnecessary. They required patients to rely on designated physicians and hospitals or charged higher copayments for using providers outside their network. They created financial incentives for physicians to reduce services. They made primary care physicians gatekeepers to specialists, with financial incentives to reduce referrals. As critics of the system noted, these practices created conflicts of interest for physicians, who were supposed to act on behalf of patients.[4]

As insurers clamped down on resource use, patient-consumers faced common problems, although their frequency and severity are disputed. When managed care health plans made physicians bear financial risk for the cost of treatment, they cut beneficial services in addition to those that were inappropriate. Utilization reviewers did not always authorize appropriate medical care, claiming that it was unnecessary. Health plans denied access to out-of-network providers when no trained provider was available in their network. They refused to reimburse emergency room care when what appeared to be an emergency to the patient turned out not to be life threatening. They limited the duration of hospital stays and restricted other medical services.[5]

As individuals, managed care patients in the 1980s and 1990s were ill equipped to address these problems. The terms of their contracts allowed them to switch health plans only once a year, so short-term market choice (exit) was not an option and switching health plans the next year would not address their current situation. The risk of individuals switching health plans was insufficient to encourage health plans to cater to them, because the loss of an individual enrollee would not significantly reduce their revenue. Furthermore, if the health plan believed it was losing a high-cost patient, it might welcome

their leaving. Patients had no assurance that they would be better off in alternative health plans, since they could not tell ahead of time whether other
plans would grant requests for specific medical treatment. In addition, many
individuals did not have significant options because their employer offered
a choice of only one or two health plans.[6]

Individual complaints and grievances were also rarely an effective
option.[7] Individuals who complained incurred high costs in emotional aggra-
vation and time. Yet health plans had little incentive to heed patient appeals—
if they responded by providing additional services, they reduced their profits.
Medical directors and managers who decided such appeals were not independent actors. Their discretion was restricted by organizational policies, and
their continued employment, promotion, and salary increases depended on
their furthering the organization's goals. They were often compensated with
stock options and bonuses that rewarded them for acting in the organization's
interest.

Lawsuits were rarely a meaningful alternative because the policies of health
plans usually complied with the law. Even where there were legal grounds to sue,
the cost of individual litigation was greater than the potential benefit. Sometimes plaintiffs' lawyers filed class-action lawsuits, but most of these failed.[8]
And over half of employees receive their health benefits through employer
self-funded plans regulated by the Employer Income Retirement Security Act,
which limits the compensation to patients improperly denied medical care to
the cost of service denied. It precludes payment for disability, death, lost
income, or pain and suffering caused by the denial of medical treatment.

Patients *were* able to effect change when they asserted their interests
collectively through the political process.[9] Patient-consumers formed alliances
with physicians, hospitals, and others who would also benefit from change.
In the legislative arena they framed the debate as a contest between insurance
companies and neglected mothers, newborns, and vulnerable patients. As a
result, even legislators ideologically predisposed against state regulation of
markets could support these reforms. In this way, patient-consumers broadened the dispute, developed allies, and changed the dynamics of the conflict,
an effective approach for parties who have insufficient power alone to van-
quish an adversary.[10]

Between 1995 and 2001, patient and consumer advocacy groups pursued
state and federal legislation. The Consumer Coalition for Quality in Health Care
(which emerged as an advocacy group when the Clinton administration attempted
health care reform) organized meetings of consumer groups nationally to this
end. Families U.S.A., the leading national consumer health advocacy group,

also made it a top priority to pass patients' bill of rights legislation. Other health care consumer groups, such as Consumers Union and the Center for Health Care Rights, promoted such legislation. Provider groups chafing under restrictions from health plans threw in their support.[11]

By 2001, forty-seven states had passed patients' bill of rights statutes.[12] These new state laws regulated managed care plans in several ways. Typically, they required that plans pay for emergency room care, out-of-network access to physicians, and other services in specified situations. They mandated that health plans allow patients to consult certain specialists without receiving permission from primary care physician gatekeepers. They required insurers to cover a minimum length of hospital stay for childbirth (see also Elizabeth Mitchell Armstrong and Eugene Declercq, this volume).[13] Most important, their cornerstone was the creation of independent forums to resolve disputes when health plans claim that medical care is either unnecessary or experimental, and so not covered.

Independent Review of Decisions to Deny Services: A Legal Model without Precedent

State patients' bill of rights statutes create a right to appeal.[14] When a patient appeals a health plan claim that therapy is unnecessary or experimental, the case is assigned to an independent review organization, which chooses a physician unaffiliated with the health plan to review the case.[15] If the reviewer decides that the medical care is necessary and not experimental, then the health plan must pay for it. These appeals are referred to as independent medical review (IMR) and independent review, or alternatively, external medical review and external review. Patients must complete the health plan's own grievance process before they seek an IMR.

Ironically, IMR channels collective patient dissatisfaction regarding managed care into multiple individual forms. Rather than aggregate disparate patients with common disputes about a health plan into a group of policy actors, it makes them act as individuals seeking private redress. It thus addresses problems that affect patients nationally as separate individual disputes and removes the advantage that patients have when they act collectively.

IMR creates a remedy only for individuals who appeal. Assuming that the appeal resolves the individual patient's complaint to their satisfaction, they no longer need, or are likely, to press for changes in organizational policy. Providing an individual remedy neutralizes those individuals who are most likely to be agents of change. IMR thus dampens collective action that could lead to change for all patients.

Economist Albert O. Hirschman discusses this phenomenon in his book *Exit Voice and Loyalty.*[16] He notes that when there are multiple providers, consumers can exit to seek a better alternative and that this sometimes relieves pressure for change. In a monopoly, such exit is not an option, and consumers must relieve their problem by voicing their dissatisfaction. Since complainers can't resolve their problems without bringing about changes that will affect the organization's general performance and policies, dissatisfaction promotes change. IMR, however, is an example of voice that is like exit in that it allows the individual to escape the burden of organizational policies that affects others, rather than to change those policies for everyone.

IMR appears to graft a legal model onto medical practice because medical decisions are appealed to a neutral decision maker. However, IMR differs fundamentally from court appeals. Judicial appeals create a standard that is a precedent and binds courts and the public in similar situations. The resolution of individual disputes therefore creates policy. Unlike legal appeals, IMRs don't create a precedent that other health plans must follow. Nor do they require the health plan that lost the appeal to change its policy for other patients that request the same treatment. IMR decisions are rarely public, so patients cannot learn that they have strong grounds to appeal similar denials of service. In effect, IMRs allow health plans to preserve the status quo by making an individual exception.

Reforming Independent Medical Review
So Patient Appeals Can Affect Policy

Although IMR is designed to address only individual disputes, these appeals could yield collective benefits. Patient appeals and other complaints are a greatly underused source of valuable information about organizational problems.[17] IMR data could serve as a window into health plan performance, particularly when combined with other information to yield a fuller picture. These data could reveal when health plans address the same medical issue differently and their grounds for doing so, as well as differences in how they respond to patient complaints.

Studies show that when choosing among health plans, individuals are more interested in knowing about negative experiences that patients have had than about statistics on the health outcomes for members or other measures of health care quality.[18] This preference indicates that health plan members would value information about the incidents that give rise to patient appeals, and how health plans respond. Studies also reveal that when dissatisfied purchasers report their negative experiences, they often dissuade others from purchasing the service or product criticized. Writers on consumer behavior and marketing refer to this phenomenon as "negative word of mouth."[19] It is a potent force that businesses seek to reduce or eliminate, often by resolving individual complaints, sometimes by resolving problems systematically. Critical information from IMRs would have effects similar to negative word of mouth.

If the right kind of information from patient appeals were made public, and publicized by the press or independent groups, that would spur health plans with problems to reform in order to reduce their loss of market share or risk legal liability. Patient groups could use the information for advocacy. Ombudspersons could learn about systemic problems that would affect many patients and so probably require systemic solutions. Organizations that accredit health plans could also interpret the data as part of their evaluation. Regulatory agencies could draw on it for their oversight and investigations.

What States Do with Independent Medical Review Data

We know very little about how well IMR currently functions.[20] Most patient protection statutes do not require collection of much IMR data. Furthermore, agencies that oversee IMR collect very little data that they are not required to gather, and do little with the data they obtain. They typically report how frequently IMRs uphold health plan denials and how often they support patient appeals. They state how many disputes concerned whether requested treatment was medically necessary and how many contested whether treatment was experimental. Sometimes they report this information for individual health plans and the ratio of IMRs per ten thousand insured members. Occasionally they indicate how many reviews were expedited and the number decided in the usual time frame.

In contrast, a few state agencies that manage IMRs analyze the medical issues and therapies that were the subject of the IMR, use the information to oversee health plans, and make it public. California and Massachusetts are leaders in using IMR data but also demonstrate limitations in current best practices.

California

The California Department of Managed Health Care (DMHC) Help Center assists individuals who complain in writing or by telephone regarding their health plan. Complaints address many matters, including denial of services or treatment. Patients who believe their health plan improperly denied medical services might rectify the problem through the health plan grievance process. If their health plan denies services on the grounds that they are unnecessary or experimental, patients can seek an IMR. Often patients pursue the grievance process before starting the IMR because the health plan has not made clear that it is denying the service on the grounds that it is unnecessary or experimental.

The DMHC reports total IMRs, IMRs per ten thousand enrollees, and the percentage of decisions in favor of patients and in favor of health plans. On the DMHC Web page, the public can read summaries of the most recent five hundred IMR decisions.[21] Readers can search for decisions by clinical issue, by thirty diagnostic categories and numerous subcategories, and by thirty treatment categories and numerous subcategories.[22]

The DMHC Web page allows the public to find out if a treatment they seek has been the subject of one or more IMRs and how it was resolved. However, the Web page does not indicate the name of the health plan or medical group involved in each case because the law does not allow disclosing this information. Collecting this information would be valuable because health plans contract with numerous medical groups, each of which have varying practices and policies that affect whether they deem medical care unnecessary or experimental. Decisions to deny medical treatment may be made by either a medical group or a health plan.

In interviews, DMHC officials report that several health plans that have denied a particular treatment and have been overruled by IMR continue to deny that treatment for other patients.[23] These health plans disagree with the IMR decision and say they are not obligated to change their practice for other patients. They hold that in a subsequent IMR, another reviewer might rule in the health plan's favor. If the DMHC reported which health plans did not change their practice after an IMR reverses their denial, advocacy groups could publicize this information to warn the public and urge the health plans to change their practice.

A limitation of the California data is that they do not allow comparing information on complaints *within* a health plan with data on IMRs, or tracing the relation between them, because different categories are used to classify complaints and IMRs. The DMHC uses seven categories to group health plan complaints: (1) access; (2) benefit/coverage; (3) coordination of care; (4) claims/financial issues; (5) enrollment issues; (6) health plan service/attitude; and (7) provider service/attitude. The first five categories include many issues that could lead to an IMR if the patient is dissatisfied with the health plan's final decision and requests an IMR. Access issues include lack of referrals, as well as not obtaining timely appointments, unavailability of primary or specialty providers, and lack of access to medical records. Benefit/coverage issues include disputes over whether referrals to specialists or out-of-network providers are necessary. Coordination of care issues include failure to order sufficient treatment and early hospital discharge, as well as quality of care received and continuity of care when a provider contract terminates. Claims/ financial issues include health plans not reimbursing patients for treatment they deem unnecessary or experimental. In contrast, the DMHC classifies IMR decisions into only two categories: (1) disputes over medical necessity, and (2) disputes over whether treatment is experimental.

Regarding complaints in general, numerous studies reveal that most are settled or dropped in early stages; only a few are pursued to the point of a formal grievance or lawsuit.[24] These studies map the world of complaints as a pyramid, with the bottom representing the large dissatisfied group, above them, a small number who speak out, and at the top the few individuals who pursue their grievance as far as possible. The number who pursue a grievance process declines over time, either because of the effort and time required or because they resolve their grievance. This general pattern is borne out in studies of appeals within HMOs. One study of eleven thousand appeals in two California HMOs between 1998 and 2000 analyzed both preservice denials of service and denials of reimbursement for services. Patients did not appeal beyond the first stage of a three-level appeal process in 93 percent of cases in one HMO and in 98 percent of cases in the second.[25]

Complaints in health plans continue to follow this pattern. In 2005, the DMHC received 6,087 complaints. In over 19 percent of cases where patients complained about denial of health care to the Help Center or initiated an internal health plan appeal, the health plan reversed its decision and provided the service before the completion of the IMR.[26] This means that restrictions on access appear in patient complaints before these complaints go to an IMR and are present more frequently in complaints than in IMRs. Therefore, to identify patterns of denial of medical care, it is important to analyze not only IMR decisions but also health plan complaints resolved without an IMR.[27]

Massachusetts

The Massachusetts Department of Public Health (DPH) uses IMR data to oversee health plans and resolve problems. It reports statistics on IMR decisions using fourteen categories (experimental treatment, excluded services, and twelve practice areas). It does not publish information about what kinds of service health plans denied; however, the public can obtain reports on DPH responses to IMRs.

In 2003, the DPH noticed a high appeal rate for services denied by Magellan Behavioral Health, which administered Blue Cross Blue Shield benefits, and IMRs often decided the services were necessary.[28] The DPH enlisted the

Department of Mental Health (DMH) to review the clinical criteria that Magellan used to determine necessity. It met with Magellan personnel, the DMH, and the Department of Managed Care to review the problem. As a result, Magellan changed its clinical criteria and review process; its appeals rate decreased, as did IMR reversals of Magellan's denials.[29]

The DPH also inspected mental health grievances for five other insurers and requested that they change certain practices. Nevertheless, problems continued. Appeals jumped against Harvard Pilgrim Health Care in 2004, after it replaced Value Options with Pacificare Behavioral Health. United Health Care also generated many appeals over mental health coverage in 2004 and 2005; after an investigation, the DPH in 2006 required United to change its internal appeal process. In addition, when the DPH observed many appeals over fertility treatment due to confusion over what state law requires insurers to cover, it sent every utilization review agency and independent review organization (IRO) a summary of the law.[30]

Expanding the Value of IMR Data

When IROs grew in the 1990s, critics suggested that they were sometimes biased because health plans helped select the IRO. Unlike patients, health plans were repeat players, had the resources to monitor IROs' decisions, and could choose an IRO most likely to decide in their favor. Moreover, many IROs performed other work for health plans—utilization review, quality assurance, internal appeals—and so had incentives to favor health plans in deciding IMR cases, in order to encourage health plans to employ them for their other work.[31]

The Patient Protection and Affordable Care Act of 2010 (PPACA) requires that *all* states oversee a system of IMR and seeks to redress some of these reviews' limitations. It adopts standards from the National Association of Insurance Commissioners' Uniform Health Carrier External Review Model Act (NAIC Model Act) but authorizes the secretary of the Department of Health and Human Services (DHHS) to adopt additional standards. Under the PPACA, state agencies will assign an IRO to review each appeal from a list of accredited IROs. However, the law does not require IROs to forgo other work for health plans, and so many will have conflicts of interest growing out of their other work for health plans. In addition, even when IROs do not have conflicts of interest, they decide what services health plans cover and what technologies they adopt without these decisions being subject to public scrutiny. Moreover, IROs allow multiple private organizations and individual physician reviewers to make these decisions and thereby spawn differences among health plans rather than set a single standard based on evidence.[32]

Patients, health plans, and the public should know the coverage policies of insurers and whether IMR reviewers make sound decisions. IMR and complaint information can be used to evaluate health plan choices and IMR decisions. The DHHS can advance these goals by adopting standards that require the IROs and health plans to report more robust data about medical necessity disputes. It should require reporting of data on the medical problem of the patient who sought an IRO, the therapies or interventions that the insurer claimed were unnecessary or experimental, the evidence the insurer used to justify the denial of coverage, and the evidence the independent medical reviewer used to uphold or overrule the insurer's decision. Reports on each dispute should indicate the names of firms that perform utilization review or manage specialized benefits, such as behavioral health or prescription drugs. These data would uncover problems due to these entities, which often work for multiple health plans.

With such data, it would be possible to compare trends across states, health plans, physician groups, utilization review organizations, and benefit administrators. IMR data will have greater value if insurers also report equivalent information on all complaints, grievances, and appeals within their health plan, as well as equivalent information from their ombudsperson and arbitration. Such data would help identify problems not apparent in IMR data alone.

Some health plans modify what they deem to be medically necessary or experimental for patients after an IMR reverses their decision not to pay for a service, but others do not. Health plans that change their policy should state this with their IMR data, and also notify physicians, utilization reviewers, and managers. And health plans that do not change their policy should be required to explain why they have not. To avoid a negative decision, some health plans might decide to pay for a service only after a patient initiates an IMR but then not change their practice for other patients. To verify whether this occurs, health plans should be required to report their policy on medical necessity for particular clinical issues in cases resolved before the completion of an IMR.

Policy Lessons and Limitations

A key barrier to patients becoming policy actors is their difficulty in forming groups and taking collective action. Another obstacle is that patients prefer not to engage in overt political or policy activity. Frequently, their medical problems are acute and short term rather than chronic and long term, so they do not identify themselves primarily as patients and do not have an interest in spending time and resources organizing or participating in patient advocacy groups.

Without means to facilitate or institutionalize their involvement, patients must marshal resources anew each time.

IMR legislation was a response to patient frustration with managed care. Patient advocacy groups formed alliances with provider groups, enlisted the media, created a public issue, and framed policy debate. Health plans eventually accepted the idea of independent medical review (IMR) as preferable to other reforms that patient groups advocated, such as increased liability for insurers. Yet despite its benefits, IMR does not tap patients' voice on an ongoing basis, give patients a role in governance of health plans, facilitate their organizing, or create mechanisms that further their becoming policy actors.[33] Moreover, IMR allows health plans to make exceptions to policy restrictions only for complainers, and thereby avoid systemic change. Independent medical review substitutes an informal dispute resolution process for litigation against health insurers that could create precedent and change policy. It defuses conflict that could foster the formation of patient advocacy groups or patient involvement in health plan governance.

Reporting patient complaints and IMR data in the manner I have described, however, would allow patients to influence policy change without requiring them to engage in explicit political or organizational work. Tapping that information would expose common problems in health plans. It would foster ongoing changes in response to patient complaints, rather than waiting for a crisis or political backlash to force such changes. Patients may also be policy actors in health plans by participating in surveys or in health plan governance, directly or represented by advocacy groups.

Collective patient voice has limits. Sometimes individuals can act when groups will not or can proceed more quickly than a group, which takes time to mobilize and reach agreement. Just as it is a mistake to transform all policy issues into individual disputes, it is stifling to treat all patient problems as policy questions, ignore individual problems, and preclude physicians and health plans from making individual accommodations. Furthermore, collecting data from independent medical reviews and complaints is only one way to identify restrictions on services, problems with health plan operations, and patient concerns. We should not exclude other ways to assess quality and oversee medical practice.

Notes

1. James Q. Wilson, *The Politics of Regulation* (New York: Basic Books, 1980); Paul J. Feldstein, *The Politics of Health Legislation: An Economic Perspective* (Chicago: Health Administration Press, 1996).

2. James C. Robinson, "Consolidation and the Transformation of Competition in Health Insurance," *Health Affairs* 23, 6 (2004): 11–23.

3. John K. Galbraith, *American Capitalism: The Concept of Countervailing Power* (Boston: Houghton Mifflin, 1956); Donald W. Light, "Professionalism as Counter-vailing Power," *Journal of Health Politics, Policy, and Law* 16, 3 (1991): 499–506; and Mark Schlesinger, "Countervailing Agency: A Strategy of Principled Regulation under Managed Competition," *Milbank Quarterly* 75, 1 (1997): 35–87.

4. Marc A. Rodwin, *Conflicts of Interest and the Future of Medicine: The United States, France, and Japan* (New York: Oxford University Press, 2011). Marc A. Rodwin, *Medicine, Money, and Morals: Physicians' Conflicts of Interest* (New York: Oxford University Press, 1993).

5. Marc A. Rodwin, "Consumer Protection and Managed Care: Issues, Reform Propos-als, and Trade-Offs," *Houston Law Review* 32, 5 (1996): 1319–1381.

6. Jon Gabel, "Ten Ways HMOs Have Changed during the 1990s," *Health Affairs* 16, 3 (1997): 134–145.

7. Marc A. Rodwin, "Exit and Voice in American Health Care," *Michigan Journal of Law Reform* 34, 4 (1999): 1041–1067.

8. Clark C. Havighurst, "Consumers versus Managed Care: The New Class Actions," *Health Affairs* 20, 4 (2001): 8–27; see *Tetti v. U.S. Healthcare* U.S. Ct. of App, 3rd Cir., Judge Sloviter Order Nos. 89–2091/89–2092 (May 23, 1990); *Morris v. Health-Net of California, Inc.* 988 P.2d 940 (Utah 1999); *Pulvers v. Kaiser Foundation Health Plans*, 99 Cal. App. 3d 560 (1980).

9. Marc A. Rodwin, "Consumer Protection and Managed Care: The Need for Organized Consumers," *Health Affairs* 15, 3 (1996): 110–123; Marc A. Rodwin, "Patient Accountability and Quality of Care: Lessons from Medical Consumerism and the Patients' Rights, Women's Health, and Disability Rights Movements," *American Journal of Law and Medicine* 20, 1 and 2 (1994): 147–167.

10. See E. E. Schattschneider, *The Semisovereign People* (New York: Holt, Rinehart and Winston, 1960), chap. 1.

11. Lawrence Brown and Elizabeth Eagan, "The Paradoxical Politics of Provider Re-empowerment." *Journal of Health Politics, Policy, and Law* 29, 6 (2004): 1045–71.

12. Marc A. Rodwin, "Backlash: Prelude to Managing Managed Care," *Journal of Health Politics, Policy, and Law* 24, 5 (1999): 1115–1126; Leatrice Berman-Sandler, "Independent Medical Review: Expanding Legal Remedies to Achieve Managed Care Accountability," *Annals of Health Law* 13, 1 (2004): 233–302; special issue on managed care backlash, *Journal of Health Politics, Policy, and Law* 24, 5 (1999).

13. Geraldine Dallek, *The Best from the States: The Text of Key State HMO Consumer Protection Provisions* (Washington, D.C.: Families USA Foundation, 1997); National Conference of State Legislatures, Managed Care State Laws and Regulations, Includ-ing Consumer and Provider Protections, http://www.ncsl.org/default.aspx?tabid= 14320, accessed March 18, 2010.

14. Aaron Seth Kesselheim, "What's the Appeal? Trying to Control Managed Care Med-ical Necessity Decisionmaking through a System of External Appeals," *University of Pennsylvania Law Review* 149 (2001): 873–920; Geraldine Dallek and Karen Pollitz, *External Review of Health Plan Decisions: An Update*, Kaiser Family Foundation, 2000, http://www.kff.org/insurance/upload/External-Review.pdf; Nan Hunter, "Managed Process, Due Care: Structures of Accountability in Health Care," *Yale Journal of Health Policy and Ethics* 6, 1 (2006): 93–162; Susan J. Stayn, "Securing Access to Care in Health Maintenance Organizations: Toward a Uniform Model of

Grievance and Appeal Procedures," *Columbia Law Review* 94, 5 (1994): 1674–1720; Wendy K. Mariner, "Independent External Review of Health Maintenance Organizations' Medical-Necessity Decisions," *New England Journal of Medicine* 347, 26 (2002): 2178–2182; Eleanor Kinney, "Tapping and Resolving Consumer Concerns about Health Care," *American Journal of Law and Medicine* 26, 4 (2000): 335–399; U.S. General Accounting Office, *HMO Complaints and Appeals: Most Key Procedures in Place, but Others Valued by Consumers Largely Absent,* 1998 (GAO/HEHS-98–119), www.gao.gov/archive/1998/he98119.pdf.

15. The Medicare program has always required that any request for medical service denied be reviewed by an independent organization that it contracts with to review such claims. Some states had required such review before the patients' bill of rights legislation.

16. Albert O. Hirschman, *Exit, Voice, and Loyalty: Responses to Decline in Firms, Organizations, and States* (Cambridge, Mass.: Harvard University Press, 1970).

17. Mark Schlesinger, this volume; Marsha Rosenthal and Mark Schlesinger, "Not Afraid to Blame: The Neglected Role of Blame Attribution in Medical Consumerism and Some Implications for Health Policy," *Milbank Quarterly* 80, 1 (2002): 41–95; Mark Schlesinger, Shannon Mitchell, and Brian Elbel, "Voices Unheard: Barriers to the Expression of Dissatisfaction with Health Plans," *Milbank Quarterly* 80, 4 (2002): 709–755.

18. Judith H. Hibbard and Jacquelyn J. Jewett, "What Type of Quality Information Do Consumers Want in a Health Care Report Card?" *Medical Care Research and Review* 53, 1 (1996): 28–47; Judith H. Hibbard, Paul Slovic, and Jacquelyn J. Jewett, "Informing Consumer Decisions in Health Care: Implications from Decision-Making Research," *Milbank Quarterly* 75, 3 (1997): 395–415.

19. Jane Kolodinsky, "Complaints, Redress, and Subsequent Purchases of Medical Service by Dissatisfied Consumers," *Journal of Consumer Policy* 16, 2 (1993): 193–214; Arthur Best, *When Consumers Complain* (New York: Columbia University Press, 1981); Arthur Best and Alan R. Andreasen, "Consumer Response to Unsatisfactory Purchases: A Survey of Perceiving Defects, Voicing Complaints, and Obtaining Redress," *Law and Society Review* 11, 4 (1977): 701–742.

20. For some of the few empirical studies, see Carole Roan Gresenz and David M. Studdert, "External Review of Coverage Denials by Managed Care Organizations in California," *Journal of Empirical Legal Studies* 2, 3 (2005): 449–468; Carol Roan Gresenz, David M. Studdert, Nancy Campbell, and Deborah R. Hensler, "Patients in Conflict with Managed Care: A Profile of Appeals in Two HMOs," *Health Affairs* 21, 4 (2002): 189–196; David M. Studdert and Carol Roan Gresenz, "Enrollee Appeals of Preservice Coverage Denials at Two Health Maintenance Organizations," *JAMA* 289, 7 (2003): 864–870.

21. The California Department of Managed Health Care Web page for consumer help is http://www.hmohelp.ca.gov/. The public can search and read IMR decisions at http://wp.dmhc.ca.gov/imr/search.asp. Some health plans, such as Kaiser Permanente, require binding arbitration of claims of negligence and other matters. The public can search and read complaint and arbitration decisions at http://www.hmohelp.ca.gov/library/arbitrations/gen_default.aspx. Annual reports on IMR and arbitration are available at http://www.dmhc.ca.gov/dmhc_consumer/pc/pc_arbitration.aspx.

22. California Department of Managed Health Care annual reports, 2001–2006, http://www.hmohelp.ca.gov/.

23. Laura Dooley Beile, California Department of Managed Health Care, HMO Help Center office manager, and Nancy Wong, Senior Counsel, California Department of Managed Health Care, HMO Help Center, telephone interview with author, October 2, 2007.

24. William L. Felstiner, Richard L. Abel, and Austin Sarat, "The Emergence and Transformation of Disputes: Naming, Blaming, Claiming," *Law and Society Review* 15, 3 (1981): 631–654; Best and Andreasen, "Consumer Response to Unsatisfactory Purchases"; Kolodinsky, "Complaints, Redress, and Subsequent Purchases."

25. Gresenz et al., "Patients in Conflict with Managed Care." A follow-up study of only preservice appeals found similar results; see Studdert and Gresenz, "Enrollee Appeals of Preservice Coverage Denials."

26. California Department of Managed Health Care, *Right Care at the Right Time: Annual Report 2005*, http://www.dmhc.ca.gov/library/reports/complaint/2005.pdf, accessed October 16, 2010.

27. Furthermore, if an IMR decision indicates that a health plan should allow certain treatments as medically necessary and the health plan then changes its policy, the change should affect all complaints regarding the same treatments, not only those that have been appealed or have proceeded to IMRs.

28. Office of Patient Protection, Massachusetts Department of Public Health, *Annual Report: January 1, 2003 through December 3, 2003*, http://www.mass.gov/Eeohhs2/docs/dph/patient_protection/annual_report_03.pdf, accessed October 16, 2010.

29. Ibid., *Annual Report: January 1, 2004 through December 31, 2004*, http://www.mass.gov/Eeohhs2/docs/dph/patient_protection/annual_report_04.pdf, accessed October 16, 2010.

30. Ibid., *Annual Report: January 1, 2003 through December 31, 2003*.

31. Dallek and Pollitz, *External Review*.

32. www.naic.org/documents/committees_b_uniform_health_carrier_ext_rev_model_act.pdf, accessed May 14, 2010. Section 1001(4) of the Patient Protection and Affordable Care Act creates a new Section 2719 in the Public Health Service Act, 42 U.S.C. Ch. 6A. The federal law makes the NAIC Model Act a federal regulation that insurers and self-funded benefit plans must comply with. Marc A. Rodwin, "New Standards for Medical Review Organizations: Holding Them and Health Plans Accountable for Their Decisions," *Health Affairs* 30, 3 (2011): 519–524.

33. Marc A. Rodwin, "Representing Consumers in Managed Health Care," *Journal of Health Law* 34, 2 (2001): 223–272.

How Patients Matter

Forty years ago, it would have been difficult to anticipate—perhaps even impossible to imagine—the extent to which patient voices, actions, and representations have succeeded in changing how health policy is made and how health care is practiced, delivered, and experienced. Yet there has been no systematic examination of the overall impact of patients on the health care system, nor has there been an attempt to define what success means when it comes to patient voice and activism.

In this section of the book, authors examine the diverse and far-reaching impact patients' perspectives have had on contemporary health policy. They analyze the meaning and definition of "success" in a variety of settings, from multimillion-dollar research agencies to primary care centers. Though they describe multiple ways in which patients have influenced health policy, the writers also raise important and sometimes troubling questions about how many, how activated, and how well connected patient advocates need to be in order to have an impact on policy and practice. They also ask us to reflect on whether advocates who don the mantle of the patients' perspective have the capacity to adequately represent diverse interests.

Proclaimed Successes in the Absence of Collective Mobilization

As we have noted, patients' perspectives can have an impact even in the absence of collective mobilization. Activation can occur, for example, when individual policy entrepreneurs step forward with sufficient resources and strategic acumen. The patients with rare cancers whose stories journalist Amy Dockser Marcus tells were forced into activism when they realized that researchers had few incentives to work on rare, or orphan, diseases. Faced with dire prognoses and limited time, these patients concluded that a new model of advocacy would be required to change the way the research establishment viewed their cancers. The resulting partnerships spawned between researchers and patient activists represent a striking alternative to conventional models of funding for biomedical research. Yet Marcus warns that the potential for the entrepreneurial model of patient activism may be contingent on certain historical circumstances, and the jury is still out on the longer-term sustainability of these ad hoc partnerships. Still, these entrepreneurial efforts have laid the groundwork for networks that connect previously isolated disease-specific advocates, as exemplified by the Genetic Alliance, a pattern that could eventually extend to other politically disenfranchised groups.[1]

When conditions are less promising for entrepreneurial engagement, other actors may introduce patient perspectives into policy discourse. These potential conduits for patient voice include health care professionals, who have sought to don the mantel of patient advocacy in varying degrees and ways.[2] Historian Julie Fairman's chapter examines the nurse practitioner movement, in which an emerging clinical discipline deliberately and effectively used advocacy for patient needs to advance its own professionalization and to change modes of health care delivery. Although there was not an organized patient uprising on behalf of nurse practitioners, Fairman argues that patients who voted with their feet by showing preferences for and satisfaction with this type of care made up a different type of consumer movement: "individually-mediated, idiosyncratic, and from the bottom up." Like the chapter in part 1 by DiMatteo and colleagues, Fairman's analysis highlights the importance of primary care providers as a central conduit for interpreting patient preferences.

Success Stories with a Twist: Unexpected Consequences of Patient Mobilization

The transformational impact of patient advocates is evident in both state and federal policy making in the United States, and in a number of national policies in other countries. But with each apparent success emerge questions about the compromises required on the road to victory and the longer-term consequences for patients and for subsequent cohorts of patient advocates. These may manifest in a variety of ways, but many of the most consequential can be grouped under two general concerns.

The first concern relates to the reliability of claims about patient interests in the absence of institutional arrangements that assure substantial participation by diverse actors in how these perspectives are formulated and articulated. To be sure, the governance arrangements of professional associations or industry groups (health insurers, hospitals) fall well short of the modest requirements of transparency and due process typically expected from public sector initiatives. Yet even these minimal expectations are absent in groups that purport to represent patient interests. Ironically, these inadequacies are even more pronounced in public agencies that appoint one or more patient representatives to their advisory or oversight committees, in the apparent belief that any patient's experiences are a suitable stand-in for those of all patients.

A second concern involves the space available for patient perspectives in public discourse. Given the apparent disadvantages in terms of resources and political influence that patients face compared to other actors on the health policy stage, it is not surprising that patient advocates typically strive for as simple and coherent a presentation of patient interests as possible. Yet at what cost is this apparent coherence purchased? To what extent are advocates forced to actively suppress discordant voices for fear that heterogeneity might undermine the persuasive appeal of their policy stance? There are many impediments that silence or obscure patient interests, yet ironically patient advocates themselves may not convey a representative image of patient experiences.

The checkered consequences of success are all too evident in sociologist Rachel Grob's account of the proliferation of state-mandated genetic testing of newborns. This policy case provides a stunning example of how one group of vocal advocates—parents of children with genetic diseases—succeeds in a way that obscures crucial differences among health care conditions and parents' experiences, thereby rendering significant unintended consequences almost completely invisible. As a result of such oversimplification, policy makers and the public can lose the capacity to make crucial distinctions among the rationales for and consequences of policy proposals.

Sociologist Steven Epstein considers similar questions to construct a taxonomy of what it might mean to say a social movement has been successful and what challenges persist in the face of success. Reviewing several decades of literature on patient activism, Epstein argues that a definition of success that is confined solely to policy or legislative change is too narrow to capture the transformative power of social movements and patient actions. In addition, he shows that to measure success requires taking into account the problem of representation, of expertise, and of incorporation and cooptation.

The chapters in this book reveal that patients and consumers do not and cannot speak in a unified way. In the epilogue, we return to several questions that follow from these observations: How are we to weigh and evaluate all the competing and compelling voices against each other? How can patient-consumer participation in the health care system and its transformation be as broad, fair, and democratic as possible?

Notes

1. On the emergence of advocacy coalitions connecting disease-group represen-tatives, Jannine De Mars Cody, "An Advocate's Perspective on Newborn Screening Policy," in *Ethics and Newborn Genetic Screening: New Technologies, New Challenges*, ed. Mary Ann Baily and Thomas Murray (Baltimore: Johns Hopkins University Press, 2009), 89–105. On the growing influence of formerly disenfranchised groups, David B. Resnick, "Setting Biomedical Research Priorities: Justice, Science, and Public Participation," *Kennedy Institute of Ethics Journal* 11, 2 (June 2001): 181–204; Steven Epstein, *Inclusion: The Politics of Difference in Medical Research* (Chicago: University of Chicago Press, 2009).

2. Mary E. Barber, "The Role of the Psychiatrist As Advocate," *Psychiatric Quarterly* 79, 4 (2008): 287–292; Rebekah Hamilton, "Nursing Advocacy in a Postgenomic Age," *Nursing Clinics of North America* 44, 4 (2009): 435–446; Susanna Finlay and Jane Sandall, "Someone's Rooting for You: Continuity, Advocacy, and Street-Level Bureaucracy in UK Maternal Healthcare," *Social Science and Medicine* 69, 8 (2009): 1228–1235.

The Power of Us

A New Approach to Advocacy for Rare Cancers

The estimated 1.5 million Americans diagnosed each year with cancer have a better than ever chance of surviving the disease. The five-year survival rate for cancer diagnosed between 1996 and 2004 is 66 percent, up from 50 percent for cancer diagnosed between 1975 and 1977.[1] Scientists' growing understanding of the biology of the disease has led to the development of new drugs, such as Avastin and Herceptin. These drugs are not always able to completely eradicate a cancer, but they have dramatically improved the prognosis for many patients.

Nonetheless, a large and growing number of people with cancer have not benefited from these remarkable changes. These are people that have rare cancers, defined by the National Institutes of Health as affecting fewer than 200,000 individuals in the United States. For people with extremely rare cancers, those with 40,000 or fewer diagnoses a year, the prognosis is particularly grim. Together, these very rare cancers are estimated to be the fourth leading cause of death each year in the United States, according to data presented at a 2007 NIH-sponsored conference on the epidemiology of rare cancers. In combination, they represent 27 percent of cancer diagnoses and 25 percent of cancer mortalities.[2]

There are many reasons why the advances that transformed the treatment of so many prominent cancers have not benefited those with the rarest cancers. The pharmaceutical companies that drive most of the clinical trials for new drugs in this country do not pay attention to rare cancers because the market is so small. The cost of developing drugs is so high and the process so arduous that the companies fear they will never recoup their investment. Single institutions don't usually see enough patients to generate the statistically meaningful data that lead to new theories and approaches. There is no incentive for academic cancer centers to aggregate the data of rare-cancer patients they do see. Researchers who are interested in rare cancers and have creative ideas often find it difficult to get funding to test their theories from either the government or private foundations. Studying rare cancers is not seen as a promising avenue to publishing papers or receiving grants.

I have been covering the complex and troubling issues surrounding cancer for more than five years as a reporter for the *Wall Street Journal.* Over the course of my reporting, I became intrigued by the plight of people who get extremely rare cancers. They remained marginalized, using therapies and facing survival outcomes that went largely unchanged for decades. Their stories stood in sharp contrast to the patient advocacy movements driven by cancer survivors, which are among the most successful ever created. Breast cancer advocacy groups raise huge sums of money for research from private and government sources. Millions of people participate in races and marches to raise money for breast cancer research every year. Lance Armstrong, the biking champion and cancer survivor, made his bright yellow Livestrong bracelets ubiquitous. Stand Up To Cancer, founded by a group of women cancer survivors with ties to the entertainment industry, in its first year of operation raised over $100 million for translational cancer research.[3] Cancer advocacy groups have inspired advocates of many other diseases who seek to emulate their success.

In contrast, patients who get very rare cancers find themselves on their own. The money raised by the most powerful and well-known cancer organizations does not typically fund research into their type of cancer. Many rare cancers are lethal, so there are few survivors to create and sustain large advocacy efforts.

Moreover, even when patients, families, and friends succeed in setting up foundations to raise money for research into specific rare cancers, they often find that the rudimentary tools researchers need to unravel the mechanism of the disease don't exist. There are no repositories for patients' tumors, saliva, or plasma, all vital for testing research questions. No animal models, critical for testing potential therapies, have been created. For rare-cancer advocates, it wasn't enough to raise money or awareness. They needed to create a patient advocacy that addressed the unique obstacles faced by those with uncommon tumors.

In thinking about a new model of advocacy, rare-cancer advocates took advantage of two key cultural changes: greater openness among people in discussing personal cancer diagnoses and treatments, and the development of Internet technologies. These changes made it easier and faster than ever before to find and organize people with rare cancers online and to raise significant sums of money. Instead of adopting the model pioneered by advocates with common cancers, rare-cancer advocates identified the specific obstacles preventing drug development for their cancers and then developed strategies to overcome them. This often meant interacting with researchers, clinicians, and scientists in novel and challenging ways. Many traditional cancer advocacy groups establish scientific advisory boards that evaluate research proposals and determine what to fund based on projects initiated by the researchers themselves. Rare-cancer advocates eschewed this approach, preferring less formal relationships with scientific advisers. Often it was the patients themselves, working with key researchers, who set the strategic scientific plan and research goals rather than waiting passively to see what proposals the investigators generated. Once they determined what needed to be done, the advocates searched out scientists and researchers with expertise in the fields they needed, initiating projects designed to drive the development of new drugs.

In this chapter, I focus on case studies that illustrate a new way of patient advocacy for very rare cancers. The case study approach allows a deeper examination of potential models that can be quickly disseminated and adapted by other rare-cancer survivors. It also reveals some of the limitations and remaining challenges of the emerging strategy. The advocates described here have made a difference in drawing researchers' attention to rare cancers. Some can point to new drugs or compounds that resulted from their efforts that are currently in clinical trials. Still, very few patient advocates can raise the kind of money that is necessary to search for and develop new drugs to treat very rare cancers. The next, most critical, step is to find ways to lower the barriers for others with rare cancers so they also may help drive research and advocacy efforts.

This initiative will ultimately have to come from patients as well. Often advocates are so busy trying to advance the science in their own disease that they do not focus on finding ways to capture and share what other advocacy groups are doing. Developing and disseminating best practices is critical and will make it faster and less expensive for new groups and more patients to launch similar efforts. Only when more advocates focus on drug development will patients who get these diseases receive what people who get common cancers already have: the knowledge that there is a chance that a drug will come along in time to extend their life.

When Marnie Kaufman was diagnosed with a rare cancer in 2004, her husband, Jeffrey, wanted to find a way to spur research into the little-known

disease. Over the previous decades, patient advocates had created an effective
model: raise a large sum of money, put out a call for proposals from investigators and researchers interested in exploring important scientific questions, and
then distribute the funds. It made sense to the Kaufmans that they should apply
the same strategy in trying to advance research in adenoid cystic carcinoma
(ACC), the rare salivary gland cancer that Marnie Kaufman had.[4]

But then the Kaufmans started meeting with the researchers, scientists,
and clinicians who would be the primary beneficiaries of any funds the
Kaufmans raised. They told the Kaufmans to think about a problem they had
not considered: even if they came up with the cash to support ACC research,
they might not get any takers.[5]

Unlike breast cancer or prostate cancer—each of which affects 220,000 or
more people every year—fewer than 1,000 people in the United States are diagnosed each year with ACC, making it an extremely rare cancer.[6] The disease
had a very poor long-term prognosis because it was the kind of cancer that
frequently came back after the initial treatment of surgery and radiation. When
it did recur, there were no effective drugs for further treatment. The situation
seemed unlikely to change any time soon. Pharmaceutical companies hoping
to develop a blockbuster drug considered the market economically untenable,
too few to enable the company to recoup its investment given how long it took
to get a new drug approved and the high failure rate involved in trying to
develop new drugs. Clinicians worried about how to do clinical trials for a disease that affected such a tiny percentage of people in the country when it was
already a challenge to enroll patients with common cancers in trials. It could
take ten to twenty years to complete even the smallest study in a rare cancer.

But this was only the start of the challenges advocates like the Kaufmans
faced. The same market forces that resulted in little attention or interest in rare
cancers by drug companies or academic researchers also affected advocacy
for the disease. The traditional ways of generating huge sums of money for
diseases—marches, 10K races, glamorous evening events that attracted celebrity
names, golf tournaments—often do not work for rare cancers. For one thing,
there is a much smaller pool of family, friends, and colleagues to turn to, by far
the largest source of funding for any patient advocacy group and essential if
fund-raising is not a one-time effort and needs to be sustained year after year.
It was hard to get the broader community excited about a cancer people thought
they had a low chance of ever getting. Even the traditional funding mechanism
most advocacy groups used—collecting a sum of money and then, like the
National Institutes of Health, putting out a request for proposals—was based on
the assumption that a large pool of investigators was already studying the

particular disease. These requests asked investigators to apply for grants based on work they were already doing; success depended on researchers' coming up with their own ideas, developing experiments they wanted to run, and contributing to a body of work that might ultimately lead to finding a treatment for the disease.

But none of this was the case for a rare cancer like ACC. The Kaufmans found an online support group for patients with ACC set up by a patient. It was an important source of information about which doctors saw the most ACC patients and a place to raise challenges associated with living with the disease. The group had raised some money and sent out a request for proposals, but things moved slowly. It was a passive system, dependent on busy scientists taking time to write a grant proposal for an obscure disease. There was no real connection among grants that were funded because they were all awarded to independent investigators who did not coordinate but rather submitted questions that personally interested them. Sometimes those questions were elegant from a scientific point of view but unlikely to lead to a new therapy or make a difference in the lifespan of a newly diagnosed patient. Moreover, there was very little followup or public dissemination of results, so the community had no idea of where things stood. "It was very frustrating" when he started examining the issue, Jeffrey Kaufman said. "You felt it would be a hundred-year process to find a new drug."[7]

There was another major reason that the traditional advocacy model didn't work well when it came to rare cancers. The basic tools researchers needed to pose questions and have a chance of answering them didn't exist. No repositories stored tumors, saliva, blood, and other specimens regularly taken from patients. No researchers had created cell lines based on ACC tumor cells grown in Petri dishes, or in animal models like mice. These were the essential building blocks any researcher needed in order to figure out what was driving the cancer and to test potential drugs to treat it. A huge national cancer infrastructure had been developed that helped drive traditional cancer research forward—NIH-funded labs all over the country, cutting-edge technology that allowed the testing of hundreds of thousands of compounds against cancer cells to see if one or more were effective, the very latest in tools immediately deployed into cancer research. Researchers interested in a rare cancer like ACC had access to none of that because they had no material to run through the system, a circumstance that seemed unlikely to change, because developing cell lines or setting up a tissue bank was complicated, time-consuming work. It rarely led to the scientific publications in peer-reviewed journals that were critical to academic advancement. No one won grants for that kind of labor, so few young researchers wanted to devote the time to working on such a project;

it was an academic backwater, a career dead end. Moreover, few researchers would want to embark on such a project without knowing if the Kaufmans could provide a sustained, multiyear commitment to a project, critical to accumulating enough data to even consider applying to the NIH for larger grants.

The Kaufmans could not help seeing a connection between the lack of interest in the disease by the research community and the fifteen-year survival rate for persons with ACC of only 40 percent that had not changed in decades, despite all the remarkable advances in cancer care and the development of novel targeted therapies such as Avastin, Erbitux, and Tarceva that were making a difference in many common cancers. But the underlying assumptions that had turned breast cancer advocates into such a powerful force for change simply did not hold true in thinking about advocacy on behalf of a rare cancer like ACC. After the Kaufmans founded the Adenoid Cystic Carcinoma Research Foundation, a researcher told them: "Unless you're sitting on $25 million, don't even bother with the traditional model."[8]

Advocates for rare cancers started to realize that since the traditional model had been ineffective for them, they needed to create a new model. In January 2008, Marty Tenenbaum, an Internet entrepreneur, came to the NIH to present one new approach. Tenenbaum had metastatic melanoma, a form of skin cancer that affects fifty thousand people a year. He had just founded CollabRx, a company that developed an informatics platform that would allow people with rare and orphan diseases to run their own virtual pharmaceutical companies. It was a concept designed to take advantage of the huge marketplace of online services, technology once out of the financial reach of patients but now more affordable, and the ability of patients to form linked communities via the Internet. The idea was for patients to contract out to private companies for whatever services and technologies related to drug development that they might need, much the way people bought books from Amazon.

Tenenbaum had set out a detailed road map of his vision in a number of papers and talks, all of which he posted online so that they could be read and shared. In one talk, he called this new model "the power of us," an idea that got to the crux of what was emerging among patient-driven advocates and how it differed from what came before: the insistence that patients themselves had to be the drivers of drug development. On the face of it, this seemed unfair, almost inequitable. Many rare cancers, such as pancreatic cancer, were lethal. They killed patients within a few months; treatments were debilitating. Even in a cancer such as ACC, which was slower growing and so had a better short-term prognosis, Jeffrey Kaufman had taken a leave of absence from his job when he realized that everyone else involved in the research foundation—doctors, pathologists, scientists, clinicians—were so busy with their regular work that if he was not available to prod them, chase down leads, and set up meetings, the effort would never go forward fast enough to help save his wife's life.

Tenenbaum took his inspiration from the software industry. He often described the new model of patient advocacy as being similar to that of entrepreneurs who set a up computer company out of their garage or founded dotcom companies that ended up making a fortune. The idea was to tap into a wider community to lower the cost of drug development enough that it wouldn't totally depend on the market-driven calculations of a pharmaceutical company, long the key obstacle to drug development in rare cancers. For rare-cancer advocates, that meant agreeing to share databases across disease sites so that new leads and emerging information could quickly be disseminated, setting up patient registries to bank specimens so that researchers or pharmaceutical companies would find it easier to study the cancer, finding private labs that could be hired to perform the kind of analysis and services that pharmaceutical companies once did under one roof. "If we can get the costs of drug development down to where patients and patient advocacy groups can pay for it, and the amount of time it takes to find a new drug to be within their lifetime, then we can change the game," Tenenbaum said at the NIH meeting.[9]

There had been efforts by the government to try to address the challenges that patients with rare cancers confronted. In July 2007, the NIH announced that using a high-throughput screening strategy, researchers had identified three new classes of small molecules that may be useful in treating Gaucher disease, an inherited disease that disrupts the cell's ability to dispose of cellular waste products. The discovery could eventually lead to a new treatment to correct the defective enzyme by using an oral medication, a step forward for patients who must now rely on expensive intravenous enzyme infusions that do not control all the symptoms of the disease.[10]

The discovery was made at the NIH Chemical Genomics Center, which had been created precisely with patients like Marnie Kaufman in mind. Researchers in the public sector and at academic centers often lacked the tools that the pharmaceutical industry routinely uses to find leads for possible new treatments, and the drug companies themselves did not have a financial incentive to turn their attention to rare diseases. "What goes on here is exactly what goes on in a technical level in a large pharmaceutical company," said Christopher Austin, director of the center. "We have the same high throughput screens, but we do it for rare and orphan diseases."[11]

Austin estimated that the center was able to work on fifty projects a year. "If you do the math with rare diseases alone, that's a hundred years to get through all the rare diseases," he said. So he relied on people to come to him. "It's like in the business world," he told me in a telephone interview in January 2008. "People find us through word of mouth."[12]

This was one of the key problems advocates for rare cancers faced. They were already operating on the margins. In many cases, they either never found out about the existence of the NIH Chemical Genomics Center; if they did, it took months of networking before they arrived at Austin's offices. A scientist who was already working at the NIH brought the Gaucher project to Austin; she was inside the system and understood what it offered. Once advocates found his lab, Austin was not always able to help, even though this was his mandate. With rare cancers, he said, "the critical limiting reagent" was the lack of an assay, a cell or a protein against which the robots could test a large number of drugs. "You just can't test a lot of compounds in animals; it's not practical because of the numbers you need and the huge expenses," Austin told me over the phone. "What you need is enough knowledge about a disease to be able to model it in a single cell, and that's hard." Of the six thousand rare diseases, Austin estimated that there was sufficient basic knowledge about the diseases to develop a cell-based model that could be used in screening in only 5 percent of them.

Patient advocates "need to come to us with an assay," Austin said in our phone interview, and that was another hurdle that patients with rare cancers faced. Most assays got developed because someone in the academic world was interested in studying a disease. It usually took years to develop a good assay, and with the lack of funding available for research into rare cancers, the number of investigators in academia working on assay development was small at best. Some rare-disease foundations, like the CHDI Foundation, which focused on finding cures for Huntington's disease, and the Cystic Fibrosis Foundation, had enough resources to fund multiple investigators willing to develop assays, but that was too expensive a proposition for many advocates in the rare-cancer arena. The patient advocates who came regularly to talk to Austin, walk through his lab, and admire his robots argued that even though the NIH put all the data it gathered from the center's projects into the public domain with the hope that either academics or pharmaceutical companies would use the information to develop the data into a drug for a rare disease, "we all know it won't happen." Austin believed that, in selected cases, "we should try to move it forward ourselves," working closely with the advocates.[13]

He had started to do this on a small scale when he met Josh Sommer, who had been diagnosed with chordoma, a rare bone cancer that develops in the head or spine, in January 2006 while a freshman at Duke University. There were only three hundred new cases diagnosed every year. In May 2006, Sommer underwent surgery to remove the tumor, but there were no known effective therapies if the cancer recurred, and the average survival time was stuck at seven years after diagnosis.

In November 2006, Sommer had attended a lecture at Duke by Neil Spector, director of translational research in oncology at Duke. Spector was giving a talk about his research into the epidermal growth factor receptor, which when mutated can cause breast cancer. Sommer, researching chordoma on his own, had found that the same receptor might play a role in its development. He approached Spector about testing the drug and others he was studying in his lab against chordoma cell lines. Spector agreed.

Josh Sommer and his mother, Simone, didn't have enough resources to test huge numbers of compounds against the assays they were beginning to develop. But they had met Austin at a recent conference in Washington, D.C., and when he learned that the Sommers had engaged some labs at Duke to study chordoma, he agreed to work with them. By January 2008, the center's robots were at work on chordoma, at no charge to the foundation.

Austin saw his lab as part of an emerging infrastructure that rare-cancer advocates would be able to tap. Some of it would be available for free, supported by government funding. Patient advocacy groups could buy some of it from private vendors, depending on what was needed to move their specific cancer closer toward drug development. To make this idea work, a combination of government and private investment was needed. It would be financially impossible for "every rare disease group that gets started to recreate it on its own," Austin told me in our phone interview. Once more groups like the Chordoma Foundation figured out how to tap into this research infrastructure, the information could be collected and disseminated to other groups, lowering the barriers to entry. Such an effort would also lower the cost of drug development for other groups interested in rare diseases, because "it stands to reason that you can amortize the costs across diseases by sharing infrastructure and gathering any data and experience that is collected," Austin said.

In April 2008, one year after he first met Josh and Simone Sommer, Austin already was able to present some initial findings based on testing they had done with the chordoma cell lines. "This kind of meshing of what the public and the private sector can do can make a difference in rare cancers," Austin told me.

Austin planned to test this idea further in 2009. Working with a group of government officials, patient advocates, clinicians, and researchers, he helped create a new NIH program, Therapeutics for Rare and Neglected Diseases.[14] The idea was that government funding would pay for the expensive, labor-intensive process of taking compound leads generated by Austin's institute and then developing them into drugs that could be tested in clinical trials. But for this plan to work, the patient advocates were going to have to play a new role. First, they would have to support and encourage young researchers to want to come to Austin's institute to learn how to develop assays. Without this first step, compounds would never get developed. Once compounds were developed, a scientific advisory board would have to prioritize the order in which they were sent for further development, weighing a variety of factors to select which ones would be tested in the newly formed NIH lab. This would be a complex decision with many factors involved.

Even so, under the terms of this program, rare cancers and rare diseases in general, would be playing on a more level field. If the advocates could raise some money, they could entice more researchers to study their disease, and development of an assay would go more quickly. If they proved to be good project managers, organizing a coalition of interested parties such as clinicians, researchers, and academic centers, they could more forcefully argue that the infrastructure existed to support the lab if it generated compounds to be tested. In order to go to clinical trial, pharmaceutical companies would need patient registries so they could quickly identify potential candidates to enroll. They would need access to tissue and specimen banks so they could continue to test any drug in the lab. A network of academic centers would have to be set up to coordinate all of this at sites around the country. This was all material or information that only patient advocates had the interest and ability to collect quickly.

The strategy of the new program played to the strengths of patient advocates like the Kaufmans or the Sommers. It required people who had life-threatening illnesses—some sick and in treatment and already struggling to keep their families going—to also become project managers, to educate themselves quickly on the scientific enterprise, to put together research coalitions. If they were willing to do this, they would not only have a chance to persuade the board to green light a drug's development for their disease. They would also help demonstrate the efficacy of the idea that drug development should be based not on the size of the market—that is, not on "market opportunism"— but on "scientific opportunism," Austin told me.[15] In thinking about how to overcome the limits of market opportunism, and to increase the opportunities for scientific opportunism, the Kaufmans raised more than $700,000 for ACC in the first year after they founded the organization. They decided not to send out a request for proposals but to take matters into their own hands. They did not want a large scientific advisory board; that was too unwieldy and it would be too difficult to get that many people together frequently in order to craft a scientific strategy. So they identified four scientists and researchers, leaders in head-and-neck cancers or experts in the field of drug development, who helped them develop a scientific plan. They identified what they still did not know, and what the critical steps were if new drugs were to be discovered or developed to treat ACC. Once they knew their key areas of focus, they searched for scientists, labs, groups, or researchers that had expertise in the areas they needed. Then the Kaufmans went out and hired the people they wanted to work on specific projects. Sometimes they did it the traditional way, by offering a grant to get something done. Other times, when they wanted specific tests run on a promising compound, they simply wrote a check, buying a scientific service like they would any other. Jeffrey Kaufman had been a money manager at Putnam Investments in Boston when his wife was diagnosed. He tried as much as possible to break down the issues in terms of commodities—what could he buy in the marketplace, and what did he need to have developed from scratch?

Some of the people the Kaufmans ended up working with would never have sought grant money from the foundation on their own. They might have been too busy with other work to fill out a grant application, or decided that it wasn't worth applying for a grant that might not be available the next year. But the Kaufmans didn't just offer money to the researchers. They tried to figure out additional incentives to induce researchers to invest time and effort in the project. So when they realized that M. D. Anderson Cancer Center and the University of Virginia had each collected a significant number of ACC tumor samples, they offered to fund a lab technician in each place to work on the samples, with the condition that part of the job would be standardizing the collection of additional material to insure data could be pooled, and distributing the samples to other scientists working with the foundation and studying ACC. They provided funding to researchers at the few institutions where sporadic work on ACC had previously been done, but insisted that they focus on creating new animal models of ACC, an essential building block for testing drugs in the disease.

The approach had its own challenges. If a scientist responds to a request for proposals with a grant application, it is for something that he knows he wants to do. It is his own idea, so he brings passion to it. In the case of the Kaufmans, they knew what they wanted done, but they had to persuade researchers that they wanted to do it too. In some cases, the incentive was allowing the institution to retain the rights to any information that was generated, which could be valuable if drug development were pursued. They reached out to the Institute for Drug Development in San Antonio, whose researchers develop new treatments for cancer, and signed a contract to expand the number of mouse models and also test a number of compounds to see if any of them stopped or slowed the progression of ACC. They offered to gather the tumor samples themselves, so the project would not bog down over that lack, and let the institute keep the rights to any information that was generated during the course of the project. The Kaufmans helped organize and increase the number of fresh tumor samples that got banked. When they knew a patient was going in for surgery to have a tumor removed, they worked closely with the patient, surgeon, and pathologist to arrange for tissue banking. They came up with a protocol for standardized banking so that moving forward, each of the academic centers that they funded would follow the same steps when they did tissue banking, share the specimens they had, and pool any research that emerged.

Sometimes the price tag was lower than the Kaufmans expected. They were able to take advantage of economies of scale, just as Austin had predicted would happen. They spoke personally with scientists working with the most cutting-edge technologies about what they were doing to drive research in ACC. Intellectually intrigued about gaining access to a hard-to-obtain cell line like ACC, these researchers often agreed to add ACC to their ongoing studies. The Kaufmans were therefore able to gain access to technologies that would have been extremely expensive at a private lab, lowering their own costs.

As Jeffrey Kaufman learned more not only about ACC but also about rare cancers, he realized that although every rare cancer is at a different stage in the research process, they share similar problems. It wasn't only ACC that lacked model systems for testing leads, but most rare cancers. Researchers needed the same building blocks in order to advance the science; they all needed access to more specimens, genomic and proteomic studies to find compound leads, and xenograft models for screening potential drugs. The Kaufmans had come up with a way to get all these building blocks for ACC, but he believed that with some seed funding, the same research team he had set up to push forward research in ACC could do something similar for five other rare tumors every year, first in head-and-neck cancers, their specialties, but after that for any rare cancer that needed to make progress in drug development.

There is now a cadre of patient advocates like the Kaufmans who are able to lead this kind of work. These advocates contradict the traditional notion that only scientists can come up with important hypotheses regarding diseases. In rare diseases especially, where few if any specialists focused exclusively on just one disease, patient advocates had turned themselves into experts. They had the time and the incentive to read widely, to think outside the box, to look for connections with other diseases. Many of the patient advocates were able to come up with novel ideas to try, and with some help from their scientific advisory boards, they had a keen grasp on where the science should be headed in order to move faster toward potential new therapies to treat their diseases. Many of them through their deep immersion in a wide range of topics related to their disease are able to see connections that have eluded the scientists.

What was unique about this new model of patient advocacy was that it took a strategic approach to every aspect of the drug development process. In setting up the Adenoid Cystic Carcinoma Research Foundation, the Kaufmans cast their scientific net widely, providing funding and pushing for projects but always in three main categories: specimens and models, basic research, and translational research that would eventually get new therapies into patients' hands. It had not been easy for them, or for any of the advocates embarked on this new model. It was like running a start-up; they were advocacy entrepreneurs, and they paid a steep price. Jeffrey Kaufman had not been able to continue working full-time at Putnam. He found that being the driver, the project manager, was something he could not do in the middle of the night, or on weekends, or after he got home from work. So he took a leave of absence and eventually left his job to work on the foundation full-time. Josh Sommer had not been able to continue his full-time studies at Duke. He still got frequent headaches, and he was closely monitored for any signs of recurrence; getting the foundation up and running, pushing for the generation of so much scientific data, and then having to assess what it meant and how to continue to move it forward was something he needed to do full-time.

Advocates' paying such a price raised questions about the efficacy and equity of this new model. Not everyone could afford to leave their jobs as Jeffrey Kaufman had. Not everyone wanted to take a leave from their regular life as Josh Sommer had, to transform themselves into full-time advocates, project managers, citizen scientists. There were also those who criticized this model by pointing out that, for the vast majority of the rare cancers that had attempted this new model of advocacy, there was still no cure. Although it was true that many of the diseases were as lethal as they had been when the advocates began, now cell lines existed that had not before, and so did patient registries and tissue banks. In some cases, although the advocacy groups had not found a cure, their efforts had led to the development of new therapies that at least extended the lives of patients, and this was no small achievement in diseases where the standard treatments often had not changed in decades.[16]

There was no doubt that not everyone could muster—or should even be expected to muster—the level of resources required and the kind of commitment exacted. The Kaufmans had no medical background, so they had to educate themselves about Marnie Kaufman's disease in a substantial way in order to be able to work effectively and closely with their scientific advisers. But they understood that they were the pioneers of a new model, and that once a blueprint for how to do this kind of work was developed, it would be faster, cheaper, and easier for others to do what they had done.

The Kaufmans, the Sommers, Tenenbaum, and the other patient advocates have created some of the most innovative new models in health care. They identified the obstacles in the way of making progress toward a cure, then made strategic investments to remove them. This often meant seeking out and learning about what had been done in other diseases, and then adapting the methods to their own efforts. It also required a combination of private and public resources, fostering collaboration among a set of diverse but interested players, all with the idea of driving research and drug development faster than before.

Driven primarily by the passion of the patients themselves, these groups have been able to set up tissue and specimen banks, create new cell lines for testing lead compounds, establish patient registries, form clinical trial networks, and raise significant money for high-risk research that usually cannot secure public funding. Many times they were able to generate scientific connections and theories that have had an impact not only on their illness but also on other, more common diseases. They were able to do this by forging partnerships with people, groups, and institutions that saw something to gain— academic researchers who realized that patient advocates can be effective partners in helping advance interesting research, government officials who realized that given tight federal funding for projects, forging collaborations with patient-driven groups is an effective use of resources.

But launching a patient-driven advocacy group still took too long and was too expensive. Josh Sommer said it took him months to track down critical information he needed, such as identifying government resources, including Austin's lab, that are able to do key scientific experiments for free. Kathy Guisti, who was working in the pharmaceutical industry when she was diagnosed with the rare cancer multiple myeloma and then cofounded one of the most successful patient-driven research groups, the Multiple Myeloma Research Foundation, estimated in our December 2007 telephone interview that she spent hundreds of thousands of dollars just on legal fees in order to hammer out protocols, agreements, and contracts that are now used among the members of the consortium.[17] The high costs of doing this kind of work are prohibitive. But there is a human cost too—someone with a lethal disease and a potentially limited amount of time wastes months and months trying to learn how to do something, when so much of this knowledge is available already. Giusti gives interested patient advocacy groups who want to run clinical trials or found their own consortium free use of the protocols she spent so much money hammering out with lawyers. But too often, she told me, advocates either don't know how to find her or they don't ask for help. Sometimes groups do ask Giusti to come speak with them or serve as a kind of consultant. She estimates that she spends hours doing this kind of work, all free, because she wants to help other advocates try to replicate what she did for multiple myeloma, an effort that has led to the development of four new FDA-approved drugs for the disease and sixteen more in clinical trials.[18] But she can't spend all her time helping other advocates or she won't have enough time to devote to finding cures and more effective therapies for multiple myeloma.

As a result, despite the many impressive achievements of groups like the Adenoid Cystic Carcinoma Research Foundation or the Multiple Myeloma Research Foundation, many patient-driven groups have no idea what other patients are doing. They waste precious time and scarce resources trying to figure out what they need to do. Because there is no way for the Kathy Giustis and Jeffrey Kaufmans to share information, research, and findings, what gets lost are patterns across and between diseases, promising drug leads that might be effective in more than one drug, the results of failed and successful experiments that would prevent the enormous amount of duplication in science, and all kinds of invaluable information from off-label drugs. If such information was shared and exchanged between and among these groups, the result could be advances that would help many other patients, including patients with more common diseases.

Despite the success of these new models, "the power of us" cannot be truly harnessed unless innovative ways are created to allow patient-driven groups to get connected, share data, build on each other's insights and finds, and—most important of all—create economies of scale that will lower the cost of research, clinical trials, and drug development for everybody. There should not be tens of groups like the Kaufmans—there should be hundreds, even thousands, if change is truly going to be made. This won't happen unless more people participate in driving drug development in rare cancers by creating access to public-private partnerships to share in the cost of funding scientific research and by cutting the time it now takes to get a group off the ground. If we truly want to deepen patient involvement in their own health care—and there is no other way to improve the prognosis for patients with rare cancers unless we do just that—then we must lower the costs of these efforts by leveraging work that is already underway and taking advantage of economies of scale that do not now exist.

One of the things that Jeffrey Kaufman and many other advocates discovered when they entered the world of rare-cancer research is that many patients end up being treated with existing drugs that are used off-label. But the results of this widespread off-label use are rarely captured or shared in a rigorous way. A doctor may have a plausible hypothesis for why a drug created for the large colon cancer market might also be effective in a very rare cancer like gallbladder cancer, and that drug may in fact produce a modest response that could help other patients. But although this possibility is marked in an individual patient's medical record, that is as far as it goes. Important leads that could ultimately lead to new clinical trials and possible uses for drugs in different diseases have little impact beyond an individual doctor's office. This benefits no one. Patients who have the same disease may never learn of a possibly helpful drug, a shame in rare cancers that often have no effective therapies at all. Drug companies that could financially benefit from a new patient market end up with no data to back up these new market opportunities and no financial incentive to launch a trial in a disease that has a relatively small number of patients. Doctors who want to think outside the currently existing and often very limited standard-of-care arsenal rarely learn what other doctors are using.

Patient advocates often complain that doctors and researchers work in so-called silos, unwilling to share results outside their lab, unable to see the big picture. It turns out that patient advocates also find themselves working in silos. They meet at conferences sponsored by trade groups, umbrella organizations, think tanks. These conferences are invaluable as critical social networking opportunities. But if this new form of advocacy is going to become more widespread, then more systematic, frequent sharing of data, technologies, strategies, and methods is crucial. Even with all the remarkable achievements advocacy groups have made in the rare-cancers arena, they have failed to produce a grassroots effect from their efforts. To drive forward the search for cures, patient groups are going to be far more powerful if they work together than if they try to go it alone. If patient advocacy isn't driven by the grass roots, it ultimately isn't going to work any better than the old system it has been seeking to replace.

It is going to take time to create the systems that are necessary to support and even grow the patient-driven advocacy groups that have emerged. There are steps that can be taken to lower the barriers to pursuing this new model. A research map to help patient advocates identify existing resources inside the government needs to be developed. Too many patient advocates hear by chance about resources like the Austin lab, which exists to help patients with rare cancers and rare disease; finding such resources needs to be a faster, easier process less subject to serendipity. The NIH's Office of Rare Diseases already holds occasional workshops for patient advocates to help educate them about the NIH. These workshops should be broadened to serve as springboards for pilot projects that advocates, researchers, government officials, and pharmaceutical companies agree are the most urgent to try. It is not only about allocating more resources, but also about making existing resources available to more people.

As the number of patient-driven groups increases, an online network must be created where best practices can be disseminated and shared. There also needs to be a concerted effort to develop specimens and model systems for all cancers for which there are still no effective therapies. In contrast to the more common cancers, in rare cancers that have been understudied "just having a basic tool like a cell line can make a huge difference," says Michael Kelley, who runs a lab at Duke University where Josh Sommer worked studying chordoma.[19]

But the most important policy change that needs to take place is the development of a more systematic approach to developing drugs for rare cancers. The early drivers like the Kaufmans or the Sommers realized that they were going to have to go outside the traditional system, first finding private companies to provide services and essentially purchasing what they needed, and then going back to the government once they had some initial results and demanding that these be pushed further along. When breast cancer advocates got started, they lobbied to have the government support significant amounts of basic research through increased federal funding and new grants. The rare-cancer advocates knew right away that this strategy would be less effective in diseases that affected a few hundred or a few thousand people. Now the next step is to insure that the model that the Kaufmans and Sommers and others like them have pioneered should not be available only to people who can raise huge amounts of cash. The only way to bring down the cost of this kind of enterprise is to share information and create economies of scale. Austin argued that his lab can make drug discovery cheaper for everyone if, through a combination of government and private funding and collaboration, steps are taken to collect standardized data from each experiment his team does with patient advocates and then analyze the results for connections within and across diseases.[20] Such collaboration would drive additional projects with choices and decisions based not on market size but on scientific opportunities. That some of those opportunities have been created by the efforts of the patients themselves is one of the most important contributions these groups have made. Enough of them have gone through it to start believing that, as Jeffrey Kaufman said, "we can help others do it too."[21]

Notes

1. American Cancer Society, *Cancer Facts and Figures 2009*, http://www.cancer.org/Research/CancerFactsFigures/cancer-facts-figures-2009.

2. National Cancer Institute and Office of Rare Diseases, National Institutes of Health (sponsors), "Synergizing Epidemiologic Research on Rare Cancers" conference, May 10–11, 2007, Bethesda, Md.

3. The figure is cited by Stand Up To Cancer in a press release at http://www.standup2cancer.org/node/2718.

4. Many examples of the request-for-proposals model are listed on the Web site of the National Organization for Rare Disorders (NORD), an advocacy and umbrella group for patients with rare diseases. NORD runs its own program (www.rarediseases.org/research/requests) and also lists RFPs from member organizations (www.rarediseases.org/research/member_org_rfp).

5. Jeffrey Kaufman, interview with author, Needham, Mass. March 5, 2007. The Kaufmans' story also appears in Amy Dockser Marcus, "Coaxing Cancer Researchers to Take Your Money: Sometimes Even Large Sums Can't Attract Scientists to Investigate Rare Diseases," *Wall Street Journal*, May 22, 2007.

6. Kaufman interview. Statistics about ACC and information about the disease can be found at the Adenoid Cystic Carcinoma Research Foundation Web site, accrf.org.

7. Kaufman interview.

8. Ibid.

9. Marty Tenenbaum, interview with author, January 28, 2008, Rockville, Md. More detail about Tenenbaum's ideas appears in Amy Dockser Marcus, "Putting Drug Development in Patients' Hands: An Entrepreneur Stricken with Cancer Sets Up Firm to Develop 'Virtual' Biotechs," *Wall Street Journal*, July 29, 2008.

10. U.S. Department of Health and Human Services, "Novel Approach Targets an Inherited Disorder," *NIH News*, www.genome.gov/25522141.

11. Christopher Austin, interview with author, Rockville, Md., January 28, 2008.

12. Christopher Austin, telephone interview with author, January 16, 2008.

13. Ibid.

14. More information about the program appears in Amy Dockser Marcus, "NIH Takes on New Role in Fight against Rare Diseases," *Wall Street Journal*, July 23, 2010.

15. Austin interview, January 16, 2008.

16. Kathy Giusti, telephone interview with author, December 12, 2007.

17. Ibid.

18. Ibid.

19. Michael Kelley, telephone interview with author, October 2, 2008.

20. Christopher Austin, interview with author, Washington, D.C., May 20, 2008.

21. Kaufman interview.

Patients and the Rise of the Nurse-Practitioner Profession

Patients influence health policy in both subtle and direct ways.[1] In this chapter, I present a subtle case, one in which patients helped legitimize the growth of a new provider in the 1970s, the nurse practitioner. Nurse practitioners positioned themselves as uniquely attuned to what patients wanted—hands-on care that was personal, local, and familiar. The rise of the nurse practitioner profession shows that unanticipated forces—individual patients and nurse practitioners—provided the foundation for transforming part of the health care delivery system from a piecemeal, reductionist model based on disease to one that emphasized primary care with its focus on the patient's context of family and community. To be sure, many primary care physicians during this time also practiced in a broader context, but there were never enough of them, and the medical education system could not reassure a worried public and policy makers that medical students could be enticed into primary care in numbers large enough to meet demand.

Patient choices—their voices—supported expanding the bounds of nurses' practice, sustained this expansion, and demonstrated its relevance to the health care system. This was not unified, coordinated patient voice, but a case of individual needs coalescing in unorganized, place- and time-dependent popular support of a common idea—that nurses could provide the personalized care patients wanted. Additionally, professional nursing organizations used patient preferences as a basis for improving opportunities for professional nurses, developing a patient-focused message, and arguing for changes in the health care system. In short, patients can have a crucial influence on health policy on both a local and a broader national level—they can be essential actors—even when they are not acting with any notion of the public good in mind, even when they are not trying to influence policy making, and even when they are unaware of how their individual choices might impact the legitimacy of a profession. The patient perspective is consequential even when it is indirect or tangental to larger health policy debates.

Background: Nurse Practitioners

In 1965, University of Colorado public health nurse Loretta Ford came together serendipitously with pediatrician Henry Silver to address the lack of pediatricians in rural Colorado and to formalize and strengthen the type of services public health and pediatric nurses had been providing to the poor in rural areas of the state.[2] Ford explained that she was interested in expanding the nurse's role "not because there was a shortage of physicians . . . maybe it provided the opportunity, but to tell you the truth, I wasn't even aware of it. It wasn't in my frame to help medicine out." She saw the nurse practitioner role as a way to legitimize what she and her public health colleagues were already doing. "When it came right down to it," she said, "we were making decisions. . . . There was nobody else, and, the poor families . . . frankly expected you to make those kinds of decisions anyway."[3] Ford and Silver designed a post-baccalaureate curriculum at the University of Colorado's Schools of Medicine and Nursing that included courses such as pathophysiology, child development, and health promotion.[4] Graduates of this program, armed with deeper and broader clinical knowledge, were called nurse practitioners.

Patient Choice and Voice

That patients influenced the delivery of health care services by their acceptance and choice of nurse practitioners demonstrates a relationship between the formation of larger health policy decisions, social movements, and the role of individuals. In fact, if one considers the role of individual patients and their attempts to gain basic, personalized services to meet their health care wants and needs, the idea of an individual voice joining those of others into a chorus, however unorganized, may be a crucial democratic and participatory action. These forces coalesced in the early 1970s to support a model of care centered on patients within larger cultural and social systems rather than on the visit of one ill patient and highlighted the growing problem of a delivery system based on acute care services.

Few patients in the 1970s believed they were empowered to change the health care system, especially through their choice of provider. But patients' demand for nurse practitioners shows up directly and indirectly through their use of services in clinics and private practices, patient satisfaction surveys, and coverage in popular publications. Patients' individual actions, although difficult to document, nonetheless were a crucial driving force and leave footprints that are important for understanding the changes in health care delivery that occurred in the 1970s as the nurse practitioner movement gained momentum.

Although the cumulative effect of patient preferences may seem only tangentially linked to national health policy, it is a complex and unacknowledged source of policy change that is both reliant on and separate from market forces and payment structures. Historians have documented market forces, such as payment and supply and demand, as important factors in patient preference, but they also acknowledge the influence of place, as well as of powerful social and political contextual forces such as race, class, and gender.[5] In the 1970s, physician overextension and unavailability, along with the force of various nonmarket-based social movements (e.g., the women's and consumer movements), coupled with public dissatisfaction with the structure of medical care, motivated patients to seek services in clinics staffed by nurse practitioners or teams of practitioners and physicians.[6]

An influential medical profession erected barriers to patient access to nurse practitioners through its effort to limit their practice scope and their ability to receive payment for services from third parties. Nonetheless, patients in many areas found their way to nurse practitioners in settings as diverse as self-pay or public-supported community clinics, women's health clinics, childbirth centers, and third-party hospital clinics.[7] Despite physician opposition, patients gave legitimacy to nurses practitioners, sustained them, and demonstrated their relevance to the health care system by continuing to seek their services.

Health policy changes, including the infusion of large amounts of federal money through Nurse Training Acts, occurred over the next two decades. Private organizations such as the Robert Wood Johnson Foundation earmarked money for nursing education and practice models. Starting with Idaho in the early 1970s, states began to change their practice laws to accommodate expanded nursing practice, and many physicians integrated nurse practitioners into their practices. Hospitals reorganized services, creating, for example, nurse-managed outpatient clinics or more homelike birthing experiences that imitated nurse midwife–run birth centers.[8] All these policy changes were retrospective in nature, supporting and formalizing changes already occurring on the ground.

Patients' Reliance on Nurses' Expanding Boundaries

In the late 1960s and 1970s when medical and nursing journals began to report on nurse practitioners, the public did not realize or understand what these nurses could do. Most people interacted with nurses only when they were acutely ill and hospitalized or when they sought routine care in private physician offices. The experiences and perspectives of patients were based on occasions when they were at their most vulnerable or were in places where nurses most often took on dependent roles.

Nurse practitioners broadened patients' perspective of what nurses could do. Most patients seeking medical care, "the well and the well but worried," as well as those needing coordinated care to manage chronic illnesses, benefited from their services.[9] Nurse Loretta Ford described her work in Colorado: "We would have the whole county to cover in terms of schools, maternal and child health follow up. We would have classes that we taught for the Red Cross. We would have [disabled] children's clinics, tuberculosis clinics, school clinics, immunization clinics, the child health nursing conferences, and child health conferences. So we were doing generalized services and lots of it."[10]

In Ford's clinics, typically serving the middle class or poor in rural Colorado communities, patients had little choice of providers since few physicians practiced in these areas. But they had the best opportunity to see the kinds of services nurses could offer, their talent for anticipating patient needs, and their ability to work across multiple relationships and settings. The patient encounter become larger than the visit, as the nurse practitioner might pull in resources to help with questions about nutrition, child development, or the problems of daily living with a chronic illness.

Indeed, patients found nurse practitioners to be reasonable and safe providers of care and able to offer access when no other provider was nearby, expertise in particular skills, and hands-on, personalized services that made them more comfortable relating personal and physical problems. Such patient experiences were supported by a growing number of research studies, reports by philanthropic and federal agencies, and the popular press. Study after study documented the safety and high quality of care nurse practitioners provided groups of patients with particular problems. The long-term effects of chronic hypertension, high cholesterol, and functional disabilities (e.g., difficulty walking, dressing, or writing or sexual dysfunction) caused by treatment complications and side effects were particularly responsive to care by nurse practitioners by virtue of their broader nursing paradigm.[11] The high quality of this care was clear from a meta-analysis by the Office of Technology Assessment of studies done primarily in the 1970s that estimated nurse practitioners safely cared for more than 75 percent of patients typically seeking the services of primary care physicians.[12] Most physicians, whose education and practice focused on increasingly complex patient problems, were not trained to be particularly effective in dealing with the everyday issues of managing chronic illness, nor did they have a great deal of interest in taking on patients with these issues.[13]

Backed by public appropriations to support demonstration projects and education programs, and private support from foundations such as the Robert Wood Johnson Foundation and the Commonwealth Fund (which supported Ford and Silver's Colorado program), early nurse practitioner programs formalized and provided the skill support for expanded nursing care. Ford and Silver published accounts describing their program in 1967, as did physician Charles Lewis and nurse Barbara Resnick, who reported on their 1964 study of new models of nurse-resident teams at the University of Kansas Medical Center in Kansas City. Both studies described patients receiving care from nurses who provided services typically within the medical realm, with various levels of physician supervision. Ford's nurses worked without physician supervision with patients in rural areas where overwhelming chronic health problems like tuberculosis, malnutrition, and child development issues predominated. In contrast, the patients in Resnick's study encountered nurses working in close proximity with physicians in high-volume urban outpatient clinics dogged by problems of patient appointment cancellation, nonadherence to treatment, and lack of continuity of care. Outpatient clinics were typically staffed by residents or interns from the university medical center who changed rotations every few weeks, overseen by a range of medical faculty. Physicians rarely saw the same patient twice so could reap none of the benefits of established clinician-patient relationships like patient loyalty, inclination to follow medical orders, or commitment to the health promotion or disease prevention strategies that were becoming increasing popular.[14]

None of these experiments began by asking patients about the kind of care they wanted or who should provide it. But evidence of patient dissatisfaction, with the clinics in particular, was implicit in their failure to follow medical regimens, poor chronic illness management, and low immunization rates. Both Ford's and Resnick's programs generated high patient loyalty and satisfaction, as documented, for example, by the significant number of patients who kept their appointments and correctly took their medications. The programs generated a great deal of interest as reports of their work appeared in high-status medical journals such as the *New England Journal of Medicine* and were replicated around the country.[15]

Patient preferences and sources of information about nurse practitioners were widely reported in popular newspapers and magazines of the 1970s and 1980s as well. *Look* magazine published one of the earliest stories in the popular press in 1966, followed in 1972 by the *Saturday Evening Post*. *McCall's*, a leading women's magazine, ran articles about nurse practitioners starting in 1975. In one story, author Eleanor Clift noted that the Emory School of Nursing walk-in clinic staffed by nurse practitioners was so well received by the community that they "soon opened a satellite clinic in a downtown church, besides taking over the health programs of a local college and a high-rise apartment for retirees." *Ebony* and *Science Digest* pointed out that nurse practitioner was a desirable choice of profession because of patient loyalty and rising salaries.[16]

Sources as diverse as the *Wall Street Journal* and *Today's Health* referred to nurse practitioners as "supernurses," expressing what may have been surprise at their competence as well as recognition of their ability to provide high-quality services. A 1974 *Wall Street Journal* article noted that "supernurses worked in logging camps in Washington, and on remote Indian reservations. . . . In Cambridge, Mass, 12 pediatric nurse practitioners handle 25,000 patient visits a year at five neighborhood health centers in the poor sections of the city." A teenage patient in a New York City clinic told a *Today's Health* reporter that she really liked the nurse practitioner: "She's easy to talk to." By 1985, the *New York Times*, *Washington Post*, and *Wall Street Journal* had reported on nurse practitioners in their main or health sections and had printed more than 150 letters to the editor on the topic.[17] All these sources, accessible to the general public, reflected patient support for, and helped patients learn about, nurse practitioners.

Two other important factors influenced the growing public awareness and acceptance of nurse practitioners as providers. First, many physicians began to bring them into their practices, a move that increased the size and income of the practices in the absence of potential physician partners, and helped relieve their high patient loads. Patients met nurse practitioners in their trusted doctor's office, and the new additions helped the busy practice run smoother. A construction worker quoted in the *Today's Health* article noted earlier reported that he "asked for [the nurse practitioner] because it saves time. I can get to her faster than to the doctor," illustrating his confidence in the nurse practitioner as well as the overextension of his primary care physician.[18]

The second factor that supported expanded roles for nurse practitioners was public dissatisfaction with physicians. Receding patient loyalty, both real and perceived, toward their physicians was a much-discussed problem in the sixties and seventies.[19] The dissatisfaction seemed to focus on unsupportive physician communication patterns, their inability to be "caring," their inconsistent presence, and their inaccessibility.[20] In contrast, nurse practitioners spent time offering practical knowledge and skills to help patients care for themselves and their children. They served as knowledgeable proxies in the physician's absence or when rotations changed in an academic center clinic. As a nurse working in a Baltimore clinic in the early 1970s explained: "We are here [in the clinic] five days a week, whereas before the interns were here only one day a week—if that. When a patient has a problem, when they call, we talk to them. In the past, they didn't understand a lot of things and no one had the time to explain. We have the time to explain."[21]

Nurse Practitioners and Patient Preference

In the 1970s most nurse practitioners worked outside mainstream hospitals in the more independent, flexible environments of public health clinics, clinics of the women's health movement, medical offices, and other primary care settings. For example, in 1975 the Maternity Center Association in New York City opened a nurse midwife–directed childbearing center in response to complaints they received from middle-class women's health advocates who wanted a more active role and less medical intervention in their general health and childbearing experiences.[22] But typically there were no organized groups advocating the use of nurses, nor was there consistent lobbying by particular racial, cultural, or gender-based groups. There were no patient leaders or spokespersons. The influence at work here differed from that of traditional and larger consumer movements in that it was individually mediated, idiosyncratic, and from the bottom up. Because of the varied character of patient influence, many researchers choose to ignore it or to value more highly the efforts of large organized groups focused on particular diseases or conditions that have direct links to particular health policies. And some researchers tend to see nurses as highly dependent on physicians for their cultural and social authority, lacking the potential to personally engage patients as providers of health care. This perception is shaped by an underlying penchant to look to traditional relationships between physicians and nurses within hospitals as the paradigm. But to do so both misses the strong undercurrent of grassroots support for nurses, and disenfranchises the efforts of a highly gendered workforce and a middle- and lower-income patient constituency often composed of those most vulnerable and silent.

Much of the work of professional nursing is rhetorically situated as caregiving in response to patient needs. But what patients need may be different from what they want, depending on the sometimes conflicting interests of the individual and the community and of what is desired and what is available. This is particularly true in terms of how patients make decisions about who provides their health care at particular times and places. Patients may want physician care because it is considered normative—they may believe they are entitled to the services of a professional group that for decades set itself up as the expert in patient care. But physicians are often unavailable when patients want and need them most. In the early 1970s in Eustancia, New Mexico, nurse practitioner Martha Schwebach worked alone in a clinic built by the area's physician, who had left in 1968 and was never replaced. She communicated with six physicians sixty miles away in Albuquerque when she needed consultation. She made house calls and ran an emergency service of almost three thousand patients, twenty to twenty-five of whom she saw daily in the clinic.[23] By 1974, nurse practitioner Ruth Murphy in Elk County, Kansas, had set up a series of free clinics and estimated she made more than 4,500 house calls a year. The area had been without a physician for more than fifteen years, lacked public transportation, and was fifty miles from the nearest hospital.[24]

Patients influence the nursing profession at the nexus of historically contingent alternatives. Patients at first did not choose nurse practitioners to provide their care but came to see their value on their visits to clinics or offices, saw them working in partnership with physician colleagues, found them reasonable and even desirable providers, and returned for more services. As a patient in a Quincy, Massachusetts, practice in the late 1960s noted: "At first I questioned the doctor's assigning my baby to a nurse, but . . . I consented and now I ask for the nurse first."[25] When Lucile Kinlein opened one of the earliest nurse practices in the country in 1971 in College Park, Maryland, the practice was slow to get off the ground: the second month brought her first patient. But four months later, she had sixty patients.[26] Colorado pediatrician Lewis Day admitted that three of the five families that joined his practice every month in the late 1960s did so because of the nurse practitioner, commenting: "I even have patients call me at night for her phone number."[27] Physician James Johnson of Greencastle, Indiana, wrote in a 1977 report that even patients whom he had followed in his practice for two or three decades began to request the nurse practitioner.[28]

Some of the patient demand can be attributed to the lower cost of nurse practitioner services, but patients would not return if low cost meant low value or inadequate services, even if there were few other options available.[29] Cost and value are difficult factors to pull out retrospectively. Whatever its basis, this slow shift in patient demand is eventually captured in studies of patient satisfaction with nurse practitioner care reported by the late 1980s.[30] For example, in one frequently quoted study of a Wheat Ridge, Colorado, pediatric practice, 97 percent of patients were satisfied with the care they received from nurse practitioners, and 57 percent said the joint care from the physician and nurse practitioner was better than that provided by the doctor alone.[31]

Evidence of patient demand for nurse practitioners, albeit on the supply side, is also supported by the growing number of programs for nurse practitioners. Although increased federal support was indeed a major factor in program growth, another contributing factor was system demand, documented by the increasing number of graduates sought by clinics, hospitals, and private physicians. This evidence also indirectly points to patient acceptance and satisfaction, and physicians' perception of nurse practitioners' value to their practices. Newspapers such as the *New York Times* and the *Los Angeles Times* consistently ran advertisements by clinics, hospitals, and private practices searching for nurse practitioners.[32] "Patients obviously must like [the nurse practitioner] because the number of patients has doubled [since the nurse practitioner became part of the practice]," one physician noted in a 1977 publication.[33] Pediatrician Lewis R. Day found he was taking care of 50 percent more patients since he started working with a nurse practitioner in the late 1960s, and noted he was "not working as hard and the care is better."[34] Indirect evidence of patient acceptance and lower cost comes from the prepaid health plan Kaiser Permanente, which started hiring nurse practitioners quite early, in 1971, in Oakland, California. By 1974, Kaiser employed nearly one hundred nurse practitioners, allowing administrators to enroll more patients.[35] Many of the nurse practitioners provided services in the screening programs that saw a rapid increase in patient popularity in the 1970s. Patient satisfaction and demand for nurse practitioners in these Kaiser programs was noted by the authors of a 1974 study, who documented many patients spontaneously commenting on nurse practitioners' thoroughness and show of concern.[36]

Many requests for nurse practitioner services came from women who felt more comfortable with women providers than with male clinicians and wanted a different type of health care service than physicians offered. Physician James B. Johnson began to notice that his practice was beginning to attract a number of new female patients in the early 1970s who asked specifically for an appointment with the nurse practitioner. Most of these patients came from the practice of a recently retired woman gynecologist, and patients said they felt more comfortable with the nurse practitioner performing their pelvic examinations because she listened to their problems and better understood their bodies.[37] A patient who pointed out the reasons she came to see the nurse practitioner in an independent practice in Maryland in 1972 said: "No one will listen to me. They [physicians] talk to me like I am a two-year-old child and never once ask me—what do you think."[38]

Gender played an important part in patients' choice of provider for particular problems. Women found issues such as toilet training and breast-feeding easier to discuss with the typically female nurse practitioner than with a male physician.[39] And, because both family health care decision makers and nurse practitioners were usually women, the restructuring of health care delivery was a powerful female-gendered political force energized by other social movements within a system characterized by paternalism.[40]

Patients' influence—in this case, the influence of the women's health movement in the 1970s—on policy, specifically on the broadening range of choices for health service delivery, enlarges their traditional empowerment, as well as advocacy narratives that typically focus on particular diseases and health risks. Nurse practitioners typically participated in the women's health movement as private individuals and as providers. In the Feminist Women's Health Centers (FWHC) of the early 1970s in Los Angeles, nurse practitioners were "actually quite important as health care professionals. . . . The FWHCs promoted self-care most vigorously, but the participants also saw nurse practitioners as allies in their struggle against medical paternalism, helping provide the services that weren't quite medical, but perhaps not legally provided by lay workers."[41] Sheryl Ruzak, in *The Women's Health Movement*, also makes the case for the politicized nurse. By utilizing nurse practitioners instead of physicians, feminist health centers demonstrated the effectiveness and public acceptance of nonphysician providers.[42] Women took comfort from nurse practitioners who encouraged the participation of families in the birthing process and who supported freestanding birth centers, rooming-in after birth, and self-examination.[43] Some activists went on to enter nurse practitioner training programs in the years after their work in women's health clinics because they preferred the types of service nurse practitioners provided.[44]

Federal programs ensured that poor urban and rural patients had access to nurse practitioners, providing free care or charges based on a sliding scale. Funding from the Model Cities programs that began under the Lyndon B. Johnson administration in the mid 1960s supported the early training of nurse practitioners, typically in pediatrics and in women's health community clinics, as well as their employment in the clinics funded by these programs when their training ended. By 1976, for example, nurse practitioners in more than twenty cities were working in community adolescent health clinics.[45]

Community health clinics gave women, many by now educated in the advisability of yearly pap tests or birth control advice, access to broader health care services. When women came to a clinic for gynecological care, the nurse practitioners also offered additional primary care services: "In addition to the fact that they were there because they wanted contraception," a nurse practitioner who worked in a community clinic in the 1970s remembered, "if they couldn't afford other kinds of care, we were it."[46]

Patient influence also affected the state legislative arena, when state medical societies challenged nurse practitioners' ability to provide a full array of services to patients. Most of these conflicts occurred over the right of nurse practitioners to prescribe medications and treatments.[47]

In New Hampshire in the 1980s, nurse practitioners battling for the right to prescribe enlisted help from and were supported by local legislators who wanted nurse practitioners to provide care to their families, and by women who were patients of nurse practitioner activists as well as by wives of local physicians. This support was crucial and personal during the almost ten-year fight to finally gain prescriptive rights.[48] In California, when questions arose over medical practice act violations by a nurse practitioner in a free women's health clinic, the patients "really supported her" and helped resolve the issue through personal connections and testimony.[49] Ultimately, she was not charged with practicing medicine without a license; the charges were dropped.

Patient utilization of nurse practitioner services became essential evidence for the American Nursing Association's (ANA) health policy agenda in the 1980s and 1990s to highlight nurses as the key to improving access to high-quality care. Starting in the late 1970s, the ANA's media campaigns strategically positioned nurse practitioners as the standard for the routine care of such patient groups as children, pregnant women, healthy adults, and the elderly. The ANA also began to work with nurse practitioner organizations to organize consistent policy messages. The ANA's positioning came not only from the growing body of popular and research-based evidence showing patient satisfaction and acceptance with nurse practitioners and their altruistic efforts to improve patient care, but also from the growing strategic and political importance of the patient as the focus of professional legitimacy. The organization highlighted the nurse practitioner–patient relationship, using it as a powerful vehicle for furthering the organization's agenda for the nursing profession. This would become part of the legacy of patient influence on the nursing profession.

Conclusion

In terms of nurse practitioners, patient influence on the health care system came from patients' redefinition of standard care. Patients increasingly willing to use and pay for nurse practitioners for their health care redefined them as normative providers. The value and quality of patient experiences and the types of service they received coalesced as part of the rhetoric of patient rights and legitimized nurses' expanded practice.[50] As one patient noted: "Formerly, I always figured with respect to medical care that I got what I paid for. . . . I must admit that the understanding and empathy which you [the nurse practitioner] bring to your profession made this whole hassle easier for me, and I also wish such competence and sensitivity were available to all."[51]

Patient acceptance gave the ANA an effective strategy for redefining nursing within the health care system, for the public at large, as the most effective provider for particular populations. The ANA's message was clear: nurse practitioners successfully provided services patients wanted and needed. The influence of patients on this movement became a power nurses as a professional group could build on in their efforts to better define and expand the domain of their professional activities and gain public resources.

The demand of individual patients for different models of medical care, as this chapter indicates, can move ideas forward to coalesce into health policy change. We have also seen that these changes can be piecemeal and at times inadequate to support large-scale reform in the delivery system. But small-scale change is also important, at times the springboard for larger policy initiatives. Location-based models such as nurse-managed community clinics began in the 1960s as pilot projects or small locally based initiatives to provide safety-net services for both rural and urban residents without access to a primary care provider or to health insurance. These clinics, about 260 of them by 2006, are particularly good examples of patient influence, as the model is based on true partnerships developed from input between local community councils and nurse practitioner providers.[52] Better funding streams to increase patient access to nurse-managed health centers were included in all versions of the health reform bills of the 2009–2010 health policy reform initiatives.

In the 1960s and 1970s, patient needs for hands-on and individualized primary care and nurses' needs for legitimacy slowly and quietly meshed. Patients became a central conduit for the nursing profession's claims to legitimacy, demonstrating the political and economic benefits of such legitimacy. But there were also valid claims of patients' preference for the services nurse practitioners provided. Although the market factors of cost and the shortage of physicians influenced patient choice, patients also found that nurse practitioners provided the kind of care they wanted with the added benefits of lower cost and better access to care. These are enduring patient preferences that influence and weave themselves throughout health care reform initiatives today.

Notes

1. See Suzanne Gordon and Claire Fagin, "Hart Survey of Nursing," *American Journal of Nursing* 96, 3 (1996): 31–32; Jan Caldow, Christine Bond, Mandy Ryan, Neil C. Campbell, Fernando San Miguel, Alice Kiger, and Amanda Lee, "Treatment of Minor Illness in Primary Care: A National Survey of Patient Satisfaction, Attitudes, and Preferences Regarding a Wider Nursing Role," *Health Expectations* 10, 1 (2007): 30–45.

2. Parts of this section draw on Julie Fairman, *Making Room in the Clinic: U.S. Nurse Practitioners and the Evolution of Modern Health Care* (New Brunswick, N.J.: Rutgers University Press, 2008).

3. Loretta Ford, interview by author, January 19, 2006, Gainesville, Florida.

4. Loretta Ford, Marguerite Cobb, and Margaret Taylor, *Defining Clinical Content of Graduate Nursing Programs: Community Health Nursing* (Boulder, Colo.: Western Interstate Commission for Higher Education, 1967); Loretta Ford and Henry Silver, "The Expanded Role of the Nurse in Child Care," *Nursing Outlook* 15 (1967): 43–45.

5. Charles Rosenberg uses market forces and context to explain the rise of the medical profession in many of his publications, e.g., "The Therapeutic Revolution: Medicine, Meaning, and Social Change in Nineteenth-Century America," *Perspectives in Biology and Medicine* 20 (1977): 485–506. See also Irwin M. Rosenstock, "Why People Use Health Services" ("Part 2: Health Services Research I. Discussed at a Conference Held in Chicago, October 15–16, 1965"), *Milbank Memorial Fund Quarterly* 44, 3 (1966): 94–127; Ronald Anderson and John F. Newman, "Societal and Individual Determinants of Medical Care Utilization in the United States," *Milbank Memorial Fund Quarterly* 51, 1 (Winter 1973): 95–124.

6. Fairman, *Making Room in the Clinic.*

7. Wendy Lazarus, E. S. Levine, and L. S. Lewin, *Competition among Health Practitioners: The Influence of the Medical Profession on the Health Manpower Market* (Washington, D.C.: Federal Trade Commission, 1981).

8. Ibid.

9. Barbara Bates, "Can a Screening Unit Do It?" Rough draft of a paper presented at the Medical Society of the State of New York 165th Annual Convention, New York City, February 16 1971, 7, Barbara Bates Collection, Barbara Bates Center for the Study of the History of Nursing, University of Pennsylvania School of Nursing, Philadelphia (hereafter Bates Collection).

10. Ford interview.

11. Barbara Safriet, "Health Care Dollars and Regulatory Sense: The Role of Advanced Practice Nursing," *Yale Journal of Regulation* 9, 417 (1992): 417–488; Frances Hughes, Sean Clark, Deborah Sampson, Eileen Sullivan Marx, and Julie Fairman, "Nurse Practitioner Research: An Historical Analysis," in *Nurses, Nurse Practitioners*, ed. Mathy D. Mezey and Diane O. McGivern (New York: Springer, 2003), 84–108.

12. Office of Technology Assessment, *Nurse Practitioners, Physician Assistants, and Certified Nurse-Midwives: A Policy Analysis*, Health Technology Case Study 37 (Washington, D.C.: U.S. Government Printing Office, 1986).

13. Irving J. Lewis and Cecil G. Sheps, *The Sick Citadel: The American Academic Medical Center and the Public Interest* (Cambridge: Oelgeschlager, Gunn, and Hain, 1983); Rosemary Stevens, *American Medicine and the Public Interest* (Berkeley: University of California Press, 1998).

14. Loretta C. Ford and Henry K. Silver, "The Expanded Role of the Nurse in Child Care," *Nursing Outlook* 15 (1967): 43–45; Charles Lewis and Barbara Resnick, "Nurse Clinics and Progressive Ambulatory Patient Care," *New England Journal of Medicine* 277, 23 (1967): 1236–1241.

15. Henry Silver, "Use of New Types of Allied Health Professionals in Providing Care for Children," *American Journal of Diseases of Children* 116 (November 1968): 486–490; Lewis and Resnick, "Nurse Clinics."

16. Roland H. Berg, "More than a Nurse, Less than a Doctor," *Look*, September 6, 1966, 59–61; "Comeback of the Family Doctor," *Saturday Evening Post*, Summer 1972, 48; Eleanor Clift, "The New Family Doctor Is a Nurse," *McCall's*, October 1975, 35; Marly Present, "What is a . . . Nurse Practitioner? . . . A Team Player," *Science Digest* 54 (1979): 54; "Birth Control at School: Pass of Fail?" *Ebony*, October 1986, 37–38; Derek Reveron, "Stroke: A Sneaky Killer with a Knockout Punch," *Ebony*, May 1979, 106; "Black Women/White Men," *Ebony*, August 1979, 78–80; "Planned Parenthood Director," *Ebony*, September 1979, 6.

17. Joann S. Lublin, "Filling the Gap: 'Supernurses' Provide Care for Thousands," *Wall Street Journal*, July 3, 1974, www.wallstreetjournal.com; Claire Safran, "Their Patients Call Them Supernurses," *Today's Health Care*, July–August 1975, 21–23; *New York Times*, *Washington Post*, *Wall Street Journal* data from the ProQuest Historical Newspaper database.

18. Numerous articles highlighted studies, not for their research data but to contrast the practice of nurses and physicians. See, for examples, Pam Hollie, "Nurses with Training in Diagnosing Ills Help Ease MDs' Workloads," *Wall Street Journal*, August 4, 1969, www.wallstreetjournal.com; Harry Nelson, "Changes in Training of Health Personnel Urged," *Los Angeles Times*, February 15, 1971, www.latimes.com.

19. Adele Lash, "Public Attitudes toward Physicians," *Indiana Medicine* 79 (February 1986): 184–186; American Association of Retired Persons [AARP], *A Nationwide Survey of Opinions toward Health Care Costs and Medicare* (Washington, D.C.: AARP, 1983); The Equitable Life Insurance Society of the United States [ELIS], *The Equitable Healthcare Survey: Options for Controlling Costs* (New York: ELIS, 1983).

20. Naomi Breslau and Alvin H. Novack, "Public Attitudes toward Some Changes in the Division of Labor in Medicine," *Medical Care* 17, 8 (August 1979): 859–867; Kathleen A. Baldwin, Rebecca J. Sisk, Parris Watts, Jan McCubbin, Beth Brockschmidt, and Lucy N. Marion, "Acceptance of Nurse Practitioners and Physician Assistants in Meeting the Perceived Needs of Rural Communities," *Public Health Nursing* 15, 6 (1998): 389–397.

21. H.H., "Revolution in Baltimore," in *Together: A Casebook of Joint Practices in Primary Care*, ed. Berton Roueché (Chicago: Educational Publications and Innovative Communications for the National Joint Practice Commission), 47.

22. Lazarus, Levine, and Lewin, *Competition among Health Practitioners*.

23. Robert Oseasohn, Edward A. Mortimer Jr., Carol C. Geil, Betty J. Eberle, Ann E. Pressman, and Naomi L. Quenk, "Rural Medical Care: Physician's Assistant Linked to an Urban Medical Center," *JAMA* 218, 9 (November 1971): 1417–1419.

24. Jennings Parrott, "'Murphy' Needs a Doctor Who Likes to Travel," *Los Angeles Times*, June 13, 1974, www.latimes.com.25. Pam Hollie, "Nurses with Training in Diagnosing Ills Help Ease MDs' Workload," *Wall Street Journal*, August 4, 1969, www.wallstreetjournal.com.

26. "RN Reports on 1st Year in 'Practice,'" *Los Angeles Times*, July 6, 1972, http://proxy .library.upenn.edu:2082/, accessed June 2, 2008.

27. Lublin, "Supernurses."

28. J.S., "Hoppy and Dock," in *Together: A Casebook of Joint Practices in Primary Care*, ed. Berton Roueché (Chicago: Educational Publications and Innovative Communi- cations for the NJPC, 1977), 72.

29. Lawrence Linn, "Factors Associated with Patient Evaluation of Health Care," *Milbank Memorial Fund Quarterly* 53, 4 (Fall 1975): 531–548.

30. By the end of the 1970s more than two hundred studies had evaluated nurse prac- titioner care and patient satisfaction. See Office of Technology Assessment, *Nurse Practitioners*; Hughes et al., "Nurse Practitioner Research."

31. Lewis Day, R. Egli, and Henry K. Silver, "Acceptance of Pediatric Nurse Practition- ers: Parents' Opinion of Combined Care by a Pediatrician and a Pediatric Nurse Practitioner in Private Practice," *American Journal of Diseases of Children* 119 (1970): 204–208.

32. A search of the ProQuest Historical Newspaper database revealed more than 2,500 such ads, which typically appeared in the weekend sections.

33. J.S., "Hoppy and Dock," 67.

34. Lublin, "Filling the Gap."

35. Ibid.; History of Kaiser Permanente, http://www.kaisersantarosa.org/about/kaiser/ history, accessed January 28, 2010.

36. Stephen L. Taller and Robert Feldman, "The Training and Utilization of Nurse Prac- titioners in Adult Health Appraisal," *Medical Care* 12, 1 (January 1974): 40–48.

37. J.S., "Hoppy and Dock," 72.

38. "RN Reports on 1st Year."

39. Hollie, "Nurses with Training."

40. Joyce Jensen, "Women Generally Select Their Family's Physicians," *Modern Health- care*, January 31, 1986, 60–61.

41. Judith A. Houck, Women's Studies Department of Medical History and Bioethics, University of Wisconsin-Madison, personal communication to author, July 25, 2008.

42. Sheryl Ruzak, *The Women's Health Movement* (New York; Praeger, 1978), 172.

43. Joan E. Mulligan, "Some Effects of the Women's Health Movement," *Topics in Clin- ical Nursing* 4, 4 (January 1983): 1–9.

44. Lucy M. Candib, *Medicine and the Family: A Feminist Perspective* (New York: Basic Books, 1995); Matt Clark, "The Supernurses," *Newsweek*, December 5, 1977, 64.

45. Hyman Goldstein and Helen Wallace, "Services for and Needs of Pregnant Teens in Large Cities of the United States," *Public Health Reports* 93, 1 (1978): 46–54.

46. C.J., interview with M. J. Murphy, September 20, 1997, Bates Collection.

47. Arlene Keeling, *Nursing and the Privilege of Prescription* (Columbus: Ohio State University Press, 2007), 183–200.

48. Deborah A. Sampson, "Determinants and Determination: Negotiating Nurse Practi- tioner Prescribing Legislation in New Hampshire, 1973–1985" (PhD diss., University of Pennsylvania, 2006).

49. Houck, personal communication.

50. Nancy Tomes, "Patients or Health Consumers? Why the History of Contested Terms Matters," in *History and Health Policy in the United States: Putting the Past Back*

In, ed. Rosemary Stevens, Charles Rosenberg, and Lawton Burns (New Brunswick, N.J.: Rutgers University Press, 2006), 85; in this essay Tomes discusses the rhetoric of patient rights as a factor in patient advocacy.

51. J.S., "Suite 511," in *Together: A Casebook of Joint Practices in Primary Care*, ed. Berton Roueché (Chicago: Educational Publications and Innovative Communications for the NJPC, 1977), 11.

52. Joann Loviglio, "Nurse Practitioners Filling a Care Void," Associated Press, June 26, 2006.

A House on Fire

Newborn Screening, Parents' Advocacy, and the Discourse of Urgency

"It's not really a question of should we expand newborn screening. It's happening. It's going like a house on fire."

—Rodney Howell, physician

Dave Wyvill's son Zach has a genetic disease called glutaric acidemia type 1 (GA1). Had it been detected immediately after birth, the disorder could have been controlled with vitamins and a special diet. Now it's too late for Zach to be helped by early diagnosis, but his father wants to make sure that others don't go through the suffering he and his family have endured. "This should not have happened," says Wyvill. "It shouldn't happen again to somebody else's child."[1] Like other parents turned newborn-screening policy actors, Wyvill experienced an excruciating crisis: irreversible harm to his child from an undiagnosed yet treatable condition. His advocacy efforts draw on those painful experiences, both as motivation and as powerful anecdotal evidence to be mustered in the service of a campaign to expand the scope of newborn screening. However, the rapid expansion of screened conditions that he and others passionately advocate has, in practice, yielded substantial consequences beyond assuring that other families are spared this tragedy, since many of the newer screening tests are not for early-onset, clearly diagnosable, treatable disorders like GA1. The inspiring impulse to spare others suffering that Wyvill and other parent advocates so eloquently express thus has many unintended consequences. This case study of parent advocacy illuminates important disjunctures associated with the translation of personal experience to the policy arena and critical questions about the nature of representation and voice.

Newborn screening for heritable disorders was arguably the prime example, in the first decade of the new millennium, of the way much-touted genetic research is actually being translated from bench science to tangible changes in the health care system. As genetic mutations associated with a wide array of diseases have become identifiable, and screening technology has been developed for detecting these mutations through analysis of infants' heel blood, newborn-screening (NBS) programs have indeed expanded "like a house on fire." There is no doubt that emerging research coupled with new screening techniques created the conditions for this flame to ignite. But it is also clear that advocacy by parents of affected children—acting both as individuals and through advocacy groups—has been so instrumental to NBS expansion that many have viewed it as the prime source of combustion. As one commentator put it: "In any particular state, the disorders screened for are directly proportional to the number of proponents for that particular disorder in that . . . state."[2] Yet as this chapter indicates, parental influences have in fact been as much catalysts of policy action by others as they have been direct drivers of the conflagration, since they have acted to mobilize policy factors historically embedded in U.S. federalism, media coverage of social problems, and interest group politics.

This chapter examines how parent advocates have shaped a specific discourse around NBS, and how this discourse—which I will call here the urgency narrative—has then been used to champion expansion of state programs to include not just the diseases suffered by advocates' own children, but a range of other conditions as well. Consumer/community participation in the policy process has clearly been dominated by the emotional appeals of parents who argue that their child was, or could have been, saved by the addition of one more condition to the newborn-screening panel. However, parents' advocacy efforts—both as individuals and as leaders in formal advocacy organizations— are not limited to demands for inclusion of "their" disease in their state's panel. Instead, they often argue for the most inclusive possible screening programs, and for both policy shifts and normative shifts that would allow mandatory screening for conditions that have no proven treatment. Further, the personal experiences of tragedy suffered or averted that were originally articulated by parent advocates have been extended and leveraged by a range of policy actors to form the basis of a broader policy platform.

Refracted through the dramatic frames of life or death and of parental grief, the complex practical, ethical, and social issues associated with expanded screening are presented and understood in ways that result in overly rosy predictions about the consequences of expanded screening. The dominant discourse about "saving babies"—a discourse now deployed by politicians, private companies offering NBS, researchers, and the media, as well as by NBS advocates—has paved the way for confusing an array of critical distinctions: between expansion of screening for specific conditions and expansion of screening in general; between research, diagnosis, and treatment; between screening procedures that can result in saved lives and those that have questionable prognostic certainty or ability to improve health outcomes. Put another way, urgent calls from outside a house exhorting bystanders to run in and "save the baby" do effectively motivate action, but they make it difficult to pause and assess if the house is actually on fire in the first place.

My intent here is to create such a pause—one long enough to consider the origins, intensity, and nature of the threats posed not only by conditions screenable at birth, but by the current newborn-screening policy conflagration itself. This case study of the particular way citizen participation has been shaped in this highly publicized, emotionally charged arena also provides a useful context for exploring larger questions about the nature of representation and who gets to speak for whom; about the challenge and promise of participatory democracy where policy is informed by lay as well as expert perspectives; about how advocates' interests can both conflict and intersect with the interests of other stakeholders in policy debates; and about the role of qualitative social science research in constructing a more nuanced voice for lay actors in health policy debates.

The pain endured by parents whose children have died or become disabled because of an undetected, treatable disorder is enormous—far beyond quantification or comparison. Their tireless advocacy to spare others such suffering is testament both to their gigantic heart and to their formidable ingenuity, tenacity, and dedication. Similarly, many current beneficiaries of NBS are in the debt of parents who had successful screening experiences before them and then became NBS advocates. The analysis presented here is in no way intended to diminish either the pain or the good hard work of these parents. Rather, it is offered with the hope that parsing more carefully the complex issues surrounding the expansion of NBS will help us all better understand the implications of policy decisions, thereby facilitating more robust and more democratic parental participation in the policy process. I believe this is a goal all advocates ultimately share (or should share), just as they must share a perpetual struggle for influence, legitimization, and voice in a system that structurally disadvantages them.[3] It is also a goal that seems to me to suitably honor living and deceased children.

Newborn Screening: An Overview

Newborn screening, defined here as biochemical testing of the infant's blood for inherited disorders, began in the mid 1960s when Robert Guthrie developed a test for phenylketonuria (PKU), a metabolic disease causing severe mental retardation but effectively controlled with a phenylalanine-restricted diet introduced soon after birth.[4] Children's advocacy groups, such as the Association for Retarded Citizens and the March of Dimes Birth Defects Foundation, successfully advocated alongside Guthrie—who himself had a family member with the disorder—to make the new PKU testing procedure compulsory in every state. With relatively little public attention or debate, newborn genetic screening thus pioneered new terrain for U.S. medicine and public health: state-mandated diagnosis of noninfectious disease.[5] And though the initial laws were focused only on PKU, they established both a precedent and a convenient legal mechanism by which new mandatory conditions could be readily added.

Today more than four million infants undergo testing every year, making newborn screening the single most widely utilized form of testing for genetic disorders in the United States.[6] Despite the enactment of recent federal legislation that encourages expanding newborn screening and increasing funding for education and follow-up services (the Newborn Screening Saves Lives Act of 2008), the program remains under state authority. Although the recent extraordinary growth of the program has resulted in more uniformity across states than was the case formerly, NBS continues to differ substantially from state to state in the scope of testing, the technology used, the forms of parental education and notification, and the nature of follow-up services.[7]

Tinder for the blazing expansion of newborn screening has come from at least two substantial sources: changing technology, and changing ethical norms. Beginning in the 1990s, the first-generation technique of "growing out" bacteria in blood placed on filter paper was replaced by tandem mass spectrometry (MS/MS), which made it possible for one sample of blood to be analyzed simultaneously and at very low cost for more than thirty distinct gene mutations. As use of MS/MS technology spread (from thirteen states in 2002 to forty-nine states in 2007), so did the scope of conditions that states included in their mandatory screening panels.[8] Just between 2004 and 2005, the average number of conditions screened for across the states rose from eight to twenty; in the most aggressive states such as New York, the number of mandated conditions increased from eleven in 2002 to forty-six by late 2005.[9] Additional technological innovations, such as the DNA chip—a next iteration of diagnostic technology predicted to supersede MS/MS and already in use in the private sector—will soon make additional, exponential program expansion possible. Chip technology is capable of identifying ten thousand alleles, ten thousand "conditions" (or perhaps just variations) that each baby carries in her genetic makeup, and many believe it will soon be adapted for use in NBS.[10]

A second precipitating factor involves shifting ethical norms. Before 2005, the consensus among ethicists and policy makers was that newborn screening ought to be mandated only when conditions appeared early in life, efficacious treatments were possible, and access to such treatments was assured.[11] But all this changed with the release in 2005 of a report by the American College of Medical Genetics (ACMG), which was commissioned by the federal Department of Health and Human Services to analyze the contemporary state of newborn screening.[12] The report broke new ground by officially advocating that "benefits to family and society," in addition to the direct benefits to the child, be considered as a central criterion for assessing whether a specific screen should be mandated. The ACMG clearly opened the door for policy choices that serve the emotional, financial, or other interests of the infants' family members or of society at large.[13]

Additional normative shifts with respect to NBS have been more subtle, but have also had tremendous impact. These include: (1) labeling cases in which genetic abnormalities have unknown clinical significance as positive screens; (2) mandating screening at birth for conditions that do not represent an immediate or grave health threat to the infant; (3) reporting to parents screening results for untreatable conditions identified as byproducts of screening for treatable conditions, on the grounds that it is paternalistic to withhold this information from them; and (4) suggesting that carrier identification might itself represent a form of "treatability," if it altered parents' childbearing choices and thus prevented suffering by as-yet-unconceived children.

Taken together, all these changes have greatly expanded the number of children screening positive through NBS. In its report, ACMG recommended that a uniform national panel include fifty-four conditions: twenty-nine in the "core panel" (some of which were only partially treatable) and an additional twenty-five "secondary targets"—none of which met the ACMG's own criteria for treatability—which would be reported to physicians and families because they would inevitably be identified as part of the differential diagnosis for conditions on the core panel. Included on the uniform panel are metabolic disorders, hemoglobin disorders, endocrine disorders, hearing impairment, and a small number of other conditions that are not readily categorized, including cystic fibrosis. In the first few years after the ACMG report was released, much (though not all) state variation with respect to the twenty-nine core conditions disappeared, as the average number of conditions in state mandatory panels increased to thirty-three by the end of 2006. But there remained considerable variation in state incorporation of the secondary targets into their mandatory panels: by 2008, about a third of the states had publicly announced adoption of most or all of the secondary targets, while an equal number of states announced only a handful of this subset.

Despite recent efforts by the ACMG, the March of Dimes, and other advocacy groups to moderate geographic variation in newborn-screening practices, ultimately these policy decisions remain in the hands of state-level policy makers and are subject to the influence of states' political ideology; to the pressures of interstate competition; and to variations in the administrative capacity, fiscal circumstances, or party control of state governments. But most germane for our analysis here is how this decentralized process of policy making creates multiple openings for parent advocates in favor of expanded screening to become critical policy drivers in many states, and for the central narrative guiding that advocacy to be adopted by a range of other powerful policy actors.

Fighter Moms and Zealots: Screaming for Expanded Newborn Screening

Parent advocates have taken action around a number of health issues affecting their children over the past thirty years, pushing hard for research, services, funding, and public attention. Historically, these advocates have combined the powerful ingredients of effective techniques and searing emotion to produce impressive results—sometimes more impressive than is possible when advocating for adults, who are more likely to be blamed for their own problems and less likely to garner public sympathy. For example, in New York City in the early 1980s, parents built coalitions with community and housing groups, children's rights groups, and health workers to bring attention to the issue of lead paint poisoning. They successfully used the media and litigation to enforce the housing code, get their children screened, and allocate more resources for lead poisoning control.[14] More recently, parent advocates have been instrumental in increasing both services and public education programs for individuals with fetal alcohol syndrome in Washington State and in using litigation and public pressure to change public policy for early intensive behavioral educational intervention for children with autism.[15] Parent advocates also fueled the search for answers about what causes sudden infant death syndrome, and eventually were successful in obtaining millions of dollars in federal funding for research and establishing SIDS as a legitimate rather than suspect cause of death.[16]

Parent advocates for newborn screening today, like their predecessors and their contemporaries working for other health-related causes, use both heart-wrenching personal narratives about their children and an array of advocacy techniques to accomplish their goals. As one advocate describes it: "Anguish is why [an early NBS advocacy organization] began raising awareness among parents, the medical profession and the general public. Because our volunteers were very outspoken, they sometimes described their advocacy work as 'Newborn Screaming.'"[17] Others talk about themselves as zealots, or as fighter moms who become instant activists and experts because it's therapeutic and makes them feel like they're "working on something, and something is happening" even if they can't directly find a cure.[18]

Parent advocacy for NBS is also arguably distinctive in several ways. First, it has been explicitly organized primarily around a diagnostic process rather than around more traditional focuses such as expanded research, improved services, or creation of a support network. The group on whose behalf parents are advocating is thus the entire population of newborns, all of whom are theoretically at risk for rare but deadly genetic disorders, and all of whom must therefore be screened no matter how healthy they might appear. The policy actions of parents with respect to NBS expansion are aimed not primarily at improving the lives of already-identified patients, but rather at conceptualizing all infants as potential patients and being certain that accurate, comprehensive, efficiently implemented testing is conducted so that those with hidden disorders can be identified. This form of advocacy, though somewhat unusual for parent advocates, fits solidly within the risk discourse of what has been described as the "new public health," which focuses more and more on analyzing the inner workings of the asymptomatic body so as to identify and circumvent disease before it is manifest.[19] As Alan Petersen and Deborah Lupton put it: "All bodies are constructed as 'at risk' from one or more conditions or illnesses ... [since] all people, whether or not they are experiencing symptoms, may harbour 'risk factors' potentially leading to illness."[20]

NBS advocacy is also distinctive because the nature of the MS/MS diagnostic technology creates specific incentives and opportunities for parent advocates to work together across disease-specific lines. Because the technology makes possible relatively inexpensive testing for tens of disorders via the same heel blood spot, it can be regarded as a shared resource across specific disease categories. Rather than competing for funding and attention, then, as can often occur in advocacy arenas, NBS advocates working on an array of specific diseases have come increasingly to endorse "comprehensive" as well as "universal" screening—that is, implementation of a broad panel of other screening tests in addition to the specific one that has motivated them to action.[21]

Forms of NBS Parent Advocacy:
The Roads Most Traveled

Parent advocacy for expanded NBS has taken several distinct shapes over the past decade. The first is participation on formal advisory committees. As of 2008, at least thirty-eight of the fifty states had newborn-screening or genetic services advisory committees charged with reviewing newborn-screening program performance and making recommendations with respect to the addition of new conditions to the panel. Of those states with committees, thirty-four, or roughly 90 percent, have one or more members specifically identified as a parent or consumer. Notably, at least thirty-nine of forty-two parent-consumer representatives (more than 90 percent) on state NBS committees as of 2008 had a child with a genetic disorder that either is or could be screened on the newborn panel. The parents active on these committees thus are likely to hold a common perspective on NBS issues because of their shared experience with affected children.

The particular experiences of these parents, however, are not typical of those of most parents, whose concerns the committees are required neither to hear nor to consider. In the absence of such norms guiding committee participation, it is difficult to imagine that these lay members of committees otherwise made up entirely of professionals do otherwise than to rely primarily on their own experiences and those of other parents in similar circumstances. Parents who might have views about or experiences of the "new newborn screening" different from those of parents with affected children—such as parents who received an ambiguous, erroneous, or false-positive test result—are not yet represented on these committees.

The second form that parental NBS advocacy commonly takes is ad hoc—that is, parents going directly to their state legislators or testifying at state-level hearings about NBS. In several states (e.g., Florida), parents have also advocated directly with hospitals, requesting that they make expanded screening panels available directly to parents for a fee through private labs. Parents also submit public comments in response to draft reports and policy recommendations, appear at congressional hearings in connection with proposed federal legislation around NBS, and testify before advisory bodies such as the Advisory Committee on Heritable Disorders and Genetic Diseases in Newborns and

Children. Like parents sitting on state advisory committees, the vast majority of parents involved in this form of ad hoc advocacy have been those who tend to frame NBS policy deliberations using the urgency narrative.

A third way parents have entered the NBS arena as policy actors is through formal advocacy organizations. These include: (1) parent-driven organizations dedicated solely to expanding NBS (e.g., Save Babies Through Screening); (2) parent-driven organizations dedicated to disease-specific or multiple-disease advocacy that include expanded NBS—either through the addition of new screens to state panels, or through the development of new screening procedures able to detect additional disorders—among their strategies (e.g., CARES Foundation, Fight SMA); and (3) professionally driven organizations that include a focus on newborn screening and utilize parent advocates in their work (e.g., the March of Dimes). A Web-based search and analysis identified roughly six hundred organizations—most of them consumer-parent driven—advocating around genetic issues under the organizational umbrella of the Genetic Alliance and the National Organization of Rare Diseases. This investigation also revealed that approximately 27 percent of these six hundred groups include NBS as one of their issues. About 6.8 percent, or roughly forty organizations, make NBS part of their core mission. In addition, of large, disease-specific advocacy organizations identified in this search, four out of eighteen—or roughly 22 percent—devote significant attention to and have multiple mentions of NBS on their Web sites. Two of these groups—the March of Dimes and the Genetic Alliance itself—have made NBS a central platform in their advocacy campaigns and publicity activities.[22]

These forms of advocacy are distinct, and an accurate understanding of the NBS landscape requires appreciation of the approximate size and shape of each. But an equally important feature of the topography is that these categories are overlapping, with permeable boundaries; thus the activities of parents in each have synergistic effects. This synergy is most evident, as the media analysis I summarize later demonstrates, when explored in the context of professionalization processes that lead many advocates from more ad hoc strategies to participation in or leadership of formal organizations. The transition from layperson to organizational representative is evident in various arenas because of high-profile laypeople-turned-leaders such as Fran Visco of the National Breast Cancer Coalition and Sharon Terry of the Genetic Alliance. Furthermore, as Steven Epstein points out in this volume, this synergy is just one aspect of an overarching "problem of cooptation and incorporation" that fundamentally vexes patient advocacy. In Epstein's words: "Any inclination to celebrate the accomplishments of patient groups must make sense of two

potentially countervailing tendencies: the multivalent politics of incorporation, whereby the insights and legacies of patient advocacy are channeled back
into institutionalized biomedical practice; and cooptation, where the radical
potential of an activist critique is blunted or contained."

Most relevant for this examination of patients turned policy actors, however, is the increased visibility and legitimacy accorded to the urgency narrative over time, as its powerful assumptions about the nature of and need for
NBS moved from individual stories into the more codified arenas of organizational and then policy discourse.

Influencing Public Discourse:
Parent Advocates and the Media

The link between effective health advocacy and media coverage has always
been a strong one, and NBS advocacy is no exception.[23] Just as NBS parent
advocates have gained increasing traction and visibility in a variety of public
arenas, NBS has captured increasing amounts of media attention—particularly
post 2005, when NBS decisively entered the issue attention cycle created by
the mutually reinforcing phenomena of media focus, policy-maker response,
and public awareness.

These cycles follow a consistent pattern: events that had previously been
portrayed in the media as poignant individual anecdotes are linked by a catalyzing event that triggers an exponential increase in media coverage, validat-
ing comments by political figures and calls for immediate action to deal with
the impending crisis.[24] Certainly the intensity of media coverage for NBS fits
this pattern, with the ACMG report in 2005 as the catalyzing event. Of the 189
newspaper articles on NBS published in major U.S. national, state, and regional
papers from 1975 to 2007, fully 55 percent (104 articles) were published in
2006–2007.[25] And the presence of parents and advocates in these news stories
is substantial: the articles use parents or advocates as sources of evidence 32.4
percent of the time and describe parents or advocates as drivers of NBS expansion 30.9 percent of the time. The distinctive importance of parental advocacy
in the United States is evident by comparing U.S. newborn-screening articles
to the forty-five published in the Commonwealth countries during this same
time period. Outside the United States, parent-advocates are used as sources
of evidence and cited as policy drivers less than half as frequently—just 14.9
percent and 15.2 percent of the time, respectively.

The movement of parent NBS advocates from ad hoc to formalized advocacy roles—a trend taken for granted within the NBS field both because of the
prevalence of parent-driven advocacy organizations in the genetics arena in

general and because of the high visibility of vocal and effective exemplars
for NBS policy making in particular—is also suggested by trends over time in
the influences on policy discourse identified through the media analysis Mark
Schlesinger and I conducted.[26] Parents are cited in the media as 37.3 percent
of all sources of evidence in 2000 and earlier; this declines to 19.4 percent in
the period from 2001 through 2005, and finally to 15.8 percent in the period
from 2006 to 2007. At the same time, advocates are cited as sources of evidence
with increasing frequency: from 4.2 percent to 12.8 percent and finally to 13.5
percent over the same respective time periods. Yet while parents and advocates
are less often being cited as evidence, there is a concomitant increase in por-
trayals of parents and advocates as significant drivers of NBS expansion (from
13.8 percent to 34.2 percent over the same respective time periods). These
simultaneous trends suggest that parental influence over the policy process has
been increasingly transformed from ad hoc to more organized and consolidated
avenues of influence, and also that narratives recounted directly by parents are
quoted less often over time, even as representation of their influence—itself
a "story"—takes on a life of its own.

"Kids Are Dying Out There": Urgent Advocacy for Nonemergent Problems

The primary narrative driving parental advocacy for expanded newborn
screening—including advocacy for recently enacted federal NBS legislation—
has been both powerful and straightforward: simple, inexpensive tests at birth
save babies. "I want the state to prevent kids from being brain damaged and
dying," says one mother, in a statement that embodies succinctly the message
communicated by NBS parent advocates across the board. "Kids are dying out
there. . . . It's about time [the state expanded its panel]."[27] Or as another parent
puts it, invoking the negative iteration of the story: "It breaks my heart when
I hear of a child who died because it happened to have been born in a state run
by people who didn't believe its life was worth $20."[28]

As noted earlier, however, many of the tests now proposed for addition to
NBS panels clearly *don't* save the lives of screened babies, or even improve
them in any straightforward way. A significant number of the fifty-four conditions on the ACMG-recommended panel have no known treatment[29]—
and some experts assert that only PKU and perhaps five other conditions on
the ACMG-recommended panel have "treatments that are known to work."[30]
Existing pilot testing programs for diseases such as Type I diabetes and Fragile
X Syndrome, and proposed movement to develop screening methods for a
range of other common complex disorders with genetic components such as

autism and asthma, would further distance newborn screening from its historical lifesaving legacy.

The reality that not all screening results in immediate salvation is acknowledged, at times, in the explicit policy recommendations articulated by parent advocates. Nonetheless, the message of urgency embedded in the "save babies" narrative—that exhortation to act quickly, through newborn screening, to prevent kids from getting sick and dying—remains a central theme. For example, even when the question is whether states should test for conditions that are not now treatable, the answer can be that *of course* we should save babies' lives. As put by a spokesperson for Save Babies through Screening in a press release entitled "Treatability of Disorders Should Not Be Criterion for Inclusion of Screened Disorders":

> Until we start identifying affected children through screening and giving the doctors an opportunity to intervene early, we won't have treatments. . . . In addition, gene defects are quite variable, or can be expressed in different patterns, thus the result is that in any given disorder there is a range of mild to very serious symptoms. Therefore, it can't be said with any certainty that a disorder is 100% untreatable. And I have never met a parent that would just let a child die if there was any chance he or she could live a normal, healthy life.[31]

Similarly, the Congenital Adrenal Hyperplasia Research Education and Support Foundation (CARES) moves seamlessly from a focused argument about the need to screen in every state for the emergent and effectively treatable condition congenital adrenal hyperplasia (CAH), to a general endorsement of the broadest possible expansion of NBS. "Because failure to recognize [CAH] at birth has such dire consequences and because treated infants have the potential for a full and productive life," the site reads, "newborn screening is invaluable." Affected individuals and their families, the site goes on to say, "can truly help fellow sufferers of CAH by getting involved and urging the addition of CAH to newborn screening programs *and the importance of comprehensive newborn screening.* . . . [italics added]. All children should be screened for all diseases that technology can provide for at this time."[32]

To reiterate: newborn screening undeniably saves the lives of some infants, and the importance of this reality to those who benefit from it must never be underestimated. However, the claim—whether direct or indirect—that *all* available screening tests respond to an urgent need, and that *all* at least point the way to solving an urgent problem, profoundly oversimplifies the range of critical social, ethical, and legal issues that commentators with more distance from the urgency narrative agree must be confronted en route to responsible policy making.[33] To illustrate, I highlight here four aspects of the argument for expanded screening that borrow from the "save babies" narrative, and point to some of the issues that are elided in the process.

The therapeutic misconception writ large

As illustrated aptly by the earlier quotation from Save Babies Through Screening, the urgency narrative is easily extended to assert or imply that the *research* facilitated by early identification of babies with genetic disorders will actually benefit those same babies. This conflation of possible future benefit for others with immediate benefit to enrolled human subjects is commonplace: bioethicists have long pointed to the "therapeutic misconception" as a central concern to be addressed in the protection of human research subjects.[34]

In the case of NBS, however, it is arguable that this misconception is particularly problematic.[35] These programs were created not as research protocols, but as emergency public health measures, justified as both mandatory and universal precisely on the strength of claims that they serve the state's interest in protecting vulnerable children from death and disability. NBS thus lacks even the most basic structures for human subjects research, such as education about the protocol, informed consent, and capacity to easily withdraw from participation. Further, focus group research with parents about NBS suggests that parents appear prone to presume, even if explicitly told otherwise, that if conditions can be identified through medical technology, technology must be able to treat those conditions.[36]

Although it might be argued that some subset of the proposed research for treatment would be a voluntary next step for families to consider after successful diagnosis, the use of existing NBS public health laws to mandate a pool of potential subjects remains highly problematic. The universal and mandatory nature of NBS also clearly distinguishes research advocacy for expanded newborn screening from research advocacy on other issues—for example, HIV/AIDS[37]—where the doctrine of informed consent has not only remained fully intact but has been the cornerstone of advocates' arguments that patients should be able to take on risks related to research at their own discretion. As one critic summarized the NBS situation: "In all these cases of newborn screening gone haywire, there is usually some understandably zealous group of parents of sick kids, patient groups, advocacy groups saying 'Let's get on with it. . . .' Some ethicists asked for clinical trials, but these groups said, 'We don't have time to waste.'"[38]

Saving lives by preventing births

A second complicating strand in the argument to screen for untreatable conditions is that screening "saves" *future* lives by allowing families to "choose to
avoid having more children after having a child diagnosed with an untreatable
inherited disorder," or at least to make "educated family planning decisions."[39]
The time urgency suggested here is not the delay of days or hours that can—as
parent advocates have so passionately argued—mean the difference between
diagnosing a metabolic disorder before the child experiences a medical crisis
and diagnosing it after irreversible damage is already done. Rather, it's the rush
to be sure diagnosis is made of an existing child before conception of a subsequent child. But this distinction is easily lost when buried in the metanarrative
of saving lives—as are the facts that *voluntary* genetic testing for some of these
conditions is offered to most women during or before pregnancy, and that since
not all women consent to all tests, it cannot be assumed that reproductive risk
information delivered by mandatory screening is a universal good.[40]

Rare genetic disorders, the foremost threat
to infants' health and well-being

Most metabolic conditions screened by NBS are extremely rare—from one in
1,856 births to as few as one in 384,142 births.[41] However, the drama of the
"screening saves lives" story—complete with its showcasing of technological
innovation on the one hand and elegantly simple dietary treatments on the
other—is so compelling that it can easily claim status as a central plank in
the overall campaign to give babies the start in life that they deserve. "The
Haygoods' son died from a disease that went undetected at birth," reads the
opening paragraph of a prototypical news article. "Now they're trying to spare
others the same heartbreak."[42]

This disproportionately high profile for NBS relative to its numerical
impact is encouraged by two factors that combine with technological innovation to create a perfect storm. The first is a policy environment favoring high-
tech diagnosis and treatment over the social determinants of health. The "NBS
saves lives" narrative bolsters the more general tendency of messages about
diagnostic technologies to "exploit [parents'] hope of controlling frightening
conditions, [and] of predicting and eradicating risk."[43]

The second factor is the fierce interstate competition that has undergirded
NBS expansion, leading advocates to frequently condemn or praise their own
state's screening panel size relative to others'.[44] As one recent newspaper
article recounted: "Mississippi, the state that's perennially at the bottom of
health status charts, leads the nation when it comes to sparing children from

the ravages of rare genetic diseases." Despite this opening reference to Mississippi's overall laggard health status, the March of Dimes' president is then quoted as asserting: "If you're a baby born in the United States, Mississippi is your best bet. . . . Georgia has more work to do if it wants to catch up."[45]

The reality that the infant mortality rate in Mississippi during 2005 was 11.4 per thousand births compared to a national average of just 6.9 is neatly obscured when newborn screening is represented as *the* plan for saving young lives.[46] Advocates' assertion that "due to disparities in state newborn-screening programs, a healthy start and a healthy life is not a guarantee for all newborns" is difficult to counter with the same ponderous statistics and complex proposals for addressing structural underpinnings of health disparities that have fallen on largely deaf ears for the past several decades.[47]

Comprehensive universal screening in all states,
the antidote to "newborn roulette"

The theme of interstate competition regarding NBS has been leveraged by advocates to suggest that states' responsibilities to newborns are best discharged by expanding screening panels and also to emphasize that failure of states to match the state with the largest screening panel constitutes a violation of equal rights. As one parent advocate put it: "In one state you can live and lead a normal life, and in another state, you can die or be mentally retarded. . . . It's like newborn roulette."[48]

Advocates emphasize this point in media interviews and in testimony before legislators and national advisory committees. "The life of my Stephen . . .," one advocate argued, "should not be so devalued in a society where our constitutional rights are supposed to promise us equality. . . . States are left to their own means and only 18 have decided that children's lives are worth the effort and cost."[49] Another parent noted that she and other advocates view their most promising long-range strategy to be gradually pressuring their state to include *all* screenable conditions, including those that have little personal relevance.[50] By linking the argument that screening saves babies with the argument that all babies should have equal access to screening, advocates of expanded screening effectively set the bar for laggard states to meet at the highest possible number of screenable disorders, regardless of the utility of some of these tests.

Reports in the mass media once again provide evidence of the association of parents with the urgency narrative, revealed in the correlation between parents as sources of evidence in a given article and the appearance of the urgency

narrative in that same piece. The content analysis of newspaper articles in the
United States between 1970 and 2007 reveals that the more frequently parental
anecdotes appear in an article, the more likely that article is to include multiple mentions of NBS's purportedly lifesaving benefits. In articles with no
parental anecdotes, 14 percent have multiple references to lifesaving benefits,
whereas in articles with two or more parental anecdotes, 54 percent have multiple such references. Similarly, 39 percent of articles with no parental anecdotes portrayed conditions screened through NBS as treatable (presumed so,
without any supportive evidence), whereas a full 73 percent of articles that
included parental anecdotes implicitly embodied this assumption.

The persistence of these features of the urgency narrative, in contradiction
to the changing nature of the conditions covered in NBS panels, is also evident
in the content of these newspaper articles. The media continued to portray
NBS as lifesaving just as often after the ACMG report as it did before it, or even
as far back as the 1990s. In fact, the proportion of articles in which NBS is
presumed to be lifesaving remained the same (roughly 32 percent) from 1975
through 2007.

Multiple Conflagrations: NBS Expansion and
the Intersection of Policy Actors' Interests

Beginning in about 2004, the tide of NBS expansion began to turn and parent
advocates were no longer encountering so much resistance. Rather, as often
occurs, their policy interests began to coincide much more closely and explicitly with those of an array of other actors pursuing their own ends in shaping
newborn-screening policies and practices: private companies pushing to sell
screening technology and lab services; states coping with pressure to save
money by purportedly preventing future births of disabled children; the
research establishment, anxious to translate genetic bench science into clinical
practice; and politicians who could see political advantage in saving lives
through screening (especially when screening costs are cheap and funding
for follow-up services is not necessarily on the public radar).[51] As suggested
earlier, the combined engagement of these other actors also garnered the exponential growth in media coverage common to these early stages of the issue
attention cycle, which is driven (in large part) by the interaction of political
leaders and media outlets.

Though the urgency narrative had its origin in the experiences of parents
who suffered or averted crises related to their child's screenable and treatable
genetic disorder, both policy makers and the media have now appropriated
it to a significant extent. In the rhetoric of legislators, the narrative is visible in

several different ways. For example, the theme of interstate competition remains a major one (as of 2008), even though differences between state screening programs are shrinking rapidly as state after state adopts the ACMG-recommended panel. Nonetheless, Senator Hillary Clinton touted New York's leadership in NBS by noting that she is "proud to say that New York has been a leader in newborn screening since 1960 when Dr. Robert Guthrie developed the first newborn screening test." Further, New York's NBS panel expansion from eleven to forty-four conditions was to ensure the goal, Clinton said, "that every child born with a treatable disease should receive early diagnosis and lifesaving treatment so that they can grow up happy and healthy."[52] In Mississippi and Arkansas, legislators named new laws mandating broader screening after the deceased children of parent advocates who pushed tirelessly for NBS expansion.

Federal NBS legislation signed into law in 2008 is named, in full resonance with the urgency narrative, the Newborn Screening Saves Lives Act. Not unsurprisingly, the powerful prospect of death or disability from a preventable disorder dominated both congressional testimony and public discourse as the legislation worked its way to the president's desk. As described by Senator Christopher Dodd, one of the act's primary sponsors: "In the most direct sense, newborn screening saves lives. . . . Although the disorders that are tested for are quite rare, there is a chance that any one newborn can be affected, a sort of morbid lottery, if you will. In that sense, this is an issue that has a direct impact on the lives of every single family."[53]

The U.S. media generally portrays NBS as an uncomplicated solution to an urgent problem. Even when no parent of an affected child is cited, media articles in the United States are roughly 10 percent more likely to portray NBS in simplistically lifesaving terms than are comparable articles in the Commonwealth countries.[54] Heavy reliance on the urgency narrative in reports on broadly expanded screening can be particularly problematic, since errors of fact then become increasingly likely. The *Minneapolis Star Tribune*, for example, leads a 2007 article with the claim that "for little Ella Madison," a positive NBS screen for cystic fibrosis "may have made the difference between life and death."[55] However, cystic fibrosis—unlike the metabolic disorders that were the original targets of screening programs—does not generally result in sudden, dramatic illness in apparently healthy newborns, and thus cannot truthfully be used to exemplify a broader claim about NBS's capacity to save the lives of imminently imperiled infants.

With the ACMG report confidently recommending nationwide screening for fifty-four conditions, and the urgency narrative powerfully shaping a univocal discourse that makes it increasingly difficult to consider conditions one by one, "conflagration" really is an apt metaphor for depicting the rate of NBS expansion. Under these circumstances, states may adopt screening for conditions before they have adequate education, counseling, treatment, and follow-up procedures in place. Further, because states most often have no capacity to differentiate the new newborn screening from the earlier version of the program, they may treat all positive results as emergencies—even results that indicate a potential nonemergent condition. The experience of mistakenly believing one's child to be the tragic winner of a "morbid lottery"—and so condemned to death like the character in Shirley Jackson's famous story—is thus increasing. Ironically, at the same historical moment, the urgency narrative—with its invocation of both an early-onset, life-threatening illness and of a reliable cure—now captures the actual situation of a *decreasing* percentage of families with babies who screen positive.

Presentation and Representation: Have the Parents Really Spoken?

The "NBS saves lives" narrative is an enormously compelling one. However, its deployment in the service of broad NBS expansion, and the resulting impassioned policy activism for expanded NBS now burning hotly all around us, arguably represent what John McDonough has characterized as "the misuse of anecdote" in policy making—that is, the development of large-scale policies in response to individual narratives that may or may not accurately characterize the experience of a larger group.[56] In the case of NBS, I would argue that the larger group of relevance is *all* parents whose lives are touched by screening, not just those whose baby was saved from death or disability by a timely and fortuitous test result. This includes the increasingly large number of parents who receive disease labels at birth for asymptomatic babies because states are now testing for conditions whose onset is later than the newborn period, and because universal screening is resulting in the identification of genetic mutations that may never lead to symptoms of any kind. It includes the tens (or, with expanded screening, perhaps hundreds) of thousands of families—at least ten for every "true" positive baby identified—who are informed their baby has screened positive for a serious genetic disorder at birth, and who then undergo follow-up testing which determines that the initial screen was a false positive. And of course it includes all four million families whose babies are tested each year, all of whom are subject to an emerging future that includes extensive collection of genetic information from every newborn right at birth.

As I have suggested here, the dynamics of parental advocacy around NBS have made it very difficult to achieve polyvocal, broadly participatory advocacy. As Dresser describes it, the ideal process by which public participation in policy decisions can be fostered would include: fair distribution among interest groups of opportunities to participate; an inclusive perspective on the part of advocates about how best to serve the public; and provision of information from public health officials and others that would "assist public participants to understand and debate the values and trade-offs that are at stake in these decisions."[57] The urgency of the life-and-death narrative in NBS is so compelling, however, and the activism it ignites is so powerful, that with few exceptions, these safeguards are not in place, resulting in a situation where very little attention is paid to "not just . . . the *values* but also the *processes* by which patients' interests are defined, measured, and protected."[58] Rather, policy makers and NBS program bureaucrats hear from the usual suspects among parents, and believe that, as one public health worker told me in October 2005: "The parents have spoken, and the government has listened. Parents want to know their diagnoses no matter what."

Published research about parents' qualitative experiences with NBS programs is scanty indeed, as are reliable data regarding broader public opinion about NBS expansion, with the exception of a few focus group studies.[59] But my own research in this area clearly suggests that dramatic cases involving children's lives lost or saved are not the only diagnostic experiences that matter: even parents of children with a true positive screen have complex feelings about what Jennifer Rosner has called the "cursed blessing of newborn screening."[60] Parents whom I have interviewed speak eloquently about what is lost when the diagnosis comes so very early, or—in the case of later diagnosis—what would have been lost had the diagnosis come much earlier. They speak about how sustaining even a brief time of "blissful ignorance" during the child's infancy can be; about how overwhelming it is to care for and get to know a newborn and learn about his or her disease all at the same time; about how impossible it is to separate the diagnosis from the child's identity when knowledge of the disease comes so soon; about how much parental power and control tend to be ceded to health care providers when the parent is taken unawares by a diagnosis of a completely unsuspected genetic disorder. The parents I interviewed spoke also by their actions, by electing *not* to have their second or third babies—who were known to be at risk for genetic disease for which there is not yet a mandatory screen—evaluated at birth, despite their verbal support of newborn-screening policy in the abstract.

Parents of babies who screen positive for a genetic disorder via NBS but then prove, after follow-up testing, not to be affected at all or to be genetic "carriers" who will not manifest the disease but may pass it on to their own children, are another group whose voices remain mute in public dialog about NBS—despite their much greater number than parents of "true positive" children. We know from earlier research that, even after follow-up tests indicate to the satisfaction of *clinicians* that the infant's health is not imperiled, *parents* receiving false-positive results suffer various consequences related to the testing experience. These include increased anxiety levels, higher overall vigilance, and worry about their children's health sufficient to result in disproportionately high numbers of visits to the emergency department.[61]

Parents whose children undergo follow-up testing and *still* do not have a clear disease diagnosis—a group clinicians and NBS program directors describe as growing rapidly in the era of expanded testing—have yet another perspective that is largely absent from the NBS discourse. Although little research with this cohort of parents has yet been published, and my own qualitative interviews with them are still in process, the evidence to date suggests a heartrending poignancy embedded in their experience. As one parent in my study described the experience to me:

> I think the key thing with an asymptomatic child to me was that you are constantly [walking] the tension between saying I am in denial about this because you don't feel like anything is wrong, and feeling like you have to acknowledge it mentally, or the gods of irony, or the gods of poetic justice will make something actually wrong with your child. It is like when you get on a plane you have to acknowledge plane flying is dangerous or the plane will crash. . . . He is growing well, he is meeting all his physical and developmental milestones and so on and so forth, but you still don't know what to tell people because you don't fit into any of the groups. You don't fit into the "something is really wrong with my child group," but you don't fit into "my child is perfectly healthy group," so there is like there isn't any place for you.[62]

Statements such as this do not yet appear in the transcripts of legislative hearings, on NBS advisory committees, or in media coverage. Yet they clearly suggest that perhaps the parents, in all their diversity of experience and opinion, have not yet in fact fully spoken. The necessary research and organizing work has not yet been done, I would argue, to elicit the stories and perspectives of the majority of those who have been and will be affected by screening—people who have not gone public with a newsworthy narrative, yet whose lives are radically altered by an unsolicited early diagnosis or even a false-positive result. As Beatrix Hoffman has pointed out, the barriers to more comprehensive participation are many: "The fragmented and stratified nature of American health care makes activism equally fragmented and stratified. The massive complexity of the system means that activists can only address a tiny part of it—and that ordinary, unorganized people can do even less."[63]

Conclusion

Preventable death and disability are unmitigated tragedies. Not a single life is expendable, and no unnecessary death should pass without notice, without mourning, and without action by all who can usefully participate in change designed to protect *other* people before they suffer a similar fate. If systems need to be shaken up, if parents need to be fighters and zealots, if they need to be screamers, so be it. As Dostoyevsky's character Ivan declares to Alyosha in *The Brothers Karamazov*, imagining the response of a mother while witnessing her child's slaying: "I don't want harmony. From love for humanity I don't want it."[64]

Our health care system badly needs patients (including parents of patients or of would-be patients) to be part of creating and transforming policy—even when their inclusion results in messiness of various kinds. Our system must be responsive to those who have the courage to sacrifice harmony and give voice to both their experiences and their convictions. However, the stakes for full inclusion of patients in policy making are so high that more must be done than to simply make room at the table for those who spontaneously move from service recipient or citizen to policy activist. Indeed, we must go beyond mere responsiveness—as others in this volume have noted—to proactive solicitation of broad and democratic participation. Put another way, those with the most power to shape health policy have a duty not only to listen to what they are being told but also to ask, in various ways, for the perspective of those who may not be first to voluntarily stand up and speak. One important legacy of parents' persuasive influence over the course of newborn screening should be to remind us that as a polity, we need to pay careful attention to how our collective actions touch individuals' lives. To do this, as the NBS story illustrates, requires more than pro forma acquiescence to participation. It requires more, even, than willingness to grant entree to those who speak loudest. What is needed is a serious commitment of time, attention, and resources so that we are able to hear the quiet as well as the forceful voices of personal experience.

Qualitative social science research designed to elicit nuanced voice that might not otherwise be heard is one useful mechanism for this important work. Another is careful revisiting of operating guidelines and procedures that govern parent/patient participation in formal committee structures—in terms of both who is qualified to be a member, and how duties to truly represent a class of people are defined, encouraged, enabled, and evaluated. Civic engagement around issues in genetics, via mechanisms such as community-based participatory research and deliberative policy making, is another promising avenue.[65] Finally, at a broader level, health system reform must heed the call of advocates who insist that no new policy agenda can succeed unless it institutionalizes arrangements both for giving all individuals who interact with the health care system effective consumer voice (largely by providing access to advocates) and for ensuring that patterns in the cumulative experience of consumers are effectively identified and articulated at community and policy-making levels.

The urgency narrative has evolved from a heartfelt solo sung by those for whom it has personal meaning to a powerful chorus chanted by an ever-expanding group of actors (such as policy makers and industry representatives) whose motivations and experiences are *not* directly shaped by the death or disability of a loved one. In the process, the powerful threat of tragedy, and the promise of averting it, have reached beyond specific situations where they have established or plausible merit to a general analogy that no longer ably captures complex consequences of policy for affected groups. It is our shared responsibility to protect the integrity of both the original solo, and of the chorus that has swelled in its wake, by ensuring that as newborn-screening policy evolves over time, its changing implications and expanding scope of influence are reflected by changes in who and what is included in policy discussions. As I have suggested here, to make this aspiration a reality calls for thinking through the role of parents and of parental voice with significantly more analytic nuance and imagination than has been evidenced to date.

Notes

1. Michael Waldholz, "Testing Fate; A Drop of Blood Saves One Baby; Another Falls Ill." *Wall Street Journal*, June 17, 2004. The chapter epigraph is from Gina Kolata, "Panel to Advise Tests on Babies for 29 Diseases," *New York Times*, February 21, 2005.
2. Carey Goldberg, "Big Gap in Screening U.S. Infants for Hereditary Ills," *New York Times*, February 26, 2000.
3. Nancy Tomes, "Patients or Health-Care Consumers? Why the History of Contested Terms Matters," in *History and Health Policy in the United States: Putting the Past Back In*, ed. Rosemary Stevens, Charles Rosenberg, and Lawton Burns (New Brunswick, N.J.: Rutgers University Press, 2006), 83–110; Rachel Jewkes and Anne Murcott, "Community Representatives: Representing the Community?" *Social Science Medicine* 46, 7 (1998): 843–858.
4. American Academy of Pediatrics [AAP], "Serving the Family from Birth to the Medical Home Newborn Screening: A Blueprint for the Future A Call for a National

Agenda on State Newborn Screening Programs," *Pediatrics* 106, no. 2 (2000): 389–427.

5. Ellen W. Clayton, "Symposium: Legal and Ethical Issues Raised by Human Genome Project, Screening, and Treatment of Newborns," *Houston Law Review* 29 (1992): 85–148.

6. Diane Paul, "Contesting Consent: The Challenge to Compulsory Neonatal Screening for PKU," *Perspectives in Biology and Medicine* 42, 2 (1999): 207; AAP, "Serving the Family."

7. AAP, "Serving the Family"; American College of Obstetricians and Gynecologists [ACOG], "ACOG Committee Opinion No. 287, October: Newborn Screening," *Obstetrics and Gynecology* 102, 4 (2003): 887–889; Sarah E. Gollust, Barbara P. Fuller, Paul S. Miller, and Barbara Biesecker, "Community Involvement in Developing Policies for Genetic Testing: Assessing the Interests and Experiences of Individuals Affected by Genetic Conditions," *Health Policy and Ethics* 95, 1 (2005): 35; *Newborn Screening: Characteristics of State Programs*, No. GAO-03–449 (Washington, D.C.: U.S. General Accounting Office, 2003); Timothy Hoff and Adrienne Hoyt, "Practices and Perceptions of Long-Term Follow-up among State Newborn Screening Programs," *Pediatrics* 117, 6 (2006): 922–929; Bradford Therrell, Alissa Johnson, and Donna Williams, "Status of Newborn Screening Programs in the United States," *Pediatrics* 117, 5 (2006): S212–S252.

8. U.S. General Accounting Office, Newborn Screening, http:genes-r-us.uthscsa.edu/, accessed May 31, 2007.

9. For all states, see Hoff and Hoyt, "Practices and Perceptions"; for New York, see Al Baker, "State Will Expand Tests That Find Defects in Newborns," *New York Times*, October 8, 2004.

10. Bridget Wilcken, "Ethical Issues in Newborn Screening and the Impact of New Technologies," *European Journal of Pediatrics* 162, 1 (2003): s62–s66; ACOG, "Newborn Screening."

11. Therrell, "U.S. Newborn Screening Policy Dilemmas."

12. American College of Medical Genetics [ACMG], "Newborn Screening: Toward a Uniform Screening Panel and System," *Genetics Medicine* 8, 5 (May 2006), supp., http://www.acmg.net/resources/policies/NBS/NBS_Exec_Sum.pdf.

13. Jeffrey Botkin, Ellen W. Clayton, Norman Fost, Wylie Burke, Thomas Murray, Mary A. Baily, Benjamin Wilfond, Alfred Berg, and Lainie Friedman Ross, "Newborn Screening Technology: Proceed with Caution," *Pediatrics* 117 (2006): 1793–1799; ACMG, "Newborn Screening."

14. Nicholas Freudenberg and Maxine Golub, "Health Education, Public Policy, and Disease Prevention: A Case History of the New York City Coalition to End Lead Poisoning," *Health Education Quarterly* 14, 4 (1987): 387–388.

15. On fetal alcohol syndrome efforts, Jocie DeVries and Ann Waller, "Parent Advocacy in FAS Public Policy Change," in *Challenge of Fetal Alcohol Syndrome: Overcoming Secondary Disabilities*, ed. Ann Steissguth and Jonathon Kanter (Seattle: University of Washington Press, 1997), 171–180; on efforts for children with autism, James A. Mulick and Eric M. Butter, "Educational Advocacy for Children with Autism," *Behavioral Interventions* 17 (2002): 57–74.

16. Martine Hackett, "Unsettled Sleep: The Construction and Consequences of a Public Health Media Campaign" (Ph.D. diss., City University of New York Graduate Center, 2007).

17. Parent advocate presentation, Sarah Lawrence College, Bronxville, N.Y., May 2007, author files.

18. For "zealots," Rita Rubin, "Saved by a Drop of Blood; States Expand Routine Testing of Newborns," *USA Today*, July 11, 2006; for "fighter moms," Sharon Wynne, "A Fighting Chance," *St. Petersburg Times*, April 25, 2006.

19. Deborah Lupton, "Risk as Moral Danger: The Social and Political Functions of Risk Discourse in Public Health," in *The Sociology of Health and Illness: Critical Perspectives*, ed. Peter Conrad (New York: Worth, 2001); Alan Petersen and Deborah Lupton, *The New Public Health: Health and Self in the Age of Risk* (London: Sage Publications, 1996); Dorothy Nelkin, "The Social Dynamics of Genetic Testing: The Case of Fragile X," *Medical Anthropology Quarterly* 10, 4 (1996): 537–550.

20. Petersen and Lupton, *The New Public Health*, 48.

21. Regarding competition among advocacy causes, Rebecca Dresser, "Public Advocacy and Allocation of Federal Funds for Biomedical Research," *Milbank Quarterly* 77, 2 (1999): 257–274

22. Jennifer Howse, Marina Weis, and Nancy Green, "Critical Role of the March of Dimes in the Expansion of Newborn Screening," *Mental Retardation and Developmental Disabilities Research Reviews* 12 (2006): 280–287.

23. Makani Themba, *Making Policy/Making Change: How Communities Are Taking Law into Their Own Hands* (Berkeley, Calif.: Chardon Press, 1999); Charlotte Ryan, *Prime Time Activism: Media Strategies for Grassroots Organizing* (Boston: South End Press, 1991).

24. B. Guy Peters and Brian W. Hogwood," In Search of the Issue-Attention Cycle," *Journal of Politics* 47 (1985): 39–53.

25. Our database included, at the time of this writing, 189 articles from the U.S. and 45 from Commonwealth countries Australia, New Zealand, and the U.K. Rachel Grob and Mark Schlesinger, "Astigmatism in the Public Eye: An Analysis of Gaps in the Media Coverage of the Ethical and Social Issues Regarding Newborn Genetic Screening," paper presented at Translating ELSI: Ethical, Legal, and Social Implications of Genomics conference, Cleveland, Ohio, May 1–3, 2008.

26. Ibid.

27. Mark Somerson, "State Urged to Test Babies for More Disorders," *Columbus (Ohio) Dispatch*, February 14, 2000.

28. D. E. Dougherty, "Testing of Newborns Can Be a Lifesaver," letter to the editor, *Boston Globe*, March 4, 2000.

29. Virginia Moyer, Ned Calonge, Steven Teutsch, and Jeffrey Botkin, on behalf of the U.S. Preventive Services Task Force, "Expanding Newborn Screening: Process, Policy, and Priorities," *Hastings Center Report* 38, 3 (2008): 32–39.

30. Botkin, quoted in Kolata, "Panel to Advise Tests."

31. Save Babies Through Screening Foundation, www.savebabies.org.

32. CARES Foundation, "Newborn Screening Advocacy," http://www.caresfoundation .org/productcart/pc/advocacy_efforts_cah.html, accessed May 2007.

33. Clayton, "Symposium"; Botkin et al., "Newborn Screening Technology."

34. Adil E. Shamoo and Felix A. Kihn-Maung-Gyi, *Ethics of the Use of Human Subjects in Research* (London: Garland Science Publishing, 2002).

35. Moyer et al., "Expanding Newborn Screening."

36. Elizabeth Campbell and Lainie F. Ross, "Parental Attitudes Regarding Newborn Screening of PKU and DMD," *American Journal of Medical Genetics* 120A (2003): 209–214.

37. Steven Epstein, "The Construction of Lay Expertise: AIDS Activism and the Forging of Credibility in the Reform of Clinical Trials," *Science, Technology, and Human Values* 20, 4 (1995), special issue.

38. Fost, quoted in Kolata, "Panel to Advise Tests."

39. Save Babies Through Screening Foundation, www.savebabies.org.

40. Barbara K. Rothman, *The Tentative Pregnancy* (New York: Viking, 1986); Rayna Rapp, *Testing Women, Testing the Fetus* (New York: Routledge, 2000).

41. New York State Department of Health, "Newborn Screening in New York State: A Guide for Health Professionals, http://www.wadsworth.org/newborn/phyguidelines .pdf.

42. Susan Schindehette, "A Simple Test Could Have Saved Ben's Life: Haygood Family and Others Pushing for Expansion of Newborn Screening," *People*, August 2, 2004, 107–108.

43. Nelkin, "Social Dynamics," 546.

44. Neil Smith, "Diseases Added to Infant Testing; Cost of Screening Increases to $89.25," *Arkansas Democrat Gazette*, November 3, 2007; Todd Cooper, "Couple to Appeal Blood Test Order," *Omaha World Herald*, December 19, 2003.

45. Patricia Guthrie, "Georgia Is Behind on Newborn Tests," *Atlanta Journal-Constitution*, July 12, 2005.

46. Erik Eckholm, "In Turnabout, Infant Deaths Climb in South," *New York Times*, April 27, 2007.

47. Peter Urban, "Newborn Screening Program Boosted," *Connecticut Post Online* (local), December 14, 2007.

48. Andy Miller and Patricia Guthrie, "Newborns at Risk: How Georgia's Health Screening Practices Can Put Newborns at Risk," *Atlanta Journal-Constitution*, Feb. 2, 2003.

49. U.S. Department of Health and Human Services, Advisory Committee on Heritable Disorders in Newborns and Children, 2005, http://www.mchb.hrsa.gov/programs/ genetics/presentations/comments/Monaco.htm, accessed February 20, 2010.

50. Parent interview with author, Association of Public Health Laboratories, Newborn Screening and Genetic Testing Symposium, Minneapolis, May 7, 2007.

51. On the frequent coincidence of policy interests, Nancy Tomes, "Patient Empowerment and the Dilemmas of Late-Modern Medicalisation," *Lancet* 369 (2007): 698–700; Deena White, "Consumer and Community Participation: A Reassessment of Process, Impact, and Value" in *The Handbook of Social Studies in Health and Medicine*, ed. Gary Albrecht, Ray Fitzpatrick, and Susan Scrimshaw *Thousand Oaks, Calif.: Sage, 2000*. On newborn screening specifically, Mary A. Baily and Thomas Murray, "Ethics, Evidence, and Cost in Newborn Screening," *Hastings Center Report 38, 3* (2008): 23–31.

52. Hillary Rodham Clinton, "Statement of Senator Hillary Rodham Clinton introducing Screening for Health of Infants and Newborns (SHINE) Act of 2006 (Washington, D.C.), July 26, 2006," States News Service.

53. Senate Subcommittee on Children and Families, "Newborn Screening: Increasing Options and Awareness," statement of Senator Chris Dodd, chair, 2nd sess., June 14, 2002, http://dodd.senate.gov/index.php?q=node/3274&pr=press/Speeches/107_02/ 0614.htm.

54. Grob and Schlesinger, "Astigmatism in the Public Eye."

55. "Five Drops of Blood: Invasion of Privacy," *Star Tribune*, Nov. 10, 2007, http://www .startribune.com/lifestyle/health/11345741.html.

56. John E. McDonough, "Using and Misusing Anecdote in Policy Making," *Health Affairs* 20, 1 (2001): 207–212.

57. Dresser, "Public Advocacy," 259.

58. Tomes, "Patient Empowerment," 698.

59. Terry Davis, Sharon Humiston, Connie Arnold, Joseph Bocchini, Pat Bass, Estella Kennen, Anna Bocchini, Donna Williams, Penny Kyler, and Michelle Lloyd-Puryear, "Recommendations for Effective Newborn Screening Communication: Results of Focus Groups with Parents, Providers, and Experts," *Pediatrics* 117 (2006): 326–340; Campbell and Ross, "Parental Attitudes."

60. Jennifer Rosner, "Lullabies for Sophia," *Hastings Center Report* 34, 6 (2004): 21. Some of my own research is reported in Rachel Grob, "Parenting in the Genomic Age: The Cursed Blessing of Newborn Screening," *New Genetics and Society* 25, 2 (2006): 159–170; Rachel Grob, "Is My Sick Child Healthy? Is My Healthy Child Sick? Changing Parental Experiences of Cystic Fibrosis in the Age of Expanded Newborn Screening," *Social Science and Medicine* 67, 7 (2008): 1056–1064.

61. Suzanne Bennett Johnson, Jin-Xion She, Amy Baughcum, Desmond Schatz, and Stacy Carmichael, "Maternal Anxiety Associated with Newborn Genetic Screening for Type 1 Diabetes," *Diabetes Care* 27, 2 (2004): 392–397; Clayton, "Symposium"; Susan E. Waisbren, Simone Albers, Steve Amato, Mary Ampola, Thomas G. Brewster, Laurie Demmer, Roger B. Eaton, Robert Greenstein, Mark Korson, Cecilia Larson et al., "Effect of Expanded Newborn Screening for Biochemical Genetic Disorders on Child Outcomes and Parental Stress," *JAMA* 290, 19 (2003): 2606–2608; Paul, "Contesting Consent."

62. For a description of the full study from which this interview is drawn, see Rachel Grob, *Testing Baby: The Transformation of Newborn Screening, Parenting and Policy* (New Brunswick, N.J.: Rutgers University Press, forthcoming).

63. Beatrix Hoffman, "Bringing the Patient Back In: Health Policy History from the Bottom Up." Presentation at the Policy History Conference, Charlottesville, Va., June 1, 2006.

64. Fyodor Dostoevsky, *The Brothers Karamazov*, trans. Constance Garnett (New York: Signet Classic, 1957), 226.

65. See for example Bruce Jennings, "Genetic Literacy and Citizenship: Possibilities for Deliberative Democratic Policymaking in Science and Medicine," *Good Society* 13, 1 (2004): 38–44.

Measuring Success

Scientific, Institutional, and Cultural Effects of Patient Advocacy

In understanding the role of patients in the transformation of health care and the improvement of health, certainly one of the most pressing tasks is to assess just how effective patients have been when they have banded together.[1] The blossoming of patient groups and health movements as political actors has rightly attracted the attention of scholars seeking to understand the significance and consequences of this form of social organization.[2] The goals pursued by these groups are increasingly diverse, as are the organizational forms they take and the methods they employ. In this chapter, however, I focus on the question of results: To what extent, and in what ways, do patient groups achieve success?

Although it is important not to romanticize patient advocacy or exaggerate the impact of patient groups,[3] I argue that it is possible to point to many ways in which such actors have succeeded in bringing about change. I examine the work of a range of patient groups—some very well known, such as breast cancer and AIDS activists, and some relatively unknown—in order to analyze the consequences of their actions and the kinds of changes that they brought about. I look critically at the question of what we actually mean by "success," and I consider both the intended and unintended consequences of patient advocacy. The struggle of patient advocates to succeed is complicated by what I here categorize as problems of representation, expertise, and incorporation and cooptation. Although there can be no blueprint or checklist for success, comparisons across cases reveal patterns that merit consideration by scholars, policy makers, and health advocates alike.

The Meanings of Success

Analysts of social movements have had much to say about the question of how and why movements succeed;[4] yet in his introduction to a volume on "how social movements matter," Marco Giugni observed that "the study of the consequences of social movements is one of the most neglected topics in the literature." Giugni complained that "investigators have generally given much more attention to origins and trajectories of social movements than to their impact on routine politics, on their social environment, on other social movements, or on the participants themselves."[5] To the extent that researchers have taken up the issue of consequences, Giugni added, any possibility of a broad engagement with the question has been sidetracked by a near-exclusive concern with a restricted set of questions having to do with the preconditions of success, such as whether disruptive or moderate tactics are more effective in bringing about change, and whether success is due more to factors internal to the movement or to features of the external environment in which the movement finds itself. (As Giugni rightly points out, these questions probably have no general answers.)

It certainly seems odd that scholars of social change would neglect the study of whether and how change occurs. However, the complexities of studying success may help explain why researchers have often shied away from the topic. What does "success" mean, anyway, in terms of a social movement? The question can (and to some extent must) be approached from the perspective of a movement's stated goals. But "movements are not homogeneous entities," and "often there is little agreement within a movement as to what goals must be pursued," either at a given moment or over time as the movement evolves.[6] Moreover, the real measure of a movement's success may not be whether it achieves *for itself* the benefits that it sought, but whether its actions end up benefiting some larger social group.[7] More problematic, focusing on a movement's stated goals ignores indirect outcomes and unintended consequences. Much of what a movement brings about may be at some remove from what it formally was seeking, and, indeed, sometimes the downstream effects of activism run counter to what the movement hoped to achieve. Yet these are results all the same. Even movement failures may be an important result insofar as they serve as "antimodels" for subsequent activists.[8]

In his analysis of the limitations of the existing literature, Giugni also took social movement scholars to task for their tendency to assume that the results of activism should necessarily be sought in the domain of policy outcomes.[9] The analytical emphasis on policy is quite understandable: the passage of legislation, or the formal adoption of new policies, is much easier to observe and to tabulate than more diffuse social and cultural effects. Yet effects that may be quite difficult to measure in precise quantitative terms can have great long-term consequences: the impact of activism on the life course of activists, the creation of new collective identities and social networks, the rise of new social alignments and political alliances, the formation of new movements or countermovements in response to an existing one, shifts in public opinion, and broad changes in cultural schemas and frameworks of understanding.

Alongside the sometimes narrow emphasis on policy outcomes, scholars too often have assumed that "real" protest targets only the central organs of political authority—that is, activism matters to the extent that social movements take on the state. However, a growing number of scholars, such as Kelly Moore and Nella Van Dyke, Sarah Soule, and Verta Taylor, have challenged this presumption by promoting the study of how social movements target nonstate actors, including "institutions such as medicine, art, science, law, and education."[10] Indeed, Elizabeth Armstrong and Mary Bernstein have put forward a manifesto for a "multi-institutional" theory of social movements, precisely in opposition to the bias in the literature toward focusing on how movements challenge the state; the authors emphasize the need to examine challenges to the diverse loci of power in modern societies.[11] Clearly, an emphasis on nonstate actors has considerable relevance for any study of health activism. Moreover, knowing whom a movement targets is essential for understanding its effects. Indeed, Moore has observed an interesting paradox with regard to the possibilities for activists' success. On the one hand, nonstate institutions may be harder to crack into than state institutions because they may present a less-public face, and authority within them may be more widely dispersed. On the other hand, nonstate institutions typically lack the resources state actors can marshal to squelch opposition, which means that once activists manage to get a foot in the door, they may have a somewhat easier time transforming such institutions.[12]

This question of the relative accessibility of various institutions to protest points to broader questions about precisely how social movements are able to bring about results. Analysts have identified an array of attributes that affect the achievement of success, including the movement's ability to cause social disruption, the resources it can bring to bear, its organizational capacities, its allies, and its categorical similarities to movements that have gained access previously.[13] At times an overemphasis on the resources and organizational capacities that set the stage for successful activism has led scholars to ignore "the potential influence of cultural and ideational factors in the determination of movement outcomes," such as whether movements do a good job of

articulating and framing their diagnoses of social problems in ways that res-
onate with their audiences.[14]

In this chapter, I apply to patient groups and health movements this set of
insights about how, when, and why social movements matter, addressing the
broad question of what such groups have accomplished with an eye to both
direct and indirect, and intended and unintended, effects of patient advocacy.
I scrutinize activist engagement with health and biomedical institutions along
with a host of other social institutions, considering outcomes on politics and
policy, social structure and organization, and cultural meanings and practices.

Varieties of Success

Many commentators have noted the sheer quantitative increase in the formation of patient groups and health movements in recent years as well as their
enhanced social visibility.[15] This upsurge of health- and disease-based organizing reflects the prevalence in recent decades of more skeptical attitudes
toward doctors, scientists, and other experts, trends also manifested in new
conceptions of patients' rights and renewed concerns with bioethical
debates.[16] Many scholars also have associated recent patient groups and health
movements with the more general expansion of rights-based movements and of
so-called new social movements since the 1960s.[17] Patient groups and health
movements pursue goals that include seeking (or sometimes rejecting) medical
cures; improving the quality of life of ill people; cultivating practical advice
for the management of illness; raising funds for research; changing scientific
and medical practices, priorities, or orientations; and changing diffuse cultural
meanings associated with health, illness, the body, and expertise.

It is important not to exaggerate the effects of patient advocacy. Patient
groups may possess limited abilities to organize and engage successfully with
health professionals or other powerful actors.[18] As Constance Nathanson has
argued, health movements may spark potent opposition from countermovements, and even when they are successful the benefits may accrue mostly to
relatively privileged, middle-class activists.[19] Still, scholars have identified a range
of ways in which these groups contribute to social and biomedical change.[20]

The conceptualization of the disease

Patient organizations may sometimes shape even the basic medical understanding of a disease. For example, as Howard Kushner has described, the U.S.
Tourette Syndrome Association played an influential role in promoting the
conception of Tourette's as an organic disease; in contrast, in the absence of
a strong group of patients and their family members, Tourette's in France is

understood within a psychodynamic framework.[21] In another example, a grass-roots self-help group, the Endometriosis Association, helped reorient conceptions of the etiology of endometriosis away from purely endogenous causal factors and toward "a more holistic view that explores connections between the human body and a chemically toxic environment."[22]

Patients' management of their illnesses

Although it has become common to speak of the "educated patient," the role of patient groups in creating such patients is sometimes overlooked. Research suggests that the activities of patient groups can change the ways in which patients engage with their physicians, their medications, and their bodies.[23] The work of Janine Barbot and Nicolas Dodier is exemplary in delineating how HIV/AIDS groups in France have been associated with various "pragmatics of information gathering" and strategies of illness management on the part of patients. Barbot has identified four types of educated patients—the patient as illness manager, the empowered patient, the science-wise patient, and the experimenter—and correlated each type with a different French HIV/AIDS support or advocacy group.[24]

Attitudes and practices of health professionals

Some health movements have inspired greater sensitivity on the part of physicians and researchers, for example, in their judgments about people who are overweight.[25] In other cases, patient groups and health movements have brought about concrete changes in physician practice—though as Katrina Karkazis has noted in her analysis of intersex activism, physicians may sometimes be unwilling to concede that their embracing of new policies had anything to do with outside pressure.[26]

The research process.

Examples of the impact of patient groups and health movements on biomedical research are abundant, and scholars have been especially inclined to document them. Patient groups have raised funds for research and have doled it out to support the lines of research they deem most important; gained a seat at the table to make decisions about research directions; promoted ethical treatment of participants in clinical trials; attempted to police perceived ethical abuses such as conflicts of interest in research; challenged the techniques for conducting and interpreting clinical trials; helped create disease and treatment registries; organized conferences; coauthored publications; and pioneered new models of participatory research that joins the efforts of lay citizens with those of experts.[27]

Other effects are less tangible but no less significant. Michel Callon and Vololona Rabeharisoa have hinted at the new "entanglements" between patients and researchers by quoting a young girl with spinal muscular atrophy who told a biologist: "I'm with you in your laboratory since you're working on my genes."[28] As David Hess has suggested, such entanglements may proceed along many alternative pathways, including conversion experiences by researchers, transformations of activists into lay researchers, or the creation of "network assemblages" in which activists "help weave together networks of patients, funding sources, clinicians and potential researchers."[29]

Technological trajectories

Patient groups and health movements, acting either as users of technologies or as their representatives, can alter the path of technological development. This impact is clear in the case of contraceptive technologies and abortifacients, where women's health advocates and organizations have altered technological scripts while asserting the priorities of bodily integrity and social justice.[30]

State policies

Michael P. Johnson and Karl Hufbauer's work on how bereaved parents convinced the U.S. Congress to fund research by passing the Sudden Infant Death Syndrome Act of 1974 is just one example of how patient groups have influenced public research funding priorities.[31] But patient groups and health movements also have brought about formal changes in state policies. For example, the tobacco control movement in the United States has had a significant effect on legislation and regulatory policy; in Britain the health consumer movement has pushed the government to develop new procedures for cases where patients claim harm by health professionals; and the fat acceptance movement has prompted the U.S. Food and Drug Administration to postpone its approval of a type of weight-loss surgery.[32] In addition, I have described how a diverse coalition of health advocates in the United States successfully pressed for new federal policies on the inclusion of women, racial and ethnic minorities, children, and the elderly as research subjects, as well as for the creation of federal offices of women's health and minority health.[33]

Corporations and markets

Probably the most frequent corporate target of patient group activity has been pharmaceutical companies. Activists concerned about issues such as drug pricing and research ethics have been able to wrest concessions from drug companies on occasion; and recent global debates about access to medications

such as antiretroviral drugs have suggested the efficacy of transnational link-
ages of patient groups and health movements in affecting the marketing
practices of drug companies as well as their ability to enforce their patents.[34]
However, these are not the only ways in which patient groups have affected
market relations. Sometimes, as in the patenting of the PXE gene described by
Deborah Heath, Rayna Rapp, and Karen-Sue Taussig, patient groups have
successfully claimed intellectual property rights for themselves.[35] In addition,
Hess has examined the productive ties between civil society organizations and
companies promoting alternative health products under the banner of "nutri-
tional therapeutics."[36] Such work may be suggestive of broader patterns by
which patient groups affect the organization of industrial fields, for example,
through their alliances with start-ups.

Cultural effects

Some of the most profound and enduring effects of patient groups and health
movements may be among the most diffuse and hardest to pinpoint. Such
groups may have an important cultural impact simply by exposing prevailing
norms and power relationships and making them available for public critique.[37] For example, as suggested by the disability movement and the intersex
movement, health activists may seek to establish the legitimacy of different
sorts of bodies or bodily experiences.[38] Or patient groups and health movements may enact public performances of bodies and diseases in ways that
challenge conventional cultural codes about appropriate gender roles or
sexualities.[39] They also may reinterpret the historical record, for example, by
attributing disease prevalence in certain groups to historical legacies of social
oppression.[40] Advocacy groups may also engage in important memorialization
work—for example, Sahra Gibbon has described how breast cancer advocates
perform acts of memorialization that connect the witnessing of loss to a new
conception of research as redemption, and Lesley Sharp has shown how
groups representing the surviving relatives of organ transplant donors have
used cultural forms such as donor quilts and Web cemeteries to challenge
transplant professionals' tendencies to "obliterate donors' identities."[41] In these
various ways, patient groups and health movements, like social movements
generally, are involved in reconstructing the "cultural schemas" that define the
rules of the game by which key social institutions operate.[42]

Complications

In their quest to achieve success, patient advocates run up against an array of
obstacles. I emphasize three of them—all linked loosely to the broader

dynamics of the professionalization of social movements—which I call the problem of representation, the problem of expertise, and the problem of incorporation and co-optation.

The Problem of Representation

Who speaks for the patient? This is a crucial question in assessing the success of health advocacy, not only because the goals of representatives may diverge from those of the represented, but also because the struggle to achieve legitimacy as the recognized voice of the patient may lead to rifts and defections within health movements. Although all social movements are prone to such tensions, health movements experience them in some distinctive ways. First, quite a few health advocacy groups that researchers have studied in recent years are organized not by patients per se, but by various proxies for patients. The proxies may be parents, relatives, or partners, in cases where the patients are too young or too physically or mentally incapacitated to advance their own interests;[43] they may be activists who may or may not have the disease or condition in question, and whose interests may not precisely coincide with those of the larger group of patients or users of medical technologies;[44] or they may be advocates speaking on behalf of broad constituencies (such as women, in the case of "women's health") whose interests transcend any specific disease.[45] All these cases call attention to the symbolic practices of representation by which spokespersons come to stand in for a group.[46]

Establishing oneself as a credible representative can endow an activist with considerable power. A clear case is that of AIDS treatment activists in the late 1980s, who presented themselves as the legitimate, organized voice of people with AIDS or HIV infection (or, more specifically, the current or potential clinical trial subject population). Once activists had monopolized the capacity to say what patients wanted, researchers could be forced to deal with them in order to ensure that research subjects would both enroll in their trials in sufficient numbers and comply with the study protocols.[47] Yet, ironically, the very success of AIDS treatment activists in establishing their representational authority helped pave the way for representational struggles within the ranks of the activists themselves. Women and people of color within groups such as ACT UP argued that relatively privileged white gay men had monopolized the public voice of the movement, to the detriment of the health concerns of underprivileged groups. Such charges helped provoke splits and secessions within a number of ACT UP organizations in the early 1990s.[48]

The politics of representation is perhaps even more complicated when political actors seek to voice the health needs of large, identity-based constituencies, such as women or people of color, who constitute large chunks of the population. For example, in calling for the increased inclusion of women, racial and ethnic minorities, children, and the elderly as research subjects in medical research, scientific and political spokespersons from each of the affected communities had to successfully position themselves as representing the interests of these various underrepresented groups. To do so—to speak credibly for such groups as "women" or "people of color"—these spokespersons hardened their claims by bridging or conflating different meanings of "representation" in medical research. They argued from a statistical standpoint that groups needed to be numerically included in studies, but at the same time they argued for representation in the sense of political voice: they saw it as their right to insist that researchers study their particular needs and conditions, and not just those of more privileged social groups. In essence, through what I have called "multi-representational politics," reformers demanded something that went well beyond the demographics of research populations: what they sought was full citizenship. Biomedical inclusion was not just a matter of counting up bodies; it also was a broader indicator of who counted.[49]

The Problem of Expertise

Patient groups and health movements have become noteworthy for their manufacture and deployment of various sorts of informal knowledge and for the development of alternative bases of expertise. Drawing on concepts such as local knowledge, subjugated knowledges, situated knowledges, and ways of knowing, scholars have explored in considerable detail the capacities of organized collectives of lay actors to assess medical knowledge claims and engage with the practices of biomedical knowledge production.[50] More generally, it is increasingly evident that being the sufferer of an illness—or a member of an affected community—can serve as epistemic grounding for developing distinctive, embodied knowledge claims.[51]

Such studies raise important questions about the character and utility of knowledge that grows out of the lived experience of sufferers of health risks. On one hand, the literature amply details the practical benefits of incorporating the experiential knowledge of the patient, not only within the doctor-patient relationship but also within the researcher-subject relationship. On the other hand, most work to date has been insufficiently critical of the tendency to valorize or romanticize lived experience as a basis for reliable knowledge, or to treat experience as a sort of bedrock resistant to critical interpretation.[52] As Michelle Murphy has observed in a study of occupational health: "'Experience' is a category of knowledge that is just as historical as other forms of knowledge. . . . It is only through particular methods rooted historically in time and space that experience becomes a kind of evidence imbued with certain truth-telling qualities."[53]

In addition to, or instead of, mobilizing experiential knowledge, patient groups and health movements also have laid claim to the formal knowledge more typically monopolized by credentialed experts, sometimes through systematic practices of self-education or community-based education.[54] In contrast to groups that are dismissive of formal knowledge, those that learn the biomedical science relevant to their condition adopt (according to Paula Treichler, in an early analysis of AIDS treatment activism) "not . . . a resistance to orthodox science but . . . strategic conceptions of 'scientific truth' that leave room for action in the face of contradictions."[55] In practice, many patient groups and health movements have combined experiential knowledge with varying degrees of mastery of formal knowledge, often producing interestingly hybrid or "translocal" ways of knowing or varieties of expertise.[56] Patient groups and health movements may also employ specific tools and technologies in their epistemic work. For example, some genetic support groups "collect family narratives, genealogical inscriptions and family trees . . . , which are first translated by genetic counselors and researchers into various forms of medical pedigrees for clinical and laboratory work, and then circulated as published pedigrees among lay and medical practitioners."[57] Callon and Rabeharisoa describe members of the French muscular dystrophy organization (the AFM) who have used "proto-instruments" that include "cameras, camcorders for taking films and photos, accounts written by patients or their parents in the form of books for the general public, requested testimonies, spontaneous letters, and lectures given by patients or their relatives." The authors note that such tools permit the production of knowledge that is "formal, transportable, cumulative, and debatable"—characteristics associated with the products of more traditional biomedical research. By this pathway, laboratory research and research conducted "in the wild" are brought together in the form of new cross-fertilizations.[58]

However, these successes on the part of activists in creating and employing hybrid and translocal expertise may be accompanied by a "scientization" of the social movement that can have unanticipated consequences. The case of AIDS treatment activism suggested that the emergence of a specialist group of activist-experts accentuated various existing divisions within the movement by creating a cleavage between the new lay experts and the "lay lay" activists left behind in the knowledge-acquisition process.[59] To the extent that facility with scientific and technical knowledge or tools becomes a de facto criterion for leadership within a movement, then scientization may reshape the movement, potentially reducing its participatory potential. In addition, scientization may raise the barriers to entry, making it harder to recruit new members and replenish leadership positions—an especially critical issue for health movements, sadly, as leaders not infrequently are at personal risk of illness or death.[60]

The Problem of Incorporation and Co-optation

Any inclination to celebrate the accomplishments of patient groups must make sense of two potentially countervailing tendencies: incorporation, whereby the insights and legacies of patient advocacy are channeled back into institutionalized biomedical practice; and cooptation, where the radical potential of an activist critique is blunted or contained. Biomedical institutions are highly flexible and resilient, according to Ilana Löwy—one might say omnivorous—and the peculiar thing about the phenomenon of incorporation is that it may be hard to judge in principle whether it should be counted as victory or defeat: Does it mark the successful transformation of biomedicine by outside forces, or the taming of a radical challenge, or even both at once?[61] Similarly, when activists come to moderate their critiques or adopt more conventional biomedical understanding, it is often hard to say whether they have allowed themselves to be co-opted or have made a well-advised shift in tactics.

Scholars have pointed to instances of outright manipulation of patients in order to co-opt them, for example through the creation by pharmaceutical companies of front groups masquerading as patient advocacy groups that are intended to build demand for a company's products or garner support for drug approval.[62] However, this extreme case is one end of a continuum of relations to pharmaceutical companies Orla O'Donovan describes that includes many other instances in which patient groups receive pharmaceutical industry financing. O'Donovan rightly cautions against assumptions of creeping "corporate colonisation," calling for detailed study of whether corporations indeed have increased their influence over patient groups' "cultures of action."[63] It is important to ask whether symbiotic relationships between patient groups and industry may sometimes usefully magnify patients' voices and extend the impact of their message—but also whether the authenticity of the patient perspective can be maintained in such situations.

Scholars also have identified cases where activist intentions were co-opted in the process of partial implementation of their concerns—for example, surgeons adapting the arguments of the fat-acceptance movement to promote weight-loss surgery, or the U.S. passage of breast cancer informed-consent laws in ways that "actually advanced and protected the professional autonomy of physicians at the expense of patient rights."[64] Another tricky case—for which blunt and accusatory terms such as "cooptation" appear unhelpful—is that of AIDS treatment activists, many of whom began to soften their critiques of clinical research and regulatory practices as they learned about the complexities involved: "The more we learned, in some ways the less we were able to ask for," was how one activist expressed it.[65] By one measure, these activists became more conservative as they became inculcated within biomedical frameworks; by another measure, they changed tactics appropriately in response to an evolving political environment and as the research trajectory, and their own understanding, advanced.[66] At a minimum, their example suggests the benefits of studying expert knowledge in broadly Foucaultian terms—not as an inert tool to be acquired, but rather as something that reshapes the subjectivities of those who become subject to it.[67]

Is institutionalization possible without some measure of "capture and control"?[68] Kyra Landzelius goes so far as to conclude her analysis of the "parents of preemies" movement in two different ways, first suggesting the practical benefits of the movement's cooperative approach, then "pivoting" to highlight "the ways in which it embeds normative ideologies about maternity and likewise is comfortably embedded within and cocooned by them."[69] At the more benign end of the incorporation spectrum, Carole Joffe has remarked on the legacy of key feminist principles within present-day medical practice: "Many of the ideas about abortion and other reproductive health services that were promoted by women's health activists of the 1970s—ranging from the simple (warming the gynecological instruments) to the more complex (seeing the patient as a fully participating partner)—have now been incorporated into practice at many facilities—even those that do not think of themselves as 'feminist.'" A related example is the mainstream medical incorporation of breastfeeding, a practice that health activists once had to defend.[70]

While these latter cases might seem closer to what could simply be called victory, it is worth reflecting on the deletions of authorship and historical process that typically accompany even beneficent incorporations.[71] Who remembers, decades later, that today's ordinary standard of care was once a radical innovation promoted by activists? Yet this act of historical forgetting may have consequences: it limits the capacity of subsequent generations of activists to benefit from examples of past struggles and to be inspired to imagine how current conditions might be otherwise.

Conclusions

Drawing on the extant scholarly literature on patient groups and health movements, I have suggested that the practical efforts of such groups can have a broad range of effects on health and biomedical institutions, political processes, personal and collective identity, and society and culture more generally. Indeed, health activism seems admirably to demonstrate the more general point, made by Elizabeth Armstrong and Mary Bernstein, that social movements ought to be studied in relation to their "multi-institutional" effects in societies where power is organized around multiple sources of material and symbolic power.[72] Of course, as is often the case in historical explanations, the problem of causality complicates our interpretations: how can we be sure that any given change is due to the actions of a particular movement and not due to some other actor or phenomenon that was simultaneously present? In the future, comparative studies (either examining similar patient groups in different historical or social contexts, or different groups in similar contexts) may provide more solid evidence that biomedical, political, social, and cultural change truly can be attributed to health advocacy. At the same time, such studies will likely be of great benefit in teasing out precisely which combinations of factors, both internal and external to a movement, are most likely to culminate in substantive changes.

To say that patient groups and health movements have effects is different from arguing that they achieve success. As I noted, the literature on social movement suggests it is no easy matter to assess the latter, let alone measure it. Judging success may require comparing effects against the movement's stated goals—not always an easy task, because goals are often a divisive issue among factions within a social movement and because goals may evolve over the course of a movement's life history. Alternatively, assessing success may be approached in relation not to a movement's professed goals but to some external standard imposed by the analyst. (We might, for example, ask whether or when the particularistic efforts of disease-specific advocacy groups have resulted in demands for more universalistic measures such as guaranteed access to health care.)[73] In either case, if we broaden our consideration of success beyond easily identifiable changes in policy, as I have proposed, it often becomes tricky to determine whether success has been achieved. At times health advocacy may bring about unanticipated changes in social institutions, collective identities, or cultural schemas, or establish a path that subsequent health advocates may tread. And sometimes, as in the cases of co-optation that I described, health advocates may succeed even while bringing about effects that run counter to at least some aspects of their avowed philosophy and political commitments.

To the extent that health advocates do succeed—either on their own terms, or on terms defined by outside observers—what accounts for the possibility of success? Certainly there is no single causal story to be told. For example, in some cases patient groups may accrue advantages through internal homogeneity and a narrow and precise definition of their goals. In other cases, however, their strength may lie in their hybrid character, their social diversity, and their ability to traverse boundaries between lay and expert worlds.[74] As Giugni has observed in relation to social movements more generally, we simply cannot speak of, nor should we search for, a secret path to success or a recipe for its achievement: "Looking for general causes and invariant models is doomed to failure, for there are no such invariant patterns in social life. . . . Instead of searching for general explanations, we would do a better job by taking into account the historically contingent combinations of factors that shape the possibilities for movements to contribute to social change."[75]

As an example of the difficulties of generalizing about efficacy, we might consider the case of HIV/AIDS activism of the sort promoted famously by groups such as ACT UP. Does this provide an effective model for others to follow? The evidence is equivocal. A number of groups, such as chronic fatigue activists, have styled themselves after ACT UP's militancy, though not always with the same success.[76] Other groups explicitly have sought to distance themselves from the aggressive image of ACT UP on the assumption that less in-your-face tactics would be more effective: these include mainstream breast cancer advocacy groups in the United States, which stressed their "ordinariness" and "moral worthiness" vis-à-vis "the public stereotype of the AIDS patient, gay, male, and radical";[77] parents of premature infants, who adopted metaphors of "generativity and affinity" in place of ACT UP's militaristic imagery;[78] and advocacy groups for assisted reproductive technologies, which adopted a style of "motherly activism" that appeals both to the left ("reproductive choice") and to the right ("family building").[79] The point is not that either being militant or being unthreatening are universally efficacious tactics. Rather, different actors will perceive different strategic advantages accruing to these (and other) orientations, depending on the constraints that they face, as well as the specifics of the disease or condition in question, the stage in the movement's development, its perceived relationship to other visible movements, and the particular historical moment.

Thus analysts of patient advocacy should certainly seek to identify patterns that hold across multiple cases, but they should do so without disembedding those patterns from the contextual circumstances that established a basis for success. Similarly, policy makers should be attentive to the well-demonstrated possibility that the inclusion of organized patient voices can improve health care by making it both more effective and more equitable, but they should not assume that there is any single ideal model for the organization of patient groups and health movements.

Notes

1. There is no clear agreement about precisely what counts as a "patient group or health movement," and I use that term to gesture at a wide range of collective actors. On "health social movements," see Phil Brown and Stephen Zavestoski, "Social Movements in Health: An Introduction," *Sociology of Health and Illness* 26, 6 (2004): 679–694; David J. Hess, "Medical Modernisation, Scientific Research Fields, and the Epistemic Politics of Health Social Movements," *Sociology of Health and Illness* 26, 6 (2004): 695–709. On "consumer movements" in health, see Hilda Bastian, "Speaking Up for Ourselves: The Evolution of Consumer Advocacy in Health Care," *International Journal of Technology Assessment in Health Care* 14, 1 (1998): 3–23; Judith Allsop, Kathryn Jones, and Rob Baggott, "Health Consumer Groups in the UK: A New Social Movement?" *Sociology of Health and Illness* 26, 6 (2004): 737–756; Marsha Rosengarten, "Consumer Activism in the Pharmacology of HIV," *Body and Society* 10, 1 (2004): 91–107; Nancy Tomes, "Patients or Health-Care Consumers? Why the History of Contested Terms Matters," in *History and Health Policy in the United States: Putting the Past Back In*, ed. Rosemary A. Stevens, Charles E. Rosenberg, and Lawton R. Burns (New Brunswick, N.J.: Rutgers University Press, 2006), 83–110. On "communities of suffering," see Randall M. Packard, Peter J. Brown, Ruth L. Berkelman, and Howard Frumkin, "Introduction: Emerging Illness As Social Process," in *Emerging Illnesses and Society: Negotiating the Public Health*, ed. Randall M. Packard, Peter J. Brown, Ruth L. Berkelman, and Howard Frumkin (Baltimore: Johns Hopkins University Press, 2004), 1–35. On groups that organize around "pain and loss experiences," see Allsop, Jones, and Baggott, "Health Consumer Groups," 738. For a more extended discussion of the question of definitions and boundaries, as well as the typologies by which we might subdivide the phenomenon, see Steven Epstein, "Patient Groups and Health Movements," in *The Handbook of Science and Technology Studies*, ed. Edward J. Hackett, Olga Amsterdamska, Michael Lynch, and Judy Wajcman (Cambridge, Mass.: MIT Press, 2008), 499–539.

2. Steven Epstein, *Impure Science: AIDS, Activism, and the Politics of Knowledge* (Berkeley: University of California Press, 1996); Bastian, "Speaking Up for Ourselves"; Allsop, Jones, and Baggott, "Health Consumer Groups"; Brown and Zavestoski, "Social Movements in Health"; Phil Brown, Stephen Zavestoski, Sabrina McCormick, Brian Mayer, Rachel Morello-Frosch, and Rebecca Gasior Altman, "Embodied Health Movements: New Approaches to Social Movements in Health," *Sociology of Health and Illness* 26, 1 (2004): 50–80; David J. Hess, "Guest Editorial: Health, the Environment, and Social Movements," *Science As Culture* 13, 4 (2004): 421–427; Randall M. Packard, Peter J. Brown, Ruth L. Berkelman, and Howard Frumkin, eds., *Emerging Illnesses and Society: Negotiating the Public Health* (Baltimore: Johns Hopkins University Press, 2004); Kyra Landzelius and

Joe Dumit, eds., "Patient Organization Movements," *Social Science and Medicine* 62, 3 (2006), special issue; Epstein, "Patient Groups and Health Movements."

3. Alan Stockdale, "Waiting for the Cure: Mapping the Social Relations of Human Gene Therapy Research," *Sociology of Health and Illness* 21, 5 (1999): 594; Constance Nathanson, "The Limitations of Social Movements as Catalysts for Change," in *Social Movements and the Transformation of American Health Care*, ed. Jane Banaszak-Holl, Sandra Levitsky, and Mayer N. Zald (Oxford: Oxford University Press, 2010), 23–38.

4. William A. Gamson, *The Strategy of Social Protest*, 2nd ed. (Belmont, Calif.: Wadsworth, 1990).

5. Marco Giugni, introduction to *How Social Movements Matter*, ed. Marco Giugni, Doug McAdam, and Charles Tilly (Minneapolis: University of Minnesota Press, 1999), xiv–xv, xi. See also Daniel M. Cress and David A. Snow, "The Outcomes of Homeless Mobilization: The Influence of Organization, Disruption, Political Mediation, and Framing," *American Journal of Sociology* 105, 4 (2000): 1063.

6. Ibid., xx.

7. Cress and Snow, "Outcomes of Homeless Mobilization," 1066.

8. Kelly Moore, *Disrupting Science: Social Movements, American Scientists, and the Politics of the Military, 1945–1975* (Princeton, N.J.: Princeton University Press, 2008), 15.

9. Giugni, introduction, xxii.

10. Kelly Moore, "Political Protest and Institutional Change: The Anti-Vietnam War Movement and American Science," in *How Social Movements Matter*, ed. Marco Giugni, Doug McAdam, and Charles Tilly (Minneapolis: University of Minnesota Press, 1999), 97. See also Gerald F. Davis, Doug McAdam, W. Richard Scott, and Mayer N. Zald, eds., *Social Movements and Organization Theory* (Cambridge: Cambridge University Press, 1995); Moore, *Disrupting Science*; Nella Van Dyke, Sarah A. Soule, and Verta A. Taylor, "The Targets of Social Movements: Beyond a Focus on the State," in *Authority in Contention*, ed. Daniel J. Myers and Daniel M. Cress (Amsterdam: Elsevier, 2004), 27–51.

11. Elizabeth Armstrong and Mary Bernstein, "Culture, Power, and Institutions: A Multi-Institutional Politics Approach to Social Movements," *Sociological Theory* 26, 1 (2008): 74–99.

12. Moore, "Political Protest," 97, 114.

13. John D. Skrentny, "Policy-Elite Perceptions and Social Movement Success: Understanding Variations in Group Inclusion in Affirmative Action," *American Journal of Sociology* 111, 6 (2006): 1764.

14. Cress and Snow, "Outcomes of Homeless Mobilization," 1063.

15. Rayna Rapp, Deborah Heath, and Karen-Sue Taussig, "Genealogical Dis-Ease: Where Hereditary Abnormality, Biomedical Explanation, and Family Responsibility Meet," in *Relative Values: Reconfiguring Kinship Studies*, ed. Sarah Franklin and Susan McKinnon (Durham, N.C.: Duke University Press, 2001), 393; Vololona Rabeharisoa, "The Struggle against Neuromuscular Diseases in France and the Emergence of the 'Partnership Model' of Patient Organisation," *Social Science and Medicine* 57, 11 (2003): 2127; Allsop, Jones, and Baggott, "Health Consumer Groups," 738, 741.

16. Brown and Zavestoski, "Social Movements in Health," 682.

17. Tom Shakespeare, "Disabled People's Self-Organisation: A New Social Movement?" *Disability, Handicap, and Society* 8, 3 (1993): 249–264; Steven Epstein, "The Construction of Lay Expertise: AIDS Activism and the Forging of Credibility in the

Reform of Clinical Trials," *Science, Technology, and Human Values* 20, 4 (1995): 412–413; Epstein, *Impure Science*, 20–21; Patricia Kaufert, "Women, Resistance, and the Breast Cancer Movement," in *Pragmatic Women and Body Politics*, ed. Margaret Lock and Patricia A. Kaufert (Cambridge: Cambridge University Press, 1998), 303; Linda L. Layne, *Motherhood Lost: A Feminist Account of Pregnancy Loss in America* (New York: Routledge, 2003), 38–39; Chloe Silverman, "A Disorder of Affect: Love, Tragedy, Biomedicine, and Citizenship in American Autism Research, 1943–2003" (Ph.D. diss., University of Pennsylvania, 2004), 361, 370; Stuart Blume, "Anti-Vaccination Movements and Their Interpretations," *Social Science and Medicine* 62, 3 (2006): 630–631.

18. Alan Stockdale, "Waiting for the Cure: Mapping the Social Relations of Human Gene Therapy Research," *Sociology of Health and Illness* 21, 5 (1999): 594.

19. Nathanson, "Limitations of Social Movements."

20. Some of the material in the bullet points that follow draws upon Epstein, "Patient Groups and Health Movements."

21. Howard I. Kushner, "Competing Medical Cultures, Patient Support Groups, and the Construction of Tourette's Syndrome," in *Emerging Illnesses and Society: Negotiating the Public Health*, ed. Randall M. Packard, Peter J. Brown, Ruth L. Berkelman, and Howard Frumkin (Baltimore: Johns Hopkins University Press, 2004), 71–101.

22. Stella M. Capek, "Reframing Endometriosis: From 'Career Woman's Disease' to Environment/Body Connections," in *Illness and the Environment: A Reader in Contested Medicine*, ed. J. Stephen Kroll-Smith, Phil Brown, and Valerie J. Gunter (New York: New York University Press, 2000), 345, 351–352.

23. Madeleine Akrich and Cecile Meadel, "Prendre ses medicaments/prendre la parole: Les Usages des medicaments par les patients dans les listes de discussion electroniques," *Sciences Sociales et Sante* 20, 1 (2002): 89–115.

24. Janine Barbot and Nicolas Dodier, "Multiplicity in Scientific Medicine: The Experience of HIV-Positive Patients," *Science, Technology, and Human Values* 27, 3 (2002): 404–440; Janine Barbot, "How to Build an 'Active' Patient? The Work of AIDS Associations in France," *Social Science and Medicine* 62, 3 (2006): 538–551.

25. Abigail C. Saguy and Kevin W. Riley, "Weighing Both Sides: Morality, Mortality, and Framing Contests over Obesity," *Journal of Health Politics, Policy, and Law* 30, 5 (2005): 869–923; Natalie Boero, "Bypassing Blame: Bariatric Surgery and the Case of Biomedical Failure," manuscript, author files.

26. Katrina Karkazis, *Fixing Sex: Intersex, Medical Authority, and Lived Experience* (Durham, N.C.: Duke University Press, 2008), 236–290.

27. Epstein, "Construction of Lay Expertise"; Epstein, *Impure Science*; Steven Epstein, "Activism, Drug Regulation, and the Politics of Therapeutic Evaluation in the AIDS Era: A Case Study of ddC and the 'Surrogate Markers' Debate," *Social Studies of Science* 27, 5 (1997): 691–726; Deborah Heath, "Bodies, Antibodies, and Modest Interventions," in *Cyborgs and Citadels*, ed. Gary L. Downey and Joseph Dumit (Santa Fe, N.M.: School of American Research Press, 1997), 67–82; Deborah Heath, "Locating Genetic Knowledge: Picturing Marfan Syndrome and Its Traveling Constituencies," *Science, Technology, and Human Values* 23, 1 (1998): 71–97; Rayna Rapp, "Extra Chromosomes and Blue Tulips: Medico-Familial Interpretations," in *Living and Working with the New Medical Technologies: Intersections of Inquiry*, ed. Margaret Lock, Allen Young, and Alberto Cambrosio (Cambridge: Cambridge University Press, 2000), 184–208; Vololona Rabeharisoa and Michel Callon, "The Involvement of Patients' Associations in Research," *International Social Science*

Journal 54, 171 (2002): 57–63; Michel Callon and Vololona Rabeharisoa, "Research 'in the Wild' and the Shaping of New Social Identities," *Technology in Society* 25, 2 (2003): 193–204; Rabeharisoa, "Struggle against Neuromuscular Diseases"; Michel Callon and Vololona Rabeharisoa, "Gino's Lesson on Humanity: Genetics, Mutual Entanglements, and the Sociologist's Role," *Economy and Society* 33, 1 (2004): 1–27; Deborah Heath, Rayna Rapp, and Karen-Sue Taussig, "Genetic Citizenship," in *A Companion to the Anthropology of Politics*, ed. David Nugent and Joan Vincent (London: Blackwell, 2004), 152–167; Vololona Rabeharisoa, "From Representation to Mediation: The Shaping of Collective Mobilization on Muscular Dystrophy in France," *Social Science and Medicine* 62, 3 (2006): 564–576.

28. Callon and Rabeharisoa, "Research 'in the Wild,'" 201.

29. Hess, "Medical Modernisation," 703–704.

30. Adele Clarke and Theresa Montini, "The Many Faces of RU486: Tales of Situated Knowledges and Technological Contestations," *Science, Technology, and Human Values* 18, 1 (1993): 42–78; Adele Clarke, *Disciplining Reproduction: Modernity, American Life Sciences, and "The Problems of Sex"* (Berkeley: University of California Press, 1998); Adele E. Clarke, "Maverick Reproductive Scientists and the Production of Contraceptives, 1915–2000+," in *Bodies of Technology: Women's Involvement with Reproductive Medicine*, ed. Ann R. Saetnan, Nelly Oudshoorn, and Marta Kirejczyk (Columbus: Ohio State University Press, 2000), 37–89; Anni Dugdale, "Intrauterine Contraceptive Devices, Situated Knowledges, and the Making of Women's Bodies," *Australian Feminist Studies* 15, 32 (2000): 165–176; Susan E. Bell, "Sexual Synthetics: Women, Science, and Microbicides," in *Synthetic Planet: Chemical Politics and the Hazards of Modern Life*, ed. Monica J. Casper (New York: Routledge, 2003), 197–211; Jessica Van Kammen, "Who Represents the Users? Critical Encounters between Women's Health Advocates and Scientists in Contraceptive RandD," in *How Users Matter: The Co-Construction of Users and Technology*, ed. Nelly Oudshoorn and Trevor Pinch (Cambridge, Mass.: MIT Press, 2003), 151–171; Anita Hardon, "Contesting Contraceptive Innovation: Reinventing the Script," *Social Science and Medicine* 62, 3 (2006): 614–627.

31. Michael P. Johnson and Karl Hufbauer, "Sudden Infant Death Syndrome as a Medical Research Problem since 1945," *Social Problems* 30, 1 (1982): 65–81.

32. Constance A. Nathanson, "Social Movements as Catalysts for Policy Change: The Case of Smoking and Guns," *Journal of Health Politics, Policy, and Law* 24, 3 (1999): 421–488; Allsop, Jones, and Baggott, "Health Consumer Groups," 752; Saguy and Riley, "Weighing Both Sides," 911.

33. Steven Epstein, *Inclusion: The Politics of Difference in Medical Research* (Chicago: University of Chicago Press, 2007).

34. Epstein, *Impure Science*; Susan Reynolds Whyte, Sjaak van der Geest, and Anita Hardon, *Social Lives of Medicines* (Cambridge: Cambridge University Press, 2002), 146–160.

35. Heath, Rapp, and Taussig, "Genetic Citizenship," 163–164.

36. David J. Hess, "Technology- and Product-Oriented Movements: Approximating Social Movement Studies and Science and Technology Studies," *Science, Technology, and Human Values* 30, 4 (2005): 515–535.

37. Joshua Gamson, "Silence, Death, and the Invisible Enemy: AIDS Activism and Social Movement 'Newness,'" *Social Problems* 36, 4 (1989): 351–365; Ilana Löwy, "Trustworthy Knowledge and Desperate Patients: Clinical Tests for New Drugs from Cancer to AIDS," in *Living and Working with the New Medical*

Technologies: Intersections of Inquiry, ed. Margaret Lock, Allen Young, and Alberto Cambrosio (Cambridge: Cambridge University Press, 2000), 74.

38. Shakespeare, "Disabled People's Self-Organisation"; Tom Shakespeare, "'Losing the Plot'? Medical and Activist Discourses of Contemporary Genetics and Disability," *Sociology of Health and Illness* 21, 5 (1999): 669–688; Leanne Dowse, "Contesting Practices, Challenging Codes: Self-Advocacy, Disability Politics, and the Social Model," *Disability and Society* 16, 1 (2001): 123–141; Rayna Rapp and Faye Ginsburg, "Enabling Disability: Rewriting Kinship, Reimagining Citizenship," *Public Culture* 13, 3 (2001): 533–556; Karkazis, *Fixing Sex*.

39. Maren Klawiter, "Racing for the Cure, Walking Women, and Toxic Touring: Mapping Cultures of Action within the Bay Area Terrain of Breast Cancer," *Social Problems* 46, 1 (1999): 104–126.

40. Alondra Nelson, "Black Power, Biomedicine, and the Politics of Knowledge" (Ph.D. diss., New York University, 2003), chap. 4.

41. Sahra Gibbon, *Breast Cancer Genes and the Gendering of Knowledge : Science and Citizenship in the Cultural Context of the "New" Genetics* (Houndmills: Palgrave Macmillan, 2007); Lesley A. Sharp, "Commodified Kin: Death, Mourning, and Competing Claims on the Bodies of Organ Donors in the United States," *American Anthropologist* 103, 1 (2001): 125.

42. Francesca Polletta, "Culture in and Outside Institutions," in *Authority in Contention*, ed. Daniel J. Myers and Daniel M. Cress (Amsterdam: Elsevier, 2004), 161–183.

43. Renee L. Beard, "Advocating Voice: Organisational, Historical, and Social Milieux of the Alzheimer's Disease Movement," *Sociology of Health and Illness* 26, 6 (2004): 798.

44. Epstein, "Construction of Lay Expertise"; Epstein, *Impure Science*, 252–253; Van Kammen, "Who Represents the Users?"

45. Steven Epstein, "Inclusion, Diversity, and Biomedical Knowledge Making: The Multiple Politics of Representation," in *How Users Matter: The Co-Construction of Users and Technology*, ed. Nelly Oudshoorn and Trevor Pinch (Cambridge, Mass.: MIT Press, 2003), 173–190.

46. Pierre Bourdieu, "The Social Space and the Genesis of Groups," *Theory and Society* 14, 6 (1985): 723–744.

47. Epstein, "Construction of Lay Expertise."

48. Epstein, *Impure Science*.

49. Epstein, *Inclusion*, chaps. 3–4. While the movement for inclusion of underrepresented groups as research subjects proved successful in terms of changing policies and practices in the United States, I argue that it also has encouraged the tendency to conceive of sex and race differences in biological terms—which can make it harder in the end to address health disparities. This is a potent example of the unintended consequences of health activism.

50. Clifford Geertz, *Local Knowledge: Further Essays in Interpretive Anthropology* (New York: Basic Books, 1983); Michel Foucault, *Power/Knowledge* (New York: Pantheon 1980), 80–85; Donna J. Haraway, *Simians, Cyborgs, and Women: The Reinvention of Nature* (New York: Routledge, 1991), 183–201; John V. Pickstone, *Ways of Knowing: A New History of Science, Technology, and Medicine* (Chicago: University of Chicago Press, 2000).

51. Jeffrey Escoffier, "The Invention of Safer Sex: Vernacular Knowledge, Gay Politics, and HIV Prevention," *Berkeley Journal of Sociology* 43 (1999): 1–30.

52. Joan Scott, "The Evidence of Experience," *Critical Inquiry* 17, 4 (1991): 773–797.

53. Michelle Murphy, "Occupational Health from Below: The Women's Office Workers' Movement and the Hazardous Office," in *Emerging Illnesses and Society: Negotiating the Public Health*, ed. Randall M. Packard, Peter J. Brown, Ruth L. Berkelman, and Howard Frumkin (Baltimore: Johns Hopkins University Press, 2004), 202.

54. Epstein, "Construction of Lay Expertise"; Kay Dickersin and Lauren Schnaper, "Reinventing Medical Research," in *Man-Made Medicine: Women's Health, Public Policy, and Reform*, ed. Kary L. Moss (Durham, N.C.: Duke University Press, 1996), 57–76; Mary K. Anglin, "Working from the Inside Out: Implications of Breast Cancer Activism for Biomedical Policies and Practices," *Social Science and Medicine* 44, 9 (1997): 1403–1415; Kay Dickersin, Lundy Braun, Margaret Mead, Robert Millikan, Ana M. Wu, Jennifer Pietenpol, Susan Troyan, Benjamin Anderson, and Frances Visco, "Development and Implementation of a Science Training Course for Breast Cancer Activists: Project Lead (Leadership, Education, and Advocacy Development)," *Health Expectations* 4, 4 (2001): 213–220; Jennifer Reid Myhre, "Medical Mavens: Gender, Science, and the Consensus Politics of Breast Cancer Activism" (Ph.D. diss., University of California, Davis, 2002).

55. Paula A. Treichler, "How to Have Theory in an Epidemic: The Evolution of AIDS Treatment Activism," in *Technoculture*, ed. Constance Penley and Andrew Ross (Minneapolis: University of Minnesota Press, 1991). See also Paula A. Treichler, *How to Have Theory in an Epidemic: Cultural Chronicles of AIDS* (Durham, N.C.: Duke University Press, 1991). The term "lay expert" has been widely used to characterize the liminal or boundary-crossing qualities of those who succeed in establishing this sort of claim to formal knowledge. Hilary Arksey, "Expert and Lay Participation in the Construction of Medical Knowledge," *Sociology of Health and Illness* 16, 4 (1994): 448–468; Epstein, "Construction of Lay Expertise."

56. Heath, "Bodies, Antibodies, and Modest Interventions," 81–82.

57. Yoshio Nukaga, "Between Tradition and Innovation in New Genetics: The Continuity of Medical Pedigrees and the Development of Combination Work in the Case of Huntington's Disease," *New Genetics and Society* 21, 1 (2002): 59.

58. Callon and Rabeharisoa, "Research 'in the Wild,'" 197–198.

59. Epstein, "Construction of Lay Expertise"; Epstein, *Impure Science*, 284–294; for the term "lay lay," see Gilbert Elbaz, "The Sociology of AIDS Activism, the Case of ACT UP/New York, 1987–1992" (Ph.D. diss., City University of New York, 1992), 488.

60. Epstein, *Impure Science*, 327, 350–353.

61. Löwy, "Trustworthy Knowledge and Desperate Patients," 73. On judging incorporation, Melinda Goldner, "The Dynamic Interplay between Western Medicine and the Complementary and Alternative Medicine Movement: How Activists Perceive a Range of Responses from Physicians and Hospitals," *Sociology of Health and Illness* 26, 6 (2004): 727.

62. Stephen Zavestoski, Rachel Morello-Frosch, Phil Brown, Brian Mayer, Sabrina McCormick, and Rebecca Gasior Altman, "Embodied Health Movements and Challenges to the Dominant Epidemiological Paradigm," in *Authority in Contention*, ed. Daniel J. Myers and Daniel M. Cress (Amsterdam: Elsevier, 2004), 274.

63. Orla O'Donovan, "Corporate Colonisation of Health Activism? Irish Health Advocacy Organisations' Modes of Engagement with Pharmaceutical Corporations," *International Journal of Health Services* 37, 4 (2007): 711–733.

64. Theresa Michalak Montini, "Women's Activism for Breast Cancer Informed Consent Laws" (Ph.D. diss., University of California, San Francisco, 1991), vii; see also

Theresa Montini, "Gender and Emotion in the Advocacy for Breast Cancer Informed Consent Legislation," *Gender and Society* 10, 1 (1996): 9–23. On surgeons and fat acceptance, see Boero, "Bypassing Blame."

65. Epstein, *Impure Science*, 328.
66. Ibid., 342–344; Epstein, "Activism, Drug Regulation."
67. Foucault, *Power/Knowledge*.
68. Hess, "Medical Modernisation," 705. See also Hess, "Technology- and Product-Oriented Movements."
69. Kyra Landzelius, "The Incubation of a Social Movement: Preterm Babies, Parent Activists, and Neonatal Productions in the US Context," *Social Science and Medicine* 62, 3 (2006): 679–680. Another useful way forward in analysis has been suggested by Melinda Goldner, who took up the question of institutionalization by combining social movement perspectives with institutionalist approaches within sociology. In her analysis of the "dynamic interplay" between the complementary and alternative medicine movement and Western medicine, Goldner rejected any simple conclusion about incorporation by showing how distinctive outcomes on the ground mapped onto a typology of diverse institutional responses to external challenge. Goldner, "Dynamic Interplay."
70. Carole Joffe, "Abortion and the Women's Health Movement: Then and Now (Commentary)," *Journal of the American Medical Women's Association* 54, 1 (1999): 32; Jule DeJager Ward, *La Leche League: At the Crossroads of Medicine, Feminism, and Religion* (Chapel Hill: University of North Carolina Press, 2000).
71. Arksey, "Expert and Lay Participation," 464.
72. Armstrong and Bernstein, "Culture, Power, and Institutions."
73. Beatrix Hoffman, "Health Care Reform and Social Movements in the United States," *American Journal of Public Health* 93, 1 (2003): 75–85.
74. Steven Epstein, "The Strength of Diverse Ties: Multiple Hybridity in the Politics of Inclusion and Difference in U.S. Biomedical Research," in *Social Movements and the Transformation of American Health Care*, ed. Jane Banaszak-Holl, Sandra Levitsky, and Mayer N. Zald (Oxford: Oxford University Press, 2010), 79–95.
75. Giugni, introduction, xxv.
76. Deborah Barrett, "Illness Movements and the Medical Classification of Pain and Fatigue," in *Emerging Illnesses and Society: Negotiating the Public Health*, ed. Randall M. Packard, Peter J. Brown, Ruth L. Berkelman, and Howard Frumkin (Baltimore: Johns Hopkins University Press, 2004), 139–170.
77. Kaufert, "Women, Resistance," 102. See also Myhre, "Medical Mavens."
78. Landzelius, "Incubation of a Social Movement," 678.
79. Charis Thompson, *Making Parents: The Ontological Choreography of Reproductive Technologies* (Cambridge, Mass.: MIT Press, 2005), 238–239.

Epilogue

Principles for Engaging Patients in U.S. Health Care and Policy

Patients' experiences, behaviors, and advocacy strategies are remarkably diverse: the chapters in this volume document this diversity in no uncertain terms. The actors in these pages share status as recipients, surrogate recipients, or potential recipients of care, but their perspectives do not neatly meld into a single patient voice capable of articulating what people want and need from the health care system. The patient's perspective is not unitary; rather, it is a polyvocal phenomenon that defies easy categorization and straightforward policy response. Given the heterogeneity of patients' relationships to health, health care, and the policy process, what can be done to create a health care system that is more effective, responsive, and humane? How can reform responsibly acknowledge the complications inherent in the laudable aspiration to meet patients' needs without becoming stymied by the complexity of that task? If policy makers really want the health care system to have a sustained and meaningful relationship with patients, how can they transform their current flirtation into long-term engagement?

This epilogue is our collective effort to address these thorny questions. Working together, the editors and authors of this volume have endeavored to synthesize the insights from our individual chapters so they can inform a realistic ideal of democratic decision-making processes in health care. The principles we offer here are intended to get us beyond the patient conundrum of high visibility and low impact described in the introduction to this volume by suggesting how patient perspectives can be integrated into a pluralistic conception of health policy making that we believe will serve the American public far better than do current practices.

Although patient empowerment has been a watchword in U.S. health policy for the past twenty-five years, empowerment has generally been equated with informed consumerism. There have been some exceptions, such as initiatives to provide greater patient self-determination at the end of life. But for most U.S. policy makers, consumerism in medical settings has been—and continues to be—conceived largely in terms of giving people more choices and more information about them. When empowerment comes solely through the market, patients' capacity to exert influence is restricted to using their purchasing power to seek out preferred insurers or providers and to switch away (or exit) from unsatisfactory ones. We propose here a definition of empowerment that is rooted in the public sphere rather than in the market, that emphasizes voice over exit, and that promotes collective notions of patient well-being, identity, and representation instead of (or as well as) individual self-interest. "Voice," as used here, describes the various ways in which patients can publicly express their assessments of and aspirations for the health care system. Avenues for patient voice include contacting public officials; using grievance mechanisms; participating in membership organizations; mobilizing grassroots social movements; influencing research, clinical, and institutional practices; convening groups of patients and families; writing to or for mass media; and initiating legal actions.[1]

Although this epilogue offers a critique of and alternative to market-oriented empowerment, we acknowledge the potency of individualistic conceptions of patients' influence (see Nancy Tomes, Amy Dockser Marcus, Marc A. Rodwin, Julie Fairman, and Elizabeth Marshall Armstrong and Eugene DeClercq, this volume), and their likely persistence in U.S. health care and policy discourse. We seek to complement (and sometimes challenge) these market-based conceptions by exploring how patient perspectives can be recognized and incorporated into democratic deliberation.

There have been times in recent years when a large portion of the public has engaged around episodes of health care reform, including initiatives at the national level and referenda adopted in several states.[2] This epilogue shares the aspiration to broad inclusivity that was embodied in the most successful of these public campaigns. Its intent, however, is very different. Our goal is not to mobilize support in a one-off push to enact reform, but to identify ways of consistently incorporating patients' diverse perspectives into health care delivery and health policy formulation. Ultimately, our purpose is less to promote a set of specific new policies and more to change how policy makers, clinicians, and relevant interest groups incorporate patients' perspectives in policy making.

Let us be clear: we focus here on principles for patient participation rather than on concrete policies because we don't believe that any single static solution to patients' suffering, dissatisfaction, or disenfranchisement will remain effective for long. Despite the aspirations and well-intentioned efforts of public officials and citizen groups, health system reform is never a one-act play. Health care is extremely dynamic: technology development, emerging health threats, and ever-changing determinants of health (or at least our ever-evolving understanding of them) are just some of the factors that assure constant flux. Every reform effort—even the most lasting ones, such as Medicare—plants the seeds of its own malleability, since the reform itself induces further changes that could never have been fully anticipated.[3] Given this inherent imperfectability, sound health policy depends upon built-in mechanisms that encourage ongoing learning and adaptation, both for those who work within health care and for those who guide the system's evolution.

The principles we articulate here are offered as guide stars for these adaptive practices. Many of them have already been experimented with outside the United States, both in countries with nationalized health care/insurance and in those with a mix of public and private service delivery and financing. To anchor our aspirations for participatory policy making in the realpolitik of U.S. contemporary health policy, we have clustered these principles under four central challenges highlighted in this volume: enriching conceptions of the public good and collective patient identity; leveling the playing field with other stakeholders; representing diverse patient experiences; and addressing the challenges of a fragmented health care system. We offer both the principles and their associated challenges here with hope that the interplay between the two will spark a more robust conversation among policy makers regarding the merits, imperatives, and possibilities of a health policy that is more fully informed by those whose lives it touches most immediately.[4]

Principles and Practices: Enhancing Patients' Engagement in Health Policy

We present here thirteen principles for enhancing patients' engagement in health policy, grouped under the four challenges they are designed to address. For each principle, we have identified some concrete examples that could serve as templates, offering useful lessons (some positive, some negative) about the prospects for putting each principle into practice.

Enrich Conceptions of the Public Good and Collective Patient Identity

Unlike market notions of empowerment, which rest on the pursuit of individual self-interest, patients' collective voice depends upon a shared conception of the public good that is strengthened and protected by a diversity of patients speaking out. Currently, these collective conceptions are weak in U.S. health policy discourse. The preceding chapters identified two ways to offset this. First, policy makers can make clear that they value patient perspectives by taking them more fully into account during policy deliberation. Second, patients can develop a greater sense of shared identity with one another, and thus greater motivation to promote this group interest. We believe that both pathways to collective commitment are useful and offer three principles designed to strengthen them.

Principle 1: Clearly enunciate patients' right to voice

Following the example of New Zealand and other countries, the United States should build on its thirty-year history of national initiatives to promote patient voice by establishing a legal right to convey patient perspectives to policy makers.[5] Creating a right to voice raises the normative ante in a way that lessens patients' long-standing power disadvantage. The right to voice also implies that avenues for patient voice ought to be as universal and as freely accessible as other cherished rights, rather than conditional on how people pay for their medical care or where they receive services. Establishing the moral primacy of a right encourages patients to expect that their complaints and concerns will be taken seriously. This fosters voice, since the expectation that complaints could prevent problems from reoccurring is a central motive for patients' speaking up.[6] Finally, because those who bear rights in the United States are also assumed to have a reciprocal obligation to responsibly exercise them, establishing a right to voice also creates a moral imperative for patients to assert their collective interest.[7]

Principle 2: Commit to a health care system
that is responsive, caring, and humane

It is one thing to try to make primary care practice patient oriented, as reformers currently aspire to do. It is quite another to make the health care system responsive to patients. This transformation requires a commitment to provide timely redress for patients' concerns and misunderstandings; ensure that patients are treated with care and humaneness in the process; identify when these goals are not being met; and act quickly to make necessary improvements. Over the past decade, European and Commonwealth countries have focused increasingly on making their health systems and policy making more responsive to patient perspectives;[8] the United States thus has models from which to learn, and a useful incentive to close the rapidly widening gap between its own performance in this arena and that of other countries.[9]

Principle 3: Ensure that patients can more readily
learn from one another's experience

It's hard for patients to perceive a common identity when settlement agreements on disputes prohibit or inhibit disclosure; when public reporting of grievances reduces them to opaque statistics and masks all the meaningful details; and when disease-group advocates emphasize differences among conditions more than commonalities. Public policies could offset these tendencies. Policy could, for example, require greater transparency regarding dispute resolution as a way of encouraging patients to voice their grievances in greater detail, since other patients are more likely to learn from—and relate to— problematic episodes that are explicated with a more coherent narrative.[10]

Level the Playing Field between Patients and Other Stakeholders

Patient groups can have a potent influence on the politics of health care under specific circumstances, such as those illustrated in chapters by Steven Epstein, Marcus, Rodwin, and Grob. Nonetheless, we believe that, as other chapters document (Beatrix Hoffman, M. Robin DiMatteo et al., and Lori Andrews and Julie Burger), consumers remain persistently disadvantaged in their capacity for voice relative to other health care–related interests whose advocacy capacity is not inhibited by illness and that have more resources, better organization, greater experience, and a higher likelihood of articulating a single coherent position. Reasonable people (including the authors of this volume) can sensibly disagree over how much influence patients should have in the formulation of health policy. But there can be no disagreement that it is essential for policy makers in both public and private settings to have a more consistent and accurate sense of how Americans are experiencing health care. To mitigate inherent disadvantages, government should invest in an infrastructure that can level the playing field—as much as is realistic given the systemic imbalances of power and resources in the U.S. health system—in order to more effectively elicit and interpret patients' experiences. This investment should, we suggest, be guided by three additional principles.

Principle 4: Assure access to professional health advocates

Past efforts at empowerment made unrealistic assumptions about how much information patients could assimilate and how effectively they could sort through their options for responding to health care–related problems. Health care is simply too complex, frightening, and fraught with uncertainty for most individuals to take on these tasks alone. Some patients can turn to a trusted clinician, family member, or friend to assist them, but many cannot: 15–20 percent of all Americans report having no regular source of medical care (9 percent of those who have serious chronic health problems), and a third have no family or friends to help them sort through their health care experiences or choices.[11] These less-connected individuals could benefit from having trained patient–health advocates to assist them, expanding the formal advocacy capacity of the health care system.[12]

Principle 5: Establish a publicly financed patient support infrastructure

Patient advocacy pursued solely on a case-by-case basis may overlook shortfalls that reflect more systematic failings in the financing or delivery of care. Further, even when individual patients, clinicians, or family members identify patterns of problems, they generally lack the training, resources, and positioning to function as advocates for system- or policy-level change. By contrast, large provider systems, health insurers, and pharmaceutical companies are much better equipped to create structural change, but they often do so in a way that skews health policy away from the interests of patients. Rectifying this imbalance requires a separate coherent infrastructure to which all patient complaints and concerns would be reported and patterns of problems identified (even if resolution was pursued by other means). Channeling information in this way would make it easier to discern persisting shortfalls and pursue system-level remedies, as already evident in some existing programs targeted to the frailest patients.[13]

Principle 6: Promote coherent representation of collective patient experiences

Consumer influence will always be diluted if patients' experiences seem incoherent to policy makers—and this is nearly always the case at present since the fragmented, maddening health care system more or less guarantees diverse experiences and problems. If patients' perspectives are to be treated on a par with the more unified interests of economically powerful actors, these diverse experiences of health care users must be made coherent, while still acknowledging their heterogeneity. A group or organization that can act as interpreter, translating patient experience into policy discourse, is essential for carrying out this function. This might take the form of bringing together various patient representatives and advocacy groups into the advocacy infrastructure described earlier, including mechanisms like regular forums designed to synthesize their experiences and the aggregated records of patient advocacy interventions. Successful models along these lines exist both in the United States (for specialized populations) and in the United Kingdom and Canada.[14]

Represent Diverse Patient Experiences

Amplifying the voice of groups that purport to speak in patients' interests does not necessarily make either the health care system or health policy making more responsive to patients' true needs or preferences. Groups can fail to be adequately representative in all kinds of ways: because some health needs lend themselves to the formation of groups more easily than others; because some membership groups more readily muster resources and attract policy makers' attention than others; because all membership organizations are susceptible to dominance by a vocal minority. Individuals purporting to represent a group may also fail to apprehend, understand, or articulate issues that have little significance to them but that matter to others. And group members who have been designated representatives of patient interests in organizations or on advisory committees are more often selected to uphold the status quo than to represent heterodox patient perspectives. Given these complications, we identified four principles designed to ensure more robust and equitable representation of patient perspectives.

Principle 7: Assure representation of both group and individual perspectives

To offset the greater ease with which some patient interests can be successfully organized, the publicly funded infrastructure described earlier must be designed to elicit, report, and resolve both individual and group problems. Ombuds programs in the United States and patient liaison programs in other countries have promising track records at supporting individual patient voice but have not generally addressed the balance between individual and collective concerns.[15] By aggregating individual complaints and reports while encouraging group voice through patient organizations or other forums, the advocacy infrastructure can help translate isolated problems into broader mandates for improvement and change.

Principle 8: Actively elicit experiences from
a representative cross-section of Americans

As documented in Schlesinger's chapter, grievances initiated by patients do not reflect the complete range of patient experience. To provide a more representative portrait, there must be efforts to periodically solicit input from a cross-section of the public—especially groups who have proven most reticent, in the past, to come forward of their own accord. Past experience from the United States and abroad suggests that a concerted campaign to inform the public about the potential for patient engagement can significantly enhance the use of mechanisms for patient voice.[16] And federally funded initiatives in the United States have demonstrated that population-based surveys can reach even the most disadvantaged and disenfranchised patient groups.[17] Asking people the right questions, once their attention has been engaged, has proven to be crucial.

Principle 9: Hold advocacy groups accountable
to fully represent their members' experiences

Though patients experience health care and respond to problematic encounters in varied ways, there is a tendency among patient advocacy groups to simplify this diversity to a singular perspective in order to enhance the coherence of their message. This potential bias is sufficiently common and problematic that we would argue for a presumption of bias, unless the groups in question can establish that they have taken seriously the potential for heterogeneity. There are several ways of addressing this concern. Patient groups could periodically survey their members to more carefully explore the range of their experiences, or could ensure that their governance arrangements allow for open membership and equal influence among participants. Groups that are cosponsored by private interests, such as pharmaceutical companies, should be held to an even higher level of accountability to demonstrate representativeness.

Principle 10: Recognize the distinctive perspectives
of patients and their families

Although several chapters here (Joseph J. Fins and Jennifer Hersh, Marcus, Schlesinger, Grob, and Tomes) demonstrate that family members often advocate on a patient's behalf or otherwise facilitate patient voice, it would be unwise for policy makers to presume a complete congruence of patient and family interests. Tomes's chapter provides a case in point: family advocates favored a policy stance (medicalization) diametrically opposed by patients diagnosed with mental illness. To ignore distinctive family perspectives also fails to accord family members their fair moral standing, since they are themselves directly affected by the patient's illness in terms of medical expenses, caregiving pressures, and psychological burdens.[18] Although efforts to explicitly address the distinctive needs and concerns of family caregivers are nascent in the United States, these first experiments provide a foundation for initiatives that might enhance family voice in a more far-reaching manner.[19]

Address the Challenges of a Fragmented Health Care System

The three challenges just described are most relevant to the collective representation of patients' interests. But this aspiration is feasible only to the extent that individual patients and their surrogates have the wherewithal to publicly articulate their personal health care experiences.[20] Further, the skill and commitment required to represent the interests of others are learned by expressing one's personal narratives, preferences, and dissatisfactions.

Yet even were it not a precursor for collective representation, the *process* of expressing grievances would remain essential. By giving voice to their own experiences and seeking redress, patients begin to make sense of what happened to them in the health care system. For all its current limitations, individual voice appears far more effective than exit as a response to problems with medical care.

How effective it can prove, however, depends crucially on how patients cope with the complexity and fragmentation of U.S. health care. As has been amply demonstrated throughout this volume, neither health coverage nor health care is exempt from the complicated, often dysfunctional public/private arrangements that structure all facets of the U.S. welfare state. This complexity interferes with patients' capacity to identify with one another, in ways we have discussed here. It also means that health care and health coverage are far more varied, complicated, and inequitable than in virtually every other advanced market democracy. This, in turn, means that compared to their counterparts in other countries, Americans are far more likely to report confusions and misunderstandings related to their health insurance or health care.[21] They are also far more likely than citizens of other countries to be on the outside of the health care system looking in, disconnected from the sorts of advice and guidance that can promote patient voice. They are four to six times as likely to lack a regular source of medical care[22]—a problem that is most pronounced among precisely those patients who most disadvantaged economically and disenfranchised in other ways.

In light of this fragmentation, patient voice in the U.S. health care system faces some distinctive and persistent challenges—many of which will likely continue even after the 2010 reforms are fully implemented, since these expand the scope of insurance coverage but do little to address the discontinuities in financing and delivery arrangements. The following three principles create a baseline for fostering robust and equitable voice under these circumstances.

Principle 11: Simplify access to patient support and advocacy

When the health system is itself confusing, access to voice-enhancing arrangements must be kept simple. Ironically, patient support arrangements that now exist can be as confusing as the complex system itself. The Medicare program, for example, has eight pathways for filing grievances and complaints. Just as 911 provides universal access to emergency assistance with no forethought, arrangements to facilitate voice by individual patients should have a simple, easily accessed single point of entry, like the NHS Direct helpline in the United Kingdom.[23] This single point of entry should afford patients access to existing institutional arrangements that facilitate their ability to navigate care, such as ethics consultation services in hospitals, ombuds programs, and insurance appeals processes. It should also facilitate their capacity to connect to the new infrastructure we describe earlier.

Principle 12: Enhance patient voice in private as well as public settings
The principles articulated so far establish a public commitment to enhancing patient voice. Yet patients' well-being is shaped to a considerable degree by myriad private-sector decisions, such as those made by employers about health benefits, by health plans about definitions of medically necessary treatments, by hospitals about the allocation of charity care dollars, and by pharmaceutical companies about pricing strategies and discounting practices. Because these are every bit as relevant to health policy as are choices made by Congress or state legislatures, effective voice requires interventions that reach beyond what we conventionally deem the public sector. The precedent for such interventions was established during the managed care backlash in the mid-1990s, when a number of states required that health plans have formal grievance mechanisms in place, as discussed in Rodwin's chapter. To effectively empower patients, however, the scope of these requirements must be expanded; grievances generated within the private sector must be captured by the public infrastructure's reporting systems; and patients whose concerns are not fully addressed in private settings must have recourse to public alternatives.

Principle 13: Enhance patient voice to influence health care
delivery and policies outside the delivery system
Because (as DiMatteo and Fairman document) physicians, nurses, and other clinicians play such a crucial part in helping patients understand their health care experiences, efforts to promote patient voice must build on these professional roles. Reform initiatives such as advanced medical homes, integrated care plans, and ideal medical practices are all designed to encourage primary care providers to make the delivery system more responsive to patients.[24] Extrapolating these professional standards so that clinicians help their patients with other forms of advocacy—like those involving insurance coverage,

Table E.1　**Principles for Enhancing Patient Engagement in Health Policy**

Enrich Conceptions of the Public Good and Collective Patient Identity

Principle #1: Clearly enunciate patients' right to voice.

Principle #2: Commit to a health care system that is responsive, caring, and humane.

Principle #3: Ensure that patients can more readily learn from one another's experience.

Level the Playing Field for Patients and Other Stakeholders

Principle #4: Assure access to professional health advocates.

Principle #5: Establish a publicly financed patient support infrastructure.

Principle #6: Promote coherent representation of collective patient experiences.

Represent Diverse Patient Experiences

Principle #7: Assure representation of both group and individual perspectives.

Principle #8: Actively elicit experiences from a representative cross-section of Americans.

Principle #9: Hold advocacy groups accountable to fully represent their members' experiences.

Principle #10: Recognize the distinctive perspectives of patients and their families.

Address the Challenges of a Fragmented Health Care System

Principle #11: Simplify access to patient support and advocacy.

Principle #12: Enhance patient voice in private as well as public settings.

Principle #13: Enhance patient voice to influence health care delivery and policies outside the delivery system.

eligibility for public benefits, and complaint or ombuds mechanisms—could vastly enhance public voice. Indeed, more than a decade ago Canadian physicians identified advocacy for both individual patients and system reform as one of their core competencies for medical education.[25] But the extensive fragmentation of U.S. health care means that clinician-based efforts alone can never be sufficient, since too many patients have no regular source of medical care, no affordable access to the health care system, and no idea how best to overcome these barriers. What's needed is an infrastructure that people can access when they have been excluded, overlooked, or otherwise disconnected from health care, backed by a national, public commitment to hearing the voices of patients.

Getting engaged is all about passion and transformation—embracing new roles, new commitments, and new partnerships. And engagement seems an appropriate metaphor, since in this epilogue we've asked policy makers to envision a fresh approach to patient empowerment and a revitalized sense of collective patient identity. We aspire here not just to initiate greater patient engagement with health policy, but to lay the groundwork for a long-lasting relationship—one constituted by a strong mesh of reciprocal obligations among patients as well as between patients and policy makers. Both forms of commitment are needed if we are to create lasting forms of patient empowerment and a balanced chorus of patient voices.

Past empowerment initiatives demonstrate that such transformation is possible. But it won't come easily. The challenges we have identified here are formidable, and our conception of how they might be transcended or circumvented is still quite nascent. The principles laid out in this document are just the starting point. They require the engagement of a broader group to take on this task. To this end, we invite readers to contact the editors of this volume to further explore these issues. We welcome your participation and look forward to the collaborative ideas sure to be generated.

Acknowledgments

The principles explicated in this epilogue were extracted by Rachel Grob and Mark Schlesinger from earlier drafts of the volume, then reviewed and refined over the course of several in-person meetings of the authors and several rounds of e-mailed commentary. No endorsement of these principles by the Robert Wood Johnson Foundation is implied.

Notes

1. Albert Hirschman, *Exit, Voice, and Loyalty* (Cambridge, Mass.: Harvard University Press, 1980).
2. U.S. Department of Health and Human Services, *Americans Speak on Health Care Reform: Report on Health Care Community Discussions* (March 2009), 9, http:www.healthreform.gov?reports/hccd/. For statewide efforts, see Jenine Harris, Sarah Shelton, Sarah Moreland-Russell, and Douglas Luke, "Tobacco Coverage in Print Media: The Use of Timing and Themes by Tobacco Control Supporters and Opposition Before a Failed Tobacco Tax Initiative," *Tobacco Control* 19, 1 (2010): 37–43; Joel Adelson and Joanna Weinberg, "The California Stem Cell Initiative: Persuasion, Politics, and Public Science," *American Journal of Public Health* 100, 3 (2010): 446–451; Krista Farey and Vishwanath Lingappa, "California's Proposition 186: Lessons from a Single-Payer Health Care Reform Ballot Initiative Campaign," *Journal of Public Health Policy* 17, 2 (1996): 133–152.
3. Mark Schlesinger and Jacob Hacker, "Secret Weapon: The 'New' Medicare as a Route to Health Security," *Journal of Health Politics, Policy, and Law* 32 (2007): 247–292.
4. Although we address these principles and suggestions primarily to policy makers, rather than to patient-consumer advocates or advocacy groups themselves, we do not wish to imply that all patient activism or citizen participation requires central direction, nor that it should be channeled into institutionalized arrangements.

But we anticipate that these other forms of engagement will flourish unimpeded by the initiatives that we propose here.

5. Ronald Paterson, "The Patients' Complaints System in New Zealand," *Health Affairs* 21, 3 (2002): 70–79. In the United States, national initiatives to promote patient voice began with the long-term care ombudsman program in the 1970s and extended to mental health in the 1980s, state-administered managed care ombudsmen in the 1990s, and most recently to Medicare's ombudsman program established in 2003.

6. Roland Friele and R.D. Emily Sluijs, "Patient Expectations of Fair Complaint Handling in Hospitals: Empirical Data," *BMC Health Services Research* 6 (2006): 106.

7. Sydney Halpern, "Medical Authority and the Culture of Rights," *Journal of Health Politics, Policy, and Law* 29, 405 (2004): 835–852.

8. Angela Coulter, Suzanne Parsons, and Janet Askham, *Where Are the Patients in Decision-making about Their Own Care?* WHO Policy Brief (Copenhagen: World Health Organization, 2008); Angela Coulter and Christopher Jenkinson, "European Patients' Views on the Responsiveness of Health Systems and Healthcare Providers," *European Journal of Public Health* 15, 4 (2005): 355–360.

9. Cathy Schoen, Robin Osborn, Sabrina How, Michelle Doty, and Jordon Peugh, "In Chronic Condition: Experiences of Patients with Complex Health Needs in Eight Countries, 2008," *Health Affairs* 28, 1 (2008): w1–w16; Cathy Schoen, Robin Osborn, Michelle Doty, Meghan Bishop, Jordon Peugh, and Nandita Murukutla, "Toward Higher-Performance Health Care Systems: Adults' Health Care Experiences in Seven Countries, 2007" *Health Affairs* 26, 6 (November–December 2007): w717–w734.

10. Marc Elliott, Megan Beckett, David Kanouse, Katrin Hambarsoomians, and Shulamit Bernard, "Problem-Oriented Reporting of CAHPS Consumer Evaluations of Health Care," *Medical Care Research and Review* 64, 5 (2007): 600–614.

11. Schoen et al., "In Chronic Condition."

12. There are currently only a handful of training programs and far too few advocates to meet this need. To remedy this scarcity, the federal Health Resources and Services Administration could expand the scope of its training grants for health care professionals to include health advocates, who could practice in either government agencies or private nonprofit organizations. Marsha Hurst, Margaret Gaines, Rachel Grob, Laura Weil, and Sarah Davis, "Educating for Health Advocacy in Settings of Higher Education," in *Patient Advocacy for Health Care Quality*, ed. Jo Anne Earp, Elizabeth French, Elizabeth, and Melissa Gilkey (Sudbury, Mass.: Jones and Bartlett, 2008), 481–506.

13. Carroll Estes, Donna Zulman, Sheryl Goldberg, and Dawn Ogawa, "State Long-Term Care Ombudsman Programs: Factors Associated with Perceived Effectiveness," *Gerontologist* 44, 1 (2004): 104–115.

14. In the United States: LaVerne D. Miller and Latrease R. Moore, "State Mental Health Policy: Developing Statewide Consumer Networks," *Psychiatric Services* 60 (2009): 291–293. In the United Kingdom and Canada: Mark Learmonth, Graham Martin, and Philipp Warwick, "Ordinary and Effective: The Catch-22 in Managing the Public Voice in Health Care?" *Health Expectations* 12 (2009): 196–115; John Church, Duncan Saunders, Margaret Wanke, Raymond Pong, Carol Spooner, and Marlene Dorgan, "Citizen Participation in Health Decision-Making: Past Experience, Future Prospects," *Journal of Public Health Policy* 23, 1 (2002): 12–32.

15. David Evans, Jane Powell, and Tanya Cross, "Patient Advice and Liaison Services: Results of an Audit Survey in England," *Health Expectations* 11 (2008): 304–316.

16. In the United Kingdom, the NHS launched a concerted campaign to promote the use of NHS Direct, and surveys comparing patient experiences across countries indicate that the British are as much as twice as likely as citizens in other countries to report having used a health care hotline. Commonwealth Fund, *The Commonwealth Fund 2007 International Health Policy Survey of Sicker Adults* (New York: Commonwealth Fund, 2008).

17. Robert Weech-Maldonado, Marc Elliott, Atetokundo Oluwole, K. Cameron Schiller, and Ron Hays, "Survey Response Style and Differential Use of CAHPS Rating Scales by Hispanics," *Medical Care* 46, 9 (2008): 963–968; Doren Fredrickson, Teresa Jones, Craig Molgaard, Claudia Carman, Jay Schukman, S. Edward Dismuke, and Elizabeth Ablah, "Optimal Design Features for Surveying Low-Income Populations," *Journal of Health Care for the Poor and Underserved* 16, 4 (2005): 677–690.

18. Mary Jo Gibson and Ari Houser, "Valuing the Invaluable: A New Look at the Economic Value of Family Caregiving," *AARP Public Policy Institute Issue Brief* (Washington, D.C.: American Association of Retired Persons, 2007).

19. Examples include the Family-to-Family Health Information Centers, initiated in 2002 by the Maternal and Child Health Bureau of HRSA and the Aging and Disability Resource Centers, first established in 2003 as a collaboration between the Administration on Aging and the Centers for Medicare and Medicaid Services.

20. Paterson, "The Patients' Complaints System," 70–79.

21. Schoen et al., "In Chronic Condition," w1–w16.

22. Schoen et al., "Toward Higher-Performance Health Care Systems," 717–734.

23. Alicia O'Cathain, Jackie Goode, Donna Luff, Tim Strangleman, Gerard Hanlon, and David Greatbatch, "Does NHS Direct Empower Patients?" *Social Science and Medicine* 61, 8 (2005): 1761–1771.

24. John H. Wasson and Neil J. Baker, "Balanced Measures for Patient-Centered Care," *Journal of Ambulatory Care Management* 32, 1 (2009): 44–55; Shoshanna Sofaer, "Navigating Poorly Charted Territory: Patient Dilemmas in Health Care 'Nonsystems,'" *Medical Care Research and Review* 66, 1 (2009): s75–s93.

25. Sarita Verma, Leslie Flynn, and Rachelle Seguin, "Faculty's and Residents' Perceptions of Teaching and Evaluating the Role of Health Advocate," *Academic Medicine* 80 (2005): 103–108.

Notes on Contributors

Elizabeth Mitchell Armstrong teaches in the Department of Sociology at Princeton University. She is the author of *Conceiving Risk, Bearing Responsibility: Fetal Alcohol Syndrome and the Diagnosis of Moral Disorder* (Johns Hopkins University Press, 2003). Her current research investigates the notion of fetal personhood and its impact on the ethics and practice of obstetrics.

Lori Andrews is Distinguished Professor of Law, Chicago-Kent College of Law, and director of the Institute for Science, Law, and Technology, Illinois Institute of Technology. She has been an advisor on human subjects research, genetics, nanotechnology, and reproductive technologies to Congress, the World Health Organization, the National Institutes of Health, the Centers for Disease Control, the National Science Foundation, the federal Department of Health and Human Services, the Institute of Medicine of the National Academy of Sciences, and several foreign nations, and served as chair of the federal Working Group on the Ethical, Legal, and Social Implications of the Human Genome Project. She is the author of ten nonfiction books and more than 150 articles.

Julie Burger Chronis, J.D., is a regulatory counsel with the U.S. Food and Drug Administration. The chapter "A Pound of Flesh" was co-authored by Chronis in her private capacity before she joined the FDA. No official support or endorsement by the Food and Drug Administration is intended or should be inferred.

Eugene Declercq is a professor of community health sciences and an assistant dean for doctoral education at the Boston University School of Public Health, and serves on the faculty of obstetrics and gynecology at the Boston University School of Medicine. He has served as lead author of three national studies of women's experiences in childbirth and in the postpartum period entitled *Listening to Mothers I & II* and *New Mothers Speak Out.*

Desiree Despues received her Ph.D. in psychology from the University of California, Riverside, in 2006.

M. Robin DiMatteo is distinguished professor of psychology at the University of California, Riverside. She is the author of more than 125 research articles and eight books on the measurement and prediction of patient adherence to medication, prevention, and treatment, most recently *Health Behavior Change and Treatment Adherence: Evidence-Based Guidelines for Improving Healthcare* with Leslie Martin and Kelly Haskard-Zolnierek (Oxford University Press, 2010).

Steven Epstein is the John C. Shaffer Professor in the Humanities and professor of sociology at Northwestern University. He is the author of *Impure Science: AIDS, Activism, and the Politics of Knowledge* (University of California Press,

1996) and *Inclusion: The Politics of Difference in Medical Research* (University of Chicago Press, 2007), both of which have won numerous awards.

Julie Fairman is the class of 1940 bicentennial term chair and professor of nursing at the School of Nursing, University of Pennsylvania, and the director of the Barbara Bates Center for the Study of the History of Nursing. She is the author of two critically acclaimed books, *Critical Care Nursing: A History* (University of Pennsylvania Press, 1998) and *Making Room in the Clinic: Nurse Practitioners and the Evolution of Modern Health Care* (Rutgers University Press, 2008). She is currently focusing on the intersection of specialization in nursing and health care policy.

Joseph J. Fins is chief of the Division of Medical Ethics at Weill Cornell Medical College, where he serves as professor of medicine, professor of public health, and professor of medicine in psychiatry. He is also the director of medical ethics at New York–Presbyterian Weill Cornell Medical Center, a member of the adjunct faculty of Rockefeller University, and senior attending physician at the Rockefeller University Hospital. He is the author of more than two hundred publications in medical ethics and health policy; his most recent book is *A Palliative Ethic of Care: Clinical Wisdom at Life's End* (Jones and Bartlett, 2006). He is a coauthor of the 2007 *Nature* paper describing the first use of deep brain stimulation in the minimally conscious state.

Rachel Grob is associate dean of graduate studies, director of the Child Development Institute, and Health Advocacy Program faculty member at Sarah Lawrence College. She has served as director of policy analysis and planning, Andrus Children's Center, and as assistant to the deputy commissioner of health, Westchester County. She is author of *Testing Baby: The Transformation of Newborn Screening, Parenting, and Policymaking* (Rutgers University Press, 2011) and numerous articles.

Kelly B. Haskard-Zolnierek, Ph.D. (University of California at Riverside, 2007), is an assistant professor of psychology at Texas State University San Marcos.

Jennifer Hersh is research coordinator in the Division of Medical Ethics at Weill-Cornell Medical College. She holds a master of bioethics and a B.A. degree in the history and sociology of science and religion from the University of Pennsylvania.

Beatrix Hoffman is an associate professor and chair of the Department of History at Northern Illinois University. She is the author of *The Wages of Sickness: The Politics of Health Insurance in Progressive America* (University of North Carolina Press, 2001) and of articles and chapters on the history of health insurance, social movements, and access and rights to health care.

Amy Dockser Marcus is a reporter at the *Wall Street Journal*, where she writes regularly about patient advocacy, health, and medical issues. Her writing has won many awards, including the 2005 Pulitzer Prize for Beat Reporting for a yearlong series of stories about cancer survivors. She is also the author of two books about the Middle East, where she was based as a Middle East correspondent for the *Wall Street Journal* from 1991 to 1998.

Marc A. Rodwin, professor at Suffolk University Law School, is author of *Conflicts of Interest and the Future of Medicine: The United States, France, and Japan* (Oxford University Press, 2011), and *Medicine, Money, and Morals: Physicians' Conflicts of Interest* (Oxford University Press, 1993). He has assisted consumer groups, testified before Congress, and served on government advisory boards and as an expert in litigation involving fiduciary law, competition law, and managed care. Rodwin has been a visiting professor at Tokyo University Law School and University of Rennes Law School and a researcher at the Centre National de Recherche Scientifique. He was associate professor at the Indiana University School of Public and Environmental Affairs. He holds a Ph.D. from Brandeis University, a J.D. from the University of Virginia, a B.A./M.A. from Oxford University, and a B.A. from Brown University.

Mark Schlesinger is a professor of health policy and a fellow of the Institution for Social and Policy Studies at Yale University and past editor of the *Journal of Health Policy, Politics, and Law.* His recent research initiatives include studying how the changing availability of information on clinicians' practices alters patients' choices among doctors; assessing public perceptions of and responses to economic insecurity; explaining the recent rapid expansion in the scope of newborn screening among U.S. states; and understanding why particular collective responses are seen as more or less legitimate for addressing the spread of obesity among Americans. He has consulted to a half dozen federal agencies, several dozen state and local governments, and more than a score of nonprofit organizations concerned with health and social policy.

Nancy Tomes is a professor of history at Stony Brook University. She is the author of *A Generous Confidence: Thomas Story Kirkbride and the Art of Asylum Keeping* (Cambridge University Press, 1984); *Madness in America: Cultural and Medical Perceptions of Mental Illness before 1914*, coauthored with Lynn Gamwell (Cornell University Press, 1995); and *The Gospel of Germs: Men, Women, and the Microbe in American Life* (Harvard University Press, 1998). She is currently finishing a book on the rise of the twentieth-century health patient-consumer.

Summer L. Williams (Ph.D., University of California Riverside, 2008) is an assistant professor of psychology at Westfield State College, Westfield, Massachusetts.

Index

Note: The letter *t* after a page number denotes a table. The letter *f* after a page number denotes a figure.

Available titles in the Critical Issues in Health and Medicine series:

Lightning Source UK Ltd.
Milton Keynes UK
UKOW042021200513

210977UK00001B/77/P